Home Doctor

Know your body
& look after it

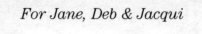

For Jane, Deb & Jacqui

HINKLER HOME MEDICAL

Home Doctor

Know your body
& look after it

HINKLER
BOOKS

Cover Design: Sam Grimmer

Home Doctor: Know Your Body and Look After It
Published in 2005 by Hinkler Books Pty Ltd
17–23 Redwood Drive
Dingley VIC 3172 Australia
www.hinklerbooks.com

This book is intended as a reference guide only, not a manual for self
treatment. If you suspect that you have a medical problem, please seek
competent medical care. The information presented here is designed to
help you make informed choices about your health. It is not intended
as a substitute for any treatment prescribed by your doctor.

ISBN 1 7412 1964 7
Printed and bound in Australia

Contents

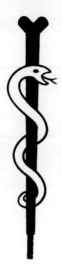

Preface

Modern society is moving at an ever increasing pace, and many people find that they just don't have time to look after themselves properly. This includes preventing mishaps and disease, as well as coping with injuries and illness whenever, and wherever, they happen.

As a result, many suffer unnecessary ills and mishaps when a little bit of prevention, taking early action or noting symptoms early rather than late could have prevented much more serious consequences.

It is far better to see a doctor and have a problem detected early, or be reassured that there no cause for concern, rather than suffer serious consequences unnecessarily or worry for no good reason.

This book is designed to be a simple guide to the most important ways in which you can look after your health, abnormal symptoms, and the health of those you care about.

Warwick Carter
Brisbane
June 2004

CURIOSITY
The most important thing in life that you can ever own is a boring medical history.

Any persistent change in bodily function,
be it pain or discomfort; a lump;
irritation; appetite, bowel or bladder habits;
or the shape, size or colour of a mole,
must be brought to the attention
of a doctor sooner rather than later.

THE TOP SIX

The most important ways to look after yourself and avoid doctor visits

---

1
Never smoke
If you have started, stop totally and completely, now!

2
Maintain a reasonable weight
This needs to be determined by your frame, age and sex.

3
Eat from a wide range of foods
Eat (in order of importance) cereals, vegetables, fruits, meat
and carbohydrates (e.g. sugar).

4
Exercise moderately and regularly
Every second day at least, get half an hour of exercise that leaves your pulse
raised and you short of breath.

5
Choose your parents carefully
Your genes and upbringing are the most important factors in determining
your long-term health.

6
Drink a moderate amount of alcohol
Those who drink a glass or two of wine on most days live a
longer and healthier life than teetotallers, but excess alcohol
markedly worsens health.

CURIOSITY
Humans are omnivores, they are designed to eat a wide range of foods, and not exclusively only one type of food.

HOW TO CHOOSE A DOCTOR

There are times, often unexpected and unwanted, when your local general practitioner can become a very important and helpful person in your life. Choosing a good family doctor can therefore be a vital decision in looking after yourself and your family.

When moving into a new area, speak to neighbours and friends to see which doctor in the area they **recommend**. Do not rely entirely on their advice though, because doctors are human and personality clashes can occur. The doctor that your neighbour can relate well to may not suit you at all.

Once you have received these recommendations, book a visit for a routine matter so that you can assess the doctor and the practice yourself. Can you communicate easily? Also check the surgery hours – do they suit you? What about after-hours cover – is it what you want? Are the surgery premises comfortable and relaxing? Is the practice too commercial or run down?

Other factors you may wish to consider are the doctor's **affiliations** such as membership of the national medical association. Not all doctors belong to their national association, but those who do, agree to abide by a strict ethical code, and the association may be able to help you if you have any problems with your doctor. They often cannot act against doctors who are not members.

Has the doctor obtained additional **qualifications** in general practice or family medicine from an academic college? These colleges encourage excellence in general practice, and doctors who belong pledge to keep up to date with the latest advances in medicine. Those doctors who belong have undertaken further study in general practice, have passed a very strict set of exams, and have been in practice for a *minimum* number of years.

Once you have decided to use a particular doctor as your family practitioner, let them know, so that appropriate files can be transferred from your old doctor and a good rapport can be established between you.

Doctor shopping is a health hazard – stay with the one practice
for all your family's medical care.

Getting the most from each visit to a doctor is also important. Any consultation will start with the doctor asking you in one way or another: 'What is wrong? How can I help you?' Having a logical answer to this question and being able to outline your problem concisely and simply helps both you and the doctor. Wisecracks such as 'You should be able to tell me that' or bland generalisations such as 'I'm not well' don't help anyone.

Most people have questions they wish to ask, but forget to ask all of them. Make up a **list**, and make sure that you have all your questions not only answered, but answered in a way that you understand. It is very easy for a doctor to use words or terms that you may not understand. If they do, let them know.

If you don't improve after the initial treatment, it is far better to **return** to the first doctor than to start shopping around. Humans are not like machines and they do not all react in the expected way. If problems arise, the original doctor will probably be in a better position to sort them out. This is more useful than confusing yourself with a multitude of opinions and treatments from several doctors.

And finally, if you are not happy with a doctor, tell them so. Many a misunderstanding can be sorted out this way, and even if you do change doctors as a result, both you and the doctor may learn something to your mutual benefit if problems are brought out in the open.

CURIOSITY

In 1950 the average worker had to work for five hours and ten minutes to earn the fee for an average general practitioner consultation, but in 2004 it took only one hour and ten minutes to earn the fee.

ABDOMINAL PAIN

A pain in the belly (abdomen) is a very common symptom, and disorders of an enormous range of organs (e.g. liver, spleen, intestine, bladder, uterus, ovaries, pancreas), glands, lymph nodes and structures (e.g. arteries, veins or nerves) may be responsible, as well as the muscles, ligaments and skin around the abdomen, or the vertebrae in the back. As a result it is important to look after yourself by paying attention to any abdominal pain, particularly pain that is severe, persistent or unexplained.

The pain may have a very serious cause, or a minor and temporary one, but any severe, persistent or recurrent abdominal pain must be checked by a doctor.

Don't be a martyr to your pain. Severe, persistent or recurrent abdominal pain must be checked by a doctor as soon as possible.

The **nature** of the pain (sharp, ache, dull), whether it is constant or intermittent; if it is affected by eating or passing urine or faeces; if it starts in one area then moves to another; what tends to make the pain better or worse; and the presence of associated symptoms such as vomiting, diarrhoea, constipation, loss of appetite, fever, pain on passing urine and menstrual period problems, may enable the doctor to make a definitive diagnosis.

Investigations to further aid a doctor may include: blood tests, X-rays (but these show only bones, and, unless a dye is injected, not soft tissue), CT scans (computerised cross sectional X-rays which show some soft tissues), ultrasound scans (using high frequency sound waves to examine organs), endoscopies (passing a flexible telescope tube in through the anus, mouth or urethra), MRIs (magnetic resonance imaging which shows many soft tissues in detail) and as a last resort, surgery.

CAUSES OF PAIN

To make it easier to differentiate the cause of the pain, the abdomen has been divided into the nine areas below. Some conditions may cause pain in two or more areas, and have been listed in each, while some conditions may cause pain almost anywhere, and have been listed in a general section.

COMMON CAUSES OF GENERALISED PAIN

Constipation may cause discomfort anywhere in the belly, but most commonly in the lower left abdomen (see area I below).

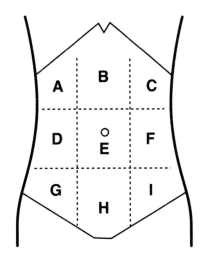

AREAS OF THE ABDOMEN

Colic in children is an intermittent, painful spasm of the gut. It is common in babies at about six weeks of age, but may occur in older children and adults as a result of overeating, swallowing air (e.g. with rapid eating or crying), anxiety and stress, or due to toxins in the food. Diarrhoea and vomiting some-times occur.

Infections of the gut by a virus (**gastroenteritis**) or bacteria (e.g. typhoid, tuber-culosis, shigellosis, brucellosis), or infestations by parasites (e.g. giardiasis, bilharzia) may cause generalised abdominal pain, diarrhoea, vomiting and fever.

A tear of a **muscle** in the belly wall, straining one of the ligaments in the groin, or inflammation of cartilages at the end of the ribs may result in pain and tenderness in the abdomen that may be difficult to differentiate from pain that is coming from inside the belly. Pain in these cases is usually aggravated by movement, and other bodily functions are unaffected.

After surgery to the abdomen, particularly for the treatment of infections (e.g. appendicitis, pelvic inflammatory disease), raw areas may be left behind on the surface of the intestine, bladder, uterus, liver or other organs. These raw areas may come into contact and adhere to each other to form adhesions. These **adhesions** may be drawn out with time to form bands, and the bowel and other organs may become twisted, distorted or inflamed by these adhesions and bands. Various symptoms may occur including quite severe abdominal pain, nausea and changes in bowel habits. Treatment is difficult as further surgery may only create more raw areas that then form more adhesions.

Nerves run between the vertebrae from the spinal cord in the back, around the body to meet at the centre front. If a nerve is pinched, pain will be felt along the course of that nerve as it runs around the belly. The most common place for a nerve to be pinched is at the point where it passes between the vertebrae, when arthritis or damage to the discs between the vertebrae may result in the nerve being trapped to cause **neuralgia**.

Shingles may cause a severe abdominal pain that is very hard to diagnose until the characteristic blistering rash appears.

Shingles is an infection of a spinal nerve caused by the virus *Herpes zoster*. This is the same virus that causes chickenpox, and once you have this infection, the virus never leaves the body, but settles at the base of nerves along the spine. At times of stress or reduced immunity, the virus may start to multiply again in one particular nerve, to cause sharp pain that gradually moves along the nerve on one side only from the back to the front of the abdomen. Shortly after the pain starts, a patchy blistering rash will appear in a line along the course of the nerve. Shingles is a medical emergency, because if treated within 72 hours of the rash first appearing, it can be cured. If diagnosis is delayed beyond this time, the pain may last for months or become permanent, particularly in elderly people.

Women who have a serious case of **salpingitis** (infection of the Fallopian tubes) may find that the infection spreads through the belly cavity to affect other organs. If the surface of the liver becomes infected, it may affect the function of the liver to cause an obstruction and abdominal pain (Fitz-Hugh-Curtis syndrome). The pain is worsened by lying down and turning, and there is often accompanying vaginal discharge, fever and pain on passing urine.

Tumours of the small intestine may cause pain anywhere in the belly, as the intestine wanders loosely throughout the belly cavity. Loss of appetite, black faeces, and nausea are other possible symptoms.

Some medications (e.g. anti-inflammatories) may have abdominal discomfort or pain as a side effect.

UNCOMMON CAUSES OF GENERALISED PAIN
Peritonitis is an infection of the membrane that lines the belly cavity (peritoneum). It usually results from a rupture of the gut (e.g. appendix, perforated peptic ulcer), a penetrating injury to the abdomen (e.g. knife wound), or spread from an infection of the fallopian tubes (salpingitis). Severe, generalised abdominal pain will occur, with acute tenderness, fever and an obviously very ill patient. Urgent medical attention is essential.

Ileus is the medical term for cessation of all contractions of the bowel. Normally the gut is constantly contracting and relaxing in waves that move the food along.

These movements may be occasionally heard as loud tummy rumbles, but can always be heard by a doctor listening through a stethoscope. An obstruction to the gut caused by a tumour, polyp, cancer or twisting of a loop of the gut may result in ileus after some hours of increasing pain as the bowel tries to overcome the obstruction. Urgent treatment is necessary to relieve the blockage and restart bowel movement before permanent damage occurs.

Patients with **coeliac disease** (sprue) are unable to digest the protein gluten which is found in cereal grains such as wheat, rye, barley and oats, but not in rice or corn. Eating any foods containing gluten will cause diarrhoea, belly discomfort, weight loss, excess wind and bloating. The disease may start at any age from childhood to mid-life and the only treatment is to exclude all these cereals from the diet.

Undiagnosed **diabetes** may first present with abdominal pains, as well as frequent passing of urine, thirst and headache.

A polyp growing in the gut may be picked up by the waves of muscular contraction that normally move food through the gut. As the polyp is pushed along, it pulls the piece of gut it is attached to along with it, to cause an infolding of the gut into itself (an **intussusception**). This inevitably leads to obstruction of the gut, severe intermittent waves of pain and ileus (see above). These obstructions may occur in the small or large gut, and are most common in children. The intussusception can be relieved by a barium enema (special X-ray) or colonoscopy (passing a flexible telescope in through the anus) if the large bowel is involved, but other cases will require surgery.

There are many more rare causes of abdominal pain than are listed here, so if in doubt, have it checked out!

CAUSES OF PAIN IN AREA A (RIGHT UPPER QUADRANT)

The main organs in this area are the liver and the gall bladder, which acts as a storage sac for the bile produced in the liver.

Inflammation or infection of the **gall bladder** (cholecystitis) and gall stones (cholelethiasis) will cause an intermittent pain that is made worse by eating, particularly fatty foods. Gall stones moving down the duct from the liver or gall bladder to the intestine will cause severe pain whenever they are pushed along by the pressure of bile behind them.

Infections of the **liver** such as hepatitis, and cysts in the liver caused by parasites (e.g. hydatid cyst from eating poorly cooked pork) may also cause pain here.

Pneumonia or pleurisy (infection of the membrane around the lungs) at the base of the lungs may irritate the diaphragm (sheet of muscle between chest and belly) to give the sensation of pain in this part of the belly, when it is actually coming from the chest.

If the vein draining blood from the liver becomes blocked by a blood clot (**thrombosis**) there will be rapid, painful and serious swelling of the liver as blood continues to be pumped into it through the hepatic artery. This condition is known as the Budd-Chiari syndrome and is usually fatal within a year or two.

CAUSES OF PAIN IN AREA B (UPPER ABDOMEN – EPIGASTRIUM)

This is probably the most common area for belly pain, as the stomach, lower end of the oesophagus (gullet) and pancreas are found here. Loops of small or large bowel may also come up into the area, particularly when lying down.

Inflammation (**gastritis**) or ulceration (**peptic ulcer**) of the stomach causes burning pain, which may be temporarily eased by eating food, but worsens after eating.

The **pancreas** produces the digestive enzymes that normally break up food to allow it to be absorbed through the gut wall. It has a duct that leads into the first part of the small intestine (duodenum). If the pancreas is damaged by infection, gall stone, alcoholism or a cancer, the digestive enzymes will leak out and start digesting the gland itself and surrounding tissue. Excruciatingly severe pain usually occurs quite rapidly, and is unrelieved by anything except narcotic injections prescribed by a doctor.

Crohn's disease is a thickening and inflammation of the small or large intestine. It is associated with variable bowel habits, belly pain and dark blood in the faeces. It is a relatively uncommon condition, but early treatment by surgical removal of the affected sections of gut can sometimes prevent it spreading.

Disorders of the **heart** may be felt as a pain in the abdomen, particularly the upper abdomen, as the heart rests on the diaphragm (sheet of muscle that separates the chest from the belly) behind the breast bone. Heart diseases as diverse as a heart attack, angina (restriction of blood flow to the heart muscle) and endocarditis (heart infection) may be responsible.

CAUSES OF PAIN IN AREA C (LEFT UPPER QUADRANT)

The only organ found entirely in this area is the spleen, but loops of both small and large intestine are also present. The spleen has three main functions – it filters blood, removing damaged cells and extracting and storing reusable elements such as iron from these cells; it stores the antibodies developed by the body during an infection, so that when a similar infection occurs in the future the antibodies can be called into play quickly; and it helps to produce new white and red blood cells.

The spleen is one of the most enigmatic organs in the body. It is essential in infants, but the older we get the less we need it, and adults who have it removed after injury can, with some precautions, live a normal life, as most of its function is taken over by bone marrow.

If the **spleen** is enlarged or inflamed, pain will be felt in the area. Common causes of this are infections (e.g. glandular fever – infectious mononucleosis, blood infections – septicaemia, tuberculosis), malaria, leukaemia (cancer of white blood cells) and severe anaemias (e.g. haemolytic anaemia). Cancer can also occur in the spleen, and it can be injured and bleed in severe accidents that involve a blow to the lower ribs on the left side.

The **irritable bowel syndrome** causes painful spasms of the large intestine that are aggravated by stress and anxiety, and associated with diarrhoea and excess wind.

Pneumonia or pleurisy (infection of the membrane around the lungs) at the base of the lungs may irritate the diaphragm (sheet of muscle between chest and belly) to give the sensation of pain in this part of the belly, when it is actually coming from the chest.

CAUSES OF PAIN IN AREA D (RIGHT SIDE)

As well as the loose loops of the small and large intestine that fill the abdomen, the organs that are found in this area are the right kidney and the fixed first part of the small intestine (duodenum).

A **peptic ulcer**, caused by excess acid production in the stomach, can develop in the duodenum to cause sharp pain and tenderness.

An infection of the right kidney (**pyelonephritis**) will cause a constant dull ache in the right side and loin, associated with frequent passing of urine, and sometimes discomfort in the lower belly (area H).

A **stone** in the kidney will cause a constant dull ache, but an excruciatingly severe pain that runs down into the groin and testes every time it moves along with the pressure of urine behind it. Blood is usually present in the urine, but sometimes can only be detected by urine test strips.

CAUSES OF PAIN IN AREA E (CENTRE)

The stomach, small and large intestine, pancreas, lymph nodes and the aorta (large main artery from the heart to the abdomen and legs) are found in this area.

A **peptic ulcer** in the stomach is caused by the concentrated hydrochloric acid in the stomach penetrating the protective mucus that normally lines the organ and eating into the stomach wall. Severe pain that is eased by eating, but is worse after eating, is common.

Appendicitis may start as a dull ache in this area due to the way the nerve supply to the appendix runs, but as the infection worsens, the pain will increase and move to the right lower abdomen (see area H). It may be associated with nausea, loss of appetite, fever and diarrhoea.

If the **small bowel** becomes obstructed by a tumour, cancer, polyp or twisting of the bowel, intense intermittent waves of pain will occur as the bowel contracts in an attempt to overcome the obstruction.

An **aneurysm** is the ballooning out of of a weakened section of an artery. If an aneurysm on the aorta starts to enlarge, leak or bursts, pain will be felt that varies from an ache to severe pain, depending on the degree of damage. A rupture of an aneurysm may cause death within minutes, so if an aneurysm is found, surgery to correct it as soon as possible is advisable.

If the main artery that supplies the intestine (mesenteric artery), or one of its branches, is blocked by a blood clot (**thrombosis**) or plaque of cholesterol, the blood supply to the gut will be partially or completely cut off. The affected part of gut will ache and not function, leading to considerable distress.

A **Meckel's diverticulum** is a side piece on the small intestine of about 3 per cent of people that forms at the point where the gut was attached to the umbilical cord before birth. This can become infected and inflamed in the same way as the appendix.

Crohn's disease (see area B) and mesenteric adenitis (see area G) may also cause pain in this area.

CAUSES OF PAIN IN AREA F (LEFT SIDE)

The left kidney, and the descending part of the large intestine (colon) are found in this area, as well as occasional loops of the small intestine. All the conditions that occur in the right side (see area D above) will occur here, but the irritable bowel syndrome (see area C above) and diverticulitis are other causes of pain.

In people who eat a low fibre diet for many years, there may be an excessive build-up of pressure in the colon (part of the large intestine). The colon has a structure of horizontal and circular muscles in its wall. This leads to a patchwork pattern of strong and weak areas, and at the weak areas the high pressure can cause a repeated bulging out of the colonic wall. These bulges eventually become permanent and form small outpocketings called diverticulae. The part of the colon most affected is that closest to the anus on the left and lower left side of the abdomen. These diverticulae may cause no trouble at all, or may become infected (**diverticulitis**) to cause pain and diarrhoea. If an infected diverticulum becomes completely blocked with faeces, an abscess may form and cause persistent trouble until it ruptures and drains. If it ruptures into the gut, the problem will settle spontaneously, but if it ruptures into the belly cavity, a very severe infection (peritonitis) will result.

Diverticulitis is a disease of the baby boomer generation, as they tended to have inadequate amounts of fibre in their diet as children and young adults.

CAUSES OF PAIN IN AREA G (RIGHT LOWER ABDOMEN)

The caecum, appendix, ureter (urine tube from the kidney to the bladder), right ovary and fallopian tube are found in this area.

The caecum is a dead end at the beginning of the large intestine. The last part of the small intestine (ileum) opens into the side of the caecum, and the appendix is a narrow ten to 15 cm long dead-end tube that attaches to the end of the caecum. If the opening from the appendix to the caecum, or the appendix itself, is blocked by a piece of faeces or indigestible food (e.g. a seed or fruit pip), it will become infected to cause **appendicitis**. Steadily worsening pain that starts in the centre of the abdomen, then moves to the right lower side, occurs in association with a fever, loss of appetite, nausea and diarrhoea.

A **stone** in the ureter will cause excruciatingly severe pain that runs down into the groin and testes or vulva every time it moves along with the pressure of urine behind it (see area D).

A **Meckel's diverticulum** is a side piece on the small intestine of about three per cent of people that forms at the point where the gut was attached to the umbilical cord before birth. This can become infected and inflamed in the same way as the appendix, and the diagnoses are easy to confuse.

Crohn's disease (see area B) may cause pain in this area.

Lymph nodes are collections of infection-fighting white cells that filter out bacteria, viruses and other organisms and abnormal cells (e.g. cancer cells) from the organs whose waste products they drain. These nodes (often incorrectly called glands) are concentrated in the neck, arm pits, groin and in the membrane that loosely connects the intestine to the back wall of the abdomen (mesentery). If those in the abdomen become infected (mesenteric adenitis), they can cause pain in the belly that may be confused with appendicitis or diverticulitis.

A hernia is merely the protrusion of an organ or tissue into an area where it is not meant to be.

A weakness in the lower muscular wall of the abdomen may allow a small loop of bowel to push through under the skin in the groin to form a **hernia**. A lump is usually obvious, and a hernia often aches. If the pain becomes intense, the gut is twisted in the hernia and cannot be supplied with blood. Food or faeces may also be trapped in the hernia. This is a medical emergency, requiring urgent surgery to relieve the obstruction before the affected piece of gut dies and becomes gangrenous.

Women may experience pain in this area due to cysts or tumours in the **ovary**, infections in the fallopian tubes (salpingitis), or an ectopic pregnancy (pregnancy developing in the Fallopian tube or beside the ovary).

Endometriosis occurs when the cells that normally line the uterus (womb) come out through the Fallopian tubes and start growing on the ovary and inside the belly. They may still bleed when a menstrual period occurs to cause pain across the lower abdomen.

Torsion of the testis is a medical emergency in which the testicle twists around and cuts off the blood vessels that supply it. Pain occurs in both the testicle and the the lower abdomen. Surgery must be performed within twelve hours or the testicle will die.

CAUSES OF PAIN IN AREA H (LOWER ABDOMEN – HYPOGASTRIUM)

The bladder, rectum (last part of the large intestine) and uterus, as well as occasional loops of small intestine, are found in this area.

Obstructions in the **large bowel** due to a polyp, abscess or cancer tend to cause a deep aching, intermittent pain in the lower abdomen, and alterations in the bowel habits.

Infections of the bladder (**cystitis**) are far more common in women than men, and result in passing urine very frequently, pain when passing urine, blood in the urine and an ache in the lower abdomen.

Muscular cramps of the **uterus** are responsible for the pain felt by women in this area during menstrual periods. Fibroids (balls of fibrous scar tissue in the muscular wall of the uterus) may worsen these cramps.

The **pelvic inflammatory disease** is an infection of the Fallopian tubes and other organs in the pelvis of a woman, often as a result of a sexually transmitted disease. A constant dull ache will be felt, that worsens with sex or menstrual periods.

Endometriosis (see area G) and an **ectopic pregnancy** (see area F) may also cause pain here.

After an **abortion**, there are often painful spasms of the muscle in the wall of the uterus, rather like bad period cramps. If the pain is more severe than this, the woman becomes feverish or develops a foul vaginal discharge, urgent medical attention should be sought.

CAUSES OF PAIN IN AREA I (LEFT LOWER ABDOMEN)

This area contains the sharply curved sigmoid colon (part of the large intestine) as well as the ureter (urine tube from the kidney to the bladder), left ovary and Fallopian tube.

Severe **constipation** will cause discomfort and aching low down in the belly on the left side. An examining doctor can often feel the hard lumps of faeces when pushing on the abdomen.

Cancer of the colon is a serious cause of discomfort and aching, that gradually worsens to a severe pain. Alterations to the normal bowel habits, loss of appetite and blood in the faeces are other symptoms.

Gastroenteritis is a viral infection of the gut that causes vomiting and diarrhoea. It may cause discomfort anywhere in the abdomen, but particularly in this area.

Diverticulitis (see area F) and hernias (see area G) are other causes of pain in this area.

Don't forget that diseases in the generalised section at the beginning of this entry may cause pain anywhere in the abdomen.

Ulcerative colitis is an inflammation of the large bowel that causes multiple shallow ulcers, pain, and a watery and bloody diarrhoea. Fever, weight loss and lack of appetite are other symptoms. It is a persistent and recurrent problem that can be controlled by medication, but not always cured.

Women may experience pain in this area due to cysts or tumours in the **ovary**, infections in the Fallopian tubes (salpingitis), or an ectopic pregnancy (pregnancy developing in the Fallopian tube or beside the ovary). Endometriosis (see area G) is another gynaecological cause of pain.

Torsion of the testes (see area G) is another possible cause.

The abdomen is an enormously complex area, and as such a huge range of diseases and conditions, from constipation to cancer, may be responsible for pain in the area. I will reiterate that it it is important to look after yourself by having any unexplained, persistent or recurrent pain in the belly thoroughly investigated.

CURIOSITY

The liver was once thought to be the seat of the soul, as it had a good blood supply connecting it to all other organs, and its true purpose was unknown.

Eighteenth century remedy – 'A rupture (hernia) is a common misfortune among children. Immediately apply a poultice of fresh cow dung and bind it on tight 'til the swelling disappears'.

ACNE

A cne, spots, pimples, zits. It doesn't matter what they are called, nobody (particularly self-conscious teenagers) likes to have them, or look at them. Look after yourself and your children by ensuring acne is treated early and effectively to prevent both psychological and skin scarring.

Acne can vary from the annual spot to a severe and distressing disease. It normally occurs in teenagers, but may develop later in life, particularly in women. It is usually more severe in teenage males, but starts earlier in females, and affects Caucasians more than African or Asian races. Your choice of parents is important, so if your father or mother had pimples, you have a greater risk of developing them.

Acne vulgaris is a severe form that almost invariably results in scarring of the face, back and chest. **Acne conglobata** affects mainly the buttocks and chest and causes skin abscesses and severe inflammation.

CAUSE

The cause is a blockage in the outflow of **oil** from a few of the millions of tiny oil glands in the skin caused by dirt, flakes of dead skin, or a thickening and excess production of oil. Once the opening of the oil duct becomes blocked, the gland becomes dilated with thick oil, inflamed and eventually infected. Hormonal changes at puberty are the major aggravating factor, as they cause changes to the thickness of the oil. Pregnancy, menopause and the oral contraceptive pill may all influence pimples in this way.

Acne may be worsened by **stress** (either psychological or physical), **illness** (e.g. a common cold), skin pressure (e.g. spectacles on the bridge of the nose or tight collars), increases in skin humidity (e.g. a fringe of hair or nylon clothing), and the excessive use of cosmetics (further blocking the oil duct openings). The severity also depends on hereditary factors. There is no evidence that diet, chocolate, vitamins or herbs have any effect on acne.

Steroid acne is caused by the excessive or inappropriate use of steroids, either as tablets or as creams.

All pimples look ten times bigger when viewed by their owner than by anyone else!

There is no evidence that **diet**, vitamins or other herbs have any effect on pimples. A small number of sufferers may find that one particular food causes a fresh crop of spots, but these people usually quickly realise this and avoid the offending substance.

Acne appears as a white- or black-headed skin eruption, with a surrounding red area of infection. The face, upper chest, upper back and neck are most commonly affected.

TREATMENT

Although a cure for acne is not normally possible, medical science can usually **control** the condition adequately. Investigations are normally unnecessary.

The first step is to ensure that the affected areas are kept clean. This does not mean scouring your face with a wire brush six times a day! Gentle **washing** with a cloth and non-perfumed non-medicated soap twice a day is quite sufficient.

The next step is a trip to your local pharmacy to discuss with the chemist the various creams and lotions available. These should be used carefully and regularly, and the instructions followed scrupulously. Most of these work by **drying** out the oil in the skin, removing any excess skin flakes, and reducing inflammation.

If your acne is very bad to start with, or the over-the-counter preparations do not adequately help you, see your general practitioner. They have many treatment combinations that can give relief to most patients. Further treatment involves combinations of **antibiotics** (e.g. tetracyclines) that may be taken in the short-term for acute flare ups or in the long-term to prevent acne, skin lotions or creams containing antibiotics and/or steroids, and changing a woman's hormonal balance by putting her on the oral contraceptive pill or using other hormones.

In rare cases it is necessary to see a skin specialist for **isotretinoin** (which can cause birth deformities if used during pregnancy), steroid injections (e.g. tri-amcinolone) into the skin around particularly bad eruptions, and abrading away the skin around scars.

The treatment of adults with maturity onset acne is more difficult than juvenile acne.

Acne may cause **complications** that include both skin and psychological scarring. Picking acne spots can cause serious secondary bacterial infections that can spread deep into the skin (cellulitis).

The main complications of acne are skin and psychological scarring.

There is no reason for anyone to put up with the full misery of recurrent acne, provided they are prepared to help themselves by following instructions carefully, and attending their doctor when necessary. Eventually acne settles with age.

CURIOSITY

There is no evidence that chocolate or other sweets cause or worsen acne.

AGEING

L ooking after yourself in younger life ensures that you will have both better quality and quantity older life.

Older people should never hold back, but get out there and live as much as they can. The old aphorism of '**use it or lose it**' holds very true. Don't act your age, act as you feel.

The most important factor in ageing is your own choice in parents. If your parents lived to a good age, you have a better chance of doing so, but with the advances in medical science and lifestyle in recent decades, even those whose parents died young can live a long life, as their blood pressure, cholesterol, diabetes, osteoporosis etc. can all be effectively controlled.

Smoking and **obesity** are factors that you can control that will affect your longevity adversely, while alcohol in small amounts actually has a beneficial effect, as does moderate regular **exercise**.

LIFESTYLE

Older people certainly have more time available to them than when they were building careers, homes and families, so they should enjoy their time by doing the travel, sports, hobbies and other activities that they always wanted to do but never got around to. Even relatively extreme activities such as abseiling, horse riding and even parachute jumps are not beyond many older people. The anticipation and organisation of these events can be more than half the fun, while recollecting and regaling your friends with the details can prolong the enjoyment for years afterwards.

It is important to **remain active** and not get into a boring routine. Vary your activities in a random way, and if an opportunity for activity presents itself, grab that opportunity, abandon any routine you may have and head off for a coffee at the local shops or a trip to the Amazon.

Even those who have had the misfortune to suffer from poor health, or don't have the financial resources to travel far, can enjoy new activities as simple as gardening, walking, music appreciation classes, learning to play bridge, research into a topic (e.g. history) that they have always wondered about, or just going to a different shopping centre to the usual one.

Never regret growing old, there is only one alternative.

SEX

Sex is often a taboo subject for the elderly, but it need not be so. Many couples have an active and rewarding sex life until the end, not necessarily involving intercourse (although doctors now have ways of helping this for both sexes), but caresses and other forms of intimacy can be just as rewarding. In fact humans are healthier and happier if they have someone to love and care about. The fact that the body is not as trim, taut and terrific as it used to be is unimportant – it is the caring and touching that counts.

There is no reason why elderly people should not maintain an active sex life until well into their seventies, but there are a number of factors which will make the task more difficult.

The main factor that can affect the elderly is the **menopause** in both men and women. Both sexes are affected, but the male menopause (andropause) is often forgotten, although there is no doubt that it does occur. From the mid-fifties onwards, the amount of male hormone in the system slowly decreases. Unlike the female menopause, where there is a relatively sudden drop in hormone levels, the drop in men is so gradual that it may not be noticed until the early seventies when sexual responsiveness and libido (desire for sex) starts to decrease. This will obviously vary from one man to another. The drop in libido in a woman may be more sudden, but a woman can still appreciate and enjoy the closeness and intimacy that sexual intercourse gives until an advanced age.

Other factors affecting the elderly can include medical problems as diverse as heart failure and arthritis, which may make sex physically more difficult, and medications (particularly those for blood pressure) that may affect a man's erection. Diseases such as diabetes and atherosclerosis cause the partial blockage of small arteries, and may also affect the ability to have an erection.

As other activities are undertaken at a slower pace in old age, so should sexual activity. Most problems can be overcome by patience, mutual understanding and sometimes the assistance of a doctor in modifying or adding medication.

Pap smears may be a concern to older women. Regular Pap smears should be continued every two or three years until age 65, and and if the last two or three have been completely normal, there may be no need to continue having them. Remember though that a Pap smear could turn up a condition of the cervix that may lead to cancer in later years. This can be treated just as well at 65 as it could at 35.

COMMON HEALTH PROBLEMS

The gradual decrease in **hearing** associated with advancing age is extraordinarily annoying, and virtually everyone in their eighties, and often much younger, has some **deafness**. This form of deafness is due to thickening of the ear drum, wear and tear on the tiny bones that conduct the vibrations of the ear drum to the hearing apparatus in the inner ear, and a loss of sensitivity in the spiral tube that senses the vibrations and turns them into nerve impulses in the brain.

The higher frequencies of sound disappear first, and this cuts out a lot of hearing discrimination, so that conversation in a noisy room melts into a constant blur of sound.

Many deaf elderly people become remarkably adept at lip reading.

Medication and surgery play no part in the treatment of this condition, but hearing aids are becoming more and more sophisticated in helping people. You can also get special hearing aids that attach to televisions and radios which may help both you and your neighbours.

The elderly often complain that they can never get enough **sleep**. It is a medical fact that you require less sleep as you grow older. Babies may need 14 hours a day, children ten hours, and adults seven to eight hours. The elderly can often feel quite comfortable with five or six hours of sleep. They are also less active than younger adults, and tend to take naps during the day, both of which reduce their need for night-time sleep. Sleeping tablets merely force artificial sleep upon elderly people who do not require it.

Sudden **falls** in the elderly may be due to a multiplicity of conditions, and often a combination of different medical and environmental factors. Poor vision and balance are common in older people, and may combine to cause falls, particularly when in unfamiliar surroundings. Anaemia, and narrowing and hardening of the arteries (arteriosclerosis from cholesterol deposits in arteries) may cause dizziness and instability.

Transient ischaemic attacks are a temporary blocking of a small artery in the brain by a blood clot, piece of plaque from a cholesterol deposit in an artery, or spasm of an artery, which results in that part of the brain failing to function for a short time. These attacks may be prevented in some cases by low dose aspirin.

Parkinson's disease causes poor muscle coordination and tremor. The limbs may not do what they are told to do as quickly as the person may wish, leading to an abnormal and unsteady style of walking.

Dementia caused by brain degeneration (e.g. Alzheimer disease) may lead to inappropriate expectations of the individual, and trying to do too much too quickly.

Arthritis may affect major joints in the limbs and back, and sudden stabs of pain or poor function may result in a fall.

Muscle **weakness** from general deterioration with age obviously makes it more difficult to remain upright. Various diseases (e.g. multiple sclerosis) may cause muscle weakness in far younger people.

Poor **nutrition** may lead to inadequate energy to walk and move properly, and a predisposition to falls.

Some elderly people develop **red palms**. They look as though they are on fire, but they feel fine. There are several dozen causes for this complaint, varying from liver disease and an overactive thyroid to blood vessel overdilation and the side effects of certain drugs. The most likely explanation is age, because the skin is thinner in older people and this allows the blood normally circulating there to show through more easily, giving a fiery red colour to the palms. If the redness doesn't worry the owner, don't worry the redness with creams that may make it worse.

Medications can have increased side effects in the elderly, and may lead to con-fusion, weakness and falling. Sedatives, blood pressure lowering medications and drugs to treat anxiety and depression are particularly likely to cause these problems.

Excess **alcohol** intake can cause anyone of any age to fall unexpectedly.

VACCINATIONS

Immunisation should also be considered in older people. Normally the word 'immunisation' makes one think of trips to exotic countries overseas, or the routine immunisation of children against diphtheria, mumps, polio etc. Immunisation is certainly important in these areas, but it is now becoming increasingly important in the complete medical care of the elderly.

Tetanus is a risk to humans of all ages, but it is often only children and young adults who receive immunisation against this ubiquitous disease. About half the victims of tetanus will die, and although it may start from any cut or puncture wound to the skin, it can be completely prevented by a vaccination that is given regularly throughout life. Many older people are keen gardeners, and it is in garden soil that the tetanus bacteria can be found, activating itself only when in a wound. They should ensure that they receive a tetanus vaccination at least once in every ten years.

The biggest risks to elderly people are falls, influenza and their complications.

Influenza epidemics reach us every winter. Some years are worse than others, but every year brings its victims, and those in the older age range are far more susceptible to the ravages of this potentially fatal disease than those who are younger and fitter. The influenza virus has the unfortunate ability to change its form slightly every year, so a flu shot will give protection for only one year. After the vaccination is given in autumn, you will have 80 per cent protection (nothing in medicine is ever 100 per cent certain) against influenza for the next year, but no protection against the common cold or other viral diseases. The side effects to the vaccine are rare, and usually include only a slight fever and muscle ache. As the vaccine is produced from eggs, those with an egg allergy should not have a flu vaccine.

Pneumonia is rare in younger people, but its incidence increases with age. Immunisation against some forms of pneumonia is now possible, and is recommended for those who have risk factors such as lung disease, heart disease, diabetes, kidney failure, reduced immunity or for those who are in nursing homes or similar institutions. The Pneumovax injection needs to be given every five years and protects those who receive it from pneumonia caused by a bacteria called *Streptococcus pneumoniae* for ten years or more. Unfortunately, there are a number of different bacteria that cause pneumonia, and although those mentioned above are the most common ones, rarer forms of pneumonia may still occur even after immunisation.

LONGEVITY

Those who are 65 years old in our modern community have a better than even chance of living until over 80, and a reasonable chance (particularly if they are female) of living until 90 or more. They should ensure that these 20 or 30 years of their life are as healthy and active as possible. Avoiding potentially debilitating diseases, such as tetanus, influenza and pneumonia, by appropriate immunisation, is one way in which they can live comfortably to a ripe old age.

No one will ever really be old, provided they continue to have something to look forward to and approach new ideas and activities with enthusiasm.

CURIOSITY
Progeria is a rare untreatable condition of very premature ageing in which a ten-year-old looks like a 70-year-old, and has similar medical problems.

ALCOHOL

You should look after yourself by ensuring that your alcohol intake is not excessive, as both binge drinking and regularly consuming excessive amounts of alcohol can be damaging to your long-term well-being.

ALCOHOL

Ethyl alcohol (C2H5OH) or ethanol, is a colourless, liquid, organic compound produced by fermentation of carbohydrates (sugars) in fruit (e.g. grapes) or grain (e.g. wheat). Less commonly, it may be produced by fermenting vegetables or even milk and honey (mead). It produces immediate effects on the human body as it is absorbed from the stomach rather than the intestine, reaching a maximum level 90 minutes after ingestion, then slowly dissipates and is excreted through the kidneys over the next 12 to 15 hours.

DRINKING

Alcohol is normally consumed in the form of intoxicating liquids that have varying strengths of alcohol. The alcohol in beer varies from below two per cent alcohol to over eight per cent. Wines vary from about eight per cent to over 14 per cent, while fortified wines (e.g. sherry, port) vary from 18 per cent to 22 per cent alcohol. Spirits (e.g. gin, whisky, brandy, rum) and liqueurs usually contain 40 per cent to 50 per cent alcohol, but some overproof spirits go much higher.

SAFE CONSUMPTION OF ALCOHOL INVOLVES:

- Two alcohol free days a week

- MEN: no more than four standard drinks a day on average, no more than six standard drinks on any one day.

- WOMEN: no more than two standard drinks a day on average, no more than four standard drinks on any one day.

One drink is not always one 'official' drink when it comes to alcohol content.

A **standard drink** contains 10 grams of alcohol.

EXAMPLES OF A STANDARD DRINK:

- Wine: small glass (100 mLs). A bottle contains seven to eight standard drinks.

- Beer full strength (five per cent) – two thirds of a stubby (250 mLs)

- Beer mid-strengh (3.5 per cent) – one stubby (375 mLs)

- Spirits (e.g. whisky, rum, vodka, brandy) – one nip (30 mLs)

- Fortified wines (e.g. port, sherry) – small glass (60 mLs).

EFFECTS

In the body, alcohol causes excitation of the brain, loss of inhibition and relief of tension and anxiety at low doses, but depresses the mood at higher doses, sedates, impairs concentration, slows reflexes, impedes learning and memory, decreases coordination, slurs speech, changes sensation, weakens muscles and increases production of urine. Other effects may include abnormalities of blood chemistry, nausea and vomiting. Self injury as a result of falls and other accidents is very common amongst those affected by alcohol.

Levels of alcohol above 0.05 per cent are considered sufficient to have significant adverse effects and impair driving. Actual legal levels of alcohol in the blood vary from country to country. A level above 0.4 per cent may be lethal.

Alcohol withdrawal (hangover) may cause tremor, headache, loss of appetite, nausea, sweating and insomnia. If the use of alcohol has been long-term, withdrawal may cause delirium tremens.

COMPLICATIONS

Many **medications** may interact with alcohol. Check with your pharmacist, doctor or check the information leaflet with the medication. Alcohol may affect the medication making it more or less effective, or the effect of alcohol may be altered by the medication.

During **pregnancy**, alcohol should be avoided, especially during the first three months when the vital organs of the foetus are developing. Later in pregnancy it is advisable to have no more than one standard drink every day with a meal. While breast feeding, do not exceed the pregnancy recommendations.

Long-term abuse of alcohol (**alcoholism**) may have other serious effects on the brain, liver and other organs.

Alcohol abuse may be a temporary problem as a reaction to anxiety or stress, but it may lead to the chronic condition of alcoholism.

Alcoholism is sometimes referred to by the slang term 'dipsomania'.

ALCOHOLISM

Alcoholism affects up to three per cent of the adult population in developed countries. It is a disease in the same way that infections and cancer are diseases. It does no good to tell an alcoholic to 'pull themselves together' or 'stop drinking before it kills them'. They need professional counselling and treatment. The biggest problem faced by families and doctors is the **denial** by so many alcoholics that they have a problem.

When alcohol is swallowed, it is absorbed very rapidly from the stomach, and commences its actions on the brain and other organs. This, of course, is one of the attractions of alcohol – it can make you very happy very quickly, and this can lead to addiction in some people. The children of alcoholics are more likely themselves to become alcoholics, and should be very wary when using alcohol.

Blood tests on liver function and alcohol levels may confirm diagnosis, and an ultrasound scan of the liver may show damage (cirrhosis).

Alcoholism has two stages of development – problem drinking and alcohol addiction. Problem drinking is the use of alcohol intermittently to ease tension and anxiety. It may be associated with the use of prescription drugs to control emotional problems. Alcohol addiction is more serious.

AN ALCOHOLIC IS SOMEONE WHO HAS **THREE** OR MORE OF THE FOLLOWING SYMPTOMS OR SIGNS:

• drinks alone

• tries to hide drinking habits from others

• continues to drink despite convincing evidence that it is damaging their health

• disrupts work or social life because of alcohol

• craves alcohol when none is available

• appears to tolerate the effects of alcohol well

• blacks out for no apparent reason

• binges on alcohol

• averages six standard alcoholic drinks a day

• has abnormal liver-function blood tests.

The social complications of alcohol are obvious and vary from the disruption of family life to poor performance at work and the risks of drink-driving.

An alcoholic has to accept that they are an alcoholic before they can be treated.

The medical effects of alcoholism can be serious to the point where they can significantly alter the quality of life and shorten the life of the alcoholic. They include:

- Cirrhosis. In this condition, the soft normal liver tissue is replaced by firm scar tissue that is unable to process the waste products of the body adequately. The other vital actions of the liver in converting and storing food products and producing chemicals essential to the body are also inhibited.

- Wernicke-Korsakoff psychosis. This syndrome causes brain damage with symptoms of depression, irrational behaviour and insanity. These conditions are related to vitamin deficiencies caused by an inadequate diet while on alcoholic binges.

- Degeneration of the cerebellum (the part of the brain that is at the back of the head) caused by alcoholism can cause permanent incoordination, difficulties in walking and performing simple tasks.

- Peripheral neuropathy is damage to the nerves supplying the body. It causes muscle cramps, pins and needles sensations and muscle pains.

Treatment involves counselling, professional treatment programs in hospital, supportive groups (e.g. Alcoholics Anonymous) and medications to ease withdrawal and prevent relapses (e.g. disulfiram, naltrexone). Withdrawal from alcohol may cause delirium tremens.

The medical effects of alcoholism can be serious to the point where they can significantly alter the quality of life and shorten the life of the alcoholic, and adversely impact on other members of the family.

CURIOSITY

Alcohol can have its uses. A generous gulp of wine, or a rapidly swallowed shot of any spirit (e.g. whisky, gin), will generally cure hiccups.

ALLERGY

L ook after yourself by becoming aware of your allergies, know how to avoid them and how to treat them without (hopefully) needing the assistance of a doctor. While most allergies are merely a nuisance, severe allergies may be life threatening.

CAUSE

An allergy is an excessive reaction to a substance that in most people causes no reaction.

An allergy may be triggered by almost any substance, including foods, pollens, dusts, plants, animals, feathers, furs, mould, drugs, natural or artificial chemicals, insect bites and gases. Some individuals are far more susceptible to a wide range of substances than others and the tendency to develop allergies may be inherited.

Allergy reactions may be very localised (e.g. at the site of an insect bite, or in just one eye), may occur suddenly or gradually, may last for a few minutes or a few months, may involve internal organs (e.g. lungs), or may be limited to the body surface (e.g. skin or nose lining).

When a person is exposed to a substance to which they are allergic, the body reacts by releasing excessive amounts of histamine from mast cells that are found in the lining of every body cavity and in the skin. Histamine is required at times to fight invading substances, but when released in excess, it causes tissue inflammation and an allergic reaction.

TESTS

Screening blood tests can determine if a patient is suffering from an allergy. An allergy to a specific substance can be detected by skin or blood tests. In the skin test, a minute amount of the suspected substance is scratched into a very small area of skin and the reaction of that skin area is then checked for a reaction a day or so later. In blood tests, specific antibodies to invading allergic substances are sought and identified. The process is one of elimination, and consequently may be very slow.

Allergy testing can be especially important for people who react violently to things such as bee stings, since they may need desensitising treatment or to carry a supply of adrenaline in case of emergency.

Significant allergies occur in 10 per cent of the population.

SYMPTOMS

The allergy reaction may cause a wide range of symptoms, including itchy skin and eyes, diarrhoea, redness and swelling of tissues, a runny nose and skin lumps, depending on the area of the body affected.

Severe allergic reactions may kill a patient by causing the throat to swell shut, acting on the heart to cause irregular beats, or inducing a critical lung spasm. A small number of highly allergic patients must carry an emergency supply of injectable adrenaline (an adrenergic stimulant) with them at all times.

TREATMENT

Treatment depends on where the allergy occurs, its severity, and its duration. Antihistamine drugs are the main treatment and may be given by tablet, mixture, injection, nose spray or cream, but some types may cause drowsiness. A severe attack may require steroid tablets or injections, adrenaline injections, or in very severe cases (anaphylaxis), emergency resuscitation. There are a number of medications (e.g. sodium cromoglycate, steroid sprays, nedocromil sodium) that can be used on a regular basis to prevent allergic reactions.

If the substance that causes an allergy can be identified, further episodes may be prevented by **desensitisation**, which involves giving extremely small doses of the allergy-causing substance to the patient by injection, and then slowly increasing the dose over many weeks or months until the patient can completely tolerate the substance.

Most allergies can be successfully treated and prevented, and some allergies can be cured by desensitisation.

Allergies may be life-threatening when a severe reaction (known as anaphylaxis) causes throat swelling bad enough to stop breathing.

ANAPHYLAXIS

Anaphylactic shock is an immediate, severe, life-threatening reaction to an allergy-causing substance. Insect stings (e.g. bees, hornets, wasps, ants) and injected drugs are the most likely causes. It is rare for inhaled, touched or eaten substances to cause this reaction, although nuts may be an exception.

The patient rapidly becomes sweaty, develops widespread pins and needles, may develop a generalised flush or red rash, or swelling in one or more parts of the body (possibly including the tongue, throat and eyelids), starts wheezing, becomes blue around the lips, may become incontinent of urine, loses consciousness, convulses and stops breathing. Swelling of the tongue and throat may cause death by suffocation if air is unable to pass into the lungs.

For **first aid** the patient is placed on their back with the neck extended to give the best possible airway, and mouth-to-mouth resuscitation and external cardiac massage are performed if necessary. The patient must be taken to a hospital as quickly as possible.

Emergency medical assistance is necessary, as injection of drugs such as adrenaline, hydrocortisone, aminophylline and an antihistamine (this is the preferred order) can reverse the reaction and save the patient's life. Patients who are aware that they may have an anaphylactic reaction often carry an adrenaline injection with them at all times to be used in an emergency.

Patients usually respond well to appropriate treatment, but death may occur within minutes if medical help is not immediately available.

CURIOSITY

Allergies may accompany a severe infection (e.g. tonsillitis) when the patient has an allergy reaction to the bacteria causing the infection.

ARTHRITIS

B y looking after your joints from a young age, you can reduce the risk of developing arthritis, and by treating any arthritis that does develop at an early stage, you can slow its progress.

CAUSES

By strict definition, arthritis is inflammation in a joint – any joint from the jaw to the big toe – and a joint is a point at which two bones come together and normally can move in relation to each other. A joint itself is made up of the bones that form it, the ligaments, tendons and muscles that support it, the cartilages that stabilise it, the synovial fluid that fills it, and the synovial membrane that lines it.

There are hundreds of reasons for a joint to become inflamed and painful. A wide range of conditions that do not affect joints directly may have arthritis as an accompanying symptom.

Any injury to a joint that causes damage to the joint surfaces, bleeding into the joint, a tear to the cartilages or ligaments, or a break of the bones forming the joint, will lead to inflammation and pain in or around that joint.

TYPES

Arthritis is not a disease definition in itself, as there are many different types of arthritis that have different symptoms and methods of treatment.

OSTEOARTHRITIS

Osteoarthritis is the most common form of arthritis. It is not, strictly speaking, a wear and tear injury to a joint, but can be considered as such without going into detailed physiology.

Osteoarthritis is a degeneration of one or more joints that affects up to 15 per cent of the population, most of them being elderly. The cartilage within joints breaks down, and inflammation of the bone exposed by the damaged cartilage occurs, which is then aggravated by injury and overuse of the joint. There is also an hereditary tendency to develop osteoarthritis.

Symptoms are usually mild at first, but slowly worsen with time and joint abuse. The knees, back, hips, feet and hands are most commonly affected. Stiffness and pain that are relieved by rest are the initial symptoms, but as the disease progresses, swelling, limitation of movement, deformity and partial dislocation (subluxation) of a joint may occur. A cracking noise may come from the joint when it is moved, and nodules may develop adjacent to joints on the fingers in severe cases.

X-rays show characteristic changes from a relatively early stage, and repeated X-rays are used to follow the course of the disease. There are no diagnostic blood tests.

Alternative treatments for all forms of arthritis abound, but there is no evidence that any of these alternative treatments do anything more than work by the placebo effect while enriching their proponents.

Patients should avoid any movement or action that causes pain in the affected joints, such as climbing stairs and carrying loads (obese patients should lose weight). Paracetamol, aspirin, heat and anti-inflammatory drugs may be used to reduce the pain in a damaged joint, and physiotherapy, acupuncture and massage have also been found to be useful.

Surgery to replace affected joints is very successful, with the most common joints replaced being the hip, knee and fingers. Surgery to fuse together the joints in the back is sometimes necessary to prevent movement between them, as they cannot be replaced. Steroid injections into an acutely inflamed joint may give rapid relief, but they cannot be repeated frequently because of the risk of damage to the joint.

The prognosis depends on the joints involved and the disease severity. Cures can be achieved by joint replacement surgery, while other patients achieve reasonable control with medications. The inflammation in some severely affected joints can sometimes 'burn out' and disappear with time.

RHEUMATOID ARTHRITIS

Rheumatoid arthritis is an inflammatory **autoimmune** disease that affects the entire body, and is not limited to the joints. The immune system is triggered off inappropriately, and the body starts to reject its own tissue. The main effect is inflammation (swelling and redness) of the smooth moist synovial membrane that lines the inside of joints. Joints most affected are in the hands and feet.

It tends to run in families from one generation to the next, and the onset may be triggered by a viral infection or stress. Rheumatoid arthritis occurs in one in every 100 people, females are three times more frequently affected than males, and it usually starts between 20 and 40 years of age. A juvenile form is known as Still's disease.

Rheumatoid arthritis is due to the body inappropriately rejecting the tissue lining some joints, in the same way that a donated organ may be rejected.

Initial **symptoms** are very mild, with early morning stiffness in the small joints of the hands and feet, loss of weight, a feeling of tiredness and being unwell, pins and needles sensations, sometimes a slight intermittent fever, and gradual deterioration over many years. Occasionally the disease has a sudden onset with severe symptoms flaring in a few days, often after emotional stress or a serious illness.

As the disease worsens, it causes increasing pain and stiffness in the small joints, progressing steadily to larger joints, the back being only rarely affected. The pain becomes more severe and constant, and the joints become swollen, tender and deformed. Additional effects can include wasting of muscle, lumps under the skin, inflamed blood vessels, heart and lung inflammation, an enlarged spleen (Felty syndrome) and lymph nodes, dry eyes and mouth, and changes to cells in the blood.

It is **diagnosed** by specific blood tests, X-rays, examination of joint fluid and the clinical findings. The level of indicators in the blood stream can give doctors a gauge to measure the severity of the disease and the response to treatment.

The condition requires constant care by doctors, physiotherapists and occupational therapists. The severity of cases varies greatly, so not all treatments are used in all patients, and the majority will only require minimal care.

In acute stages, general physical and emotional rest, and splinting the affected joints are important. Physiotherapists undertake regular passive movement of the joints to prevent permanent stiffness developing, and apply heat or cold as appropriate to reduce the inflammation.

In chronic stages, carefully graded exercise under the care of a physiotherapist is used. **Medications** for the inflammation include aspirin and other anti-inflammatory drugs. Steroids such as prednisone give dramatic, rapid relief from all the symptoms, but they may have long-term side effects (e.g. bone and skin thinning, fluid retention, weight gain, peptic ulcers, lowered resistance to infection, etc.), and their use must balance the benefits against the risks. In some cases, steroids may be injected into a particularly troublesome joint. A number of unusual drugs are also used, including gold by injection or tablet, antimalarial drugs (e.g. chloroquine), penicillamine (not the antibiotic), and cell-destroying drugs (cytotoxics).

Surgery to specific painful joints can be useful in a limited number of patients.

There is no cure, but effective controls are available for most patients, and the disease tends to burn out and become less debilitating in old age.

Some patients have irregular acute attacks throughout their lives, while others may have only one or two acute episodes at times of physical or emotional stress, while yet others steadily progress until they become totally crippled by the disease.

GOUT

Gout is caused by excess blood levels of **uric acid** (hyperuricacmia), which is produced as a normal breakdown product of protein in the diet. Normally uric acid is removed by the kidneys, but if excess is produced or the kidneys fail to work efficiently, high levels build up in the body and precipitate as crystals in the lubricating fluid of a joint. Under a microscope the crystals look like double-ended needles. An alcoholic binge or eating a lot of meat can start an attack in someone who is susceptible, and there is a tendency for the disease to run in families. Most victims are men and it usually starts between 30 and 50 years of age.

The main **symptom** is an exquisitely tender, red, swollen and painful joint. The most common joint to be involved is the ball of the foot, but almost any joint in the body may be involved. In severe attacks, a fever may develop, along with a rapid heart rate, loss of appetite and flaking of skin over the affected joint. Attacks usually start very suddenly, often at night, and may occur every week or so, or only once in a lifetime. In chronic cases uric acid crystals can form lumps (tophi) under the skin around joints and in the ear lobes. More seriously, the crystals may damage the kidneys and form kidney stones.

> *Aspirin is contraindicated in acute gout as it may elevate*
> *serum uric acid levels and aggravate the symptoms.*

High levels of uric acid found in blood tests confirm the diagnosis, and a needle may be used to take a sample of fluid from within the joint for analysis in difficult cases.

The **management** of gout takes two forms – treatment of the acute attack, and prevention of any further attacks.

Acute attacks are cured by the combination of nonsteroidal anti-inflammatory drugs (e.g. indomethacin) and colchicine (a hypouricaemic). Aspirin is contraindicated in acute gout as it may elevate serum uric acid levels and aggravate the symptoms. Rest of the affected joint to control the pain and prevent further damage is important.

Prevention involves taking tablets (e.g. allopurinol, probenecid) daily for the rest of the patient's life to prevent further attacks, not consuming excess alcohol, keeping weight under control, drinking plenty of liquids to prevent dehydration, avoiding overexposure to cold, not exercising to extremes and avoiding foods that contain high levels of purine-producing proteins which metabolise to uric acid (e.g. prawns, shellfish, liver, sardines, meat concentrates and game birds). If the prevention tablets are missed, an attack of gout can follow very quickly.

Gout can be controlled and prevented easily in most cases, provided the patient understands the problem and co-operates with treatment.

OTHER FORMS OF ARTHRITIS

There are many other types of arthritis.

Many viral and bacterial **infections** that do not infect joints directly, may nevertheless cause joint pain by inflaming surrounding tissues. Examples include influenza, Ross River fever, mumps, glandular fever (infectious mononucleosis), brucellosis (caught from cattle), German measles (rubella), hepatitis, tuberculosis (TB), Lyme disease (transmitted by tics from mice and deer), syphilis and gonorrhoea (sexually transmitted diseases).

LESS COMMON CAUSES OF ARTHRITIS MAY INCLUDE:

----

* septic arthritis (bacterial infection of a joint)

* osteomyelitis (infection of bone)

* ankylosing spondylitis (chronic inflammation of the small joints between the vertebrae in the back)

* Osgood Schlatter's disease (inflammation of the knee in teenagers)

* synovitis (inflammation of the synovial membrane lining a joint)

* psoriasis (a skin disease that may spread into joints)

- systemic lupus erythematosus and other autoimmune diseases

- bursitis (inflammation of the synovial fluid-producing sac beside a joint).

Almost any type of cancer, anywhere in the body, may cause arthritis if the cancer spreads to the joint or adjacent bones.

Damage to the nerves supplying a joint by severe diabetes, direct injury, spinal cord disease or nerve inflammation (neuralgia) may cause pain that appears to come from a joint.

And there are still more rarer causes of joint pain, so if pain persists, see your doctor.

CURIOSITY

In the nineteenth century, some medical experts believed that 'the regular monthly discharge of blood, occurring in women, wards off gout in the fairer gender'.

ASTHMA

More than three-quarters of all asthmatics do not look after themselves by adequately preventing and controlling their asthma.

CAUSE

Asthma (known decades ago as wheezy bronchitis) is a temporary narrowing of and excess production of phlegm in the small airways (bronchioles) through which air flows into and out of the lungs. The narrowing is caused by a spasm in the tiny muscles which surround the bronchioles. One in ten people in Western countries suffers from some degree of asthma, but it is uncommon in developing countries.

The absolute **cause** is unknown, but certain triggers (e.g. colds and other viral infections, temperature changes, allergies, exercise, smoke, dust and other irritants) may start an attack in susceptible individuals. Because it is more common in countries with good hygiene, there is a theory that exposure to bacteria, viruses and dirt in various forms at an early age gives some protection against asthma. The tendency to develop asthma runs in families, along with hay fever and some forms of eczema, to give a 15 times greater chance of developing the condition.

There are a number of critical **ages** in the development and disappearance of asthma. There is a tendency for asthma to start at the ages of two or seven years and at puberty, and it often goes away (often completely) at seven years and puberty, but if still present in the mid-teens, it will probably last until menopause in women and the sixties in men before fading away. Curiously, pregnancy seems to dramatically reduce the severity of asthma in most (but not all) women.

EFFECTS

Asthmatics have more trouble breathing out than breathing in. Attacks may build up slowly over many weeks and the individual may be barely aware of the deterioration in lung function, or a severe attack may start within a minute or two of exposure to a trigger. The narrowing of the airways causes shortness of breath and wheezing, coughing, particularly in children, and tightness and discomfort in the chest. Patients rarely can die rapidly from a sudden, severe asthma attack.

There is some evidence that asthma is a disease of cleanliness and reduced exposure to bacteria, as it is almost unknown in Third World countries with poor hygiene.

INVESTIGATION

Asthma is **diagnosed** by respiratory function tests, which involve blowing into a number of different machines which may be read directly, draw a graph or give an electronic reading.

The forced expiratory volume of air in one second (FEV1) is the percentage of lung air capacity that can be expelled in one second by forcibly breathing out. It is an effective measure of lung function and may be measured in a machine called a spirometer that many asthmatics use at home to check the severity of their disease. The normal range depends on age, height and sex. Values are reduced by airway narrowing in asthma. The patient's response to medication is also checked on these machines.

Once diagnosed it is important to identify any trigger substances, if possible by trial and error, or with blood and skin tests.

MANAGEMENT

The management of asthma is divided into two areas – prevention and treatment:
Prevention – prevention is far more important than treatment, as most patients tend to under-treat or treat too late. Regular use of the appropriate preventer should mean that asthma treatment is rarely necessary. Prevention can be by means of steroid sprays, which reduce inflammation in the airways, or the almost inert allergy preventers.

Steroid sprays include beclomethasone (Aldecin, Becloforte, Becotide), budesonide (Pulmicort) and fluticasone (Flixotide). Side effects may include thrush infection of the mouth, sore mouth and throat, and a dry mouth. Rinsing the mouth after use prevents most of these problems. They should be used with caution in tuberculosis cases and while pregnant. Doctors should check the patient's lung function regularly to ensure an adequate dose. Many steroid sprays are now being combined in a one-delivery device with beta-2 agonists (which treat asthma).

Airway allergy preventers are used less commonly and include sodium cromoglycate (Intal) and nedocromil sodium (Tilade). Side effects may include a hoarse voice and bad taste, but they are safe in pregnancy.

Modern preventative sprays mean that the regular use of treatments such as Ventolin should be a therapy of the past.

Treatment – the best method is by aerosol inhalations which take the medication directly into the lungs where they act to dilate the airways and liquefy the thick mucus. Many of these can have their effectiveness and ease of use improved, particularly in children, if a spacing device or machine nebuliser is used. Mixtures and tablets are also available, but they work more slowly and have greater side effects. Very severe attacks may require oxygen by mask and injections of adrenaline, theophylline or steroids.

Asthma cannot be cured, but doctors can control the disease very effectively in the vast majority of patients.

CURIOSITY

How times change. A medical textbook printed in 1832 states that 'The chronic cough of asthma can be much benefited by the regular smoking of cigars'.

BACK PAIN

L ook after your back and it will look after you. This dictum must apply from youth as even excessive back strain in a child can come back decades later to cause chronic back pain in an adult.

ANATOMY

The back is made from 24 bones, called **vertebrae**, that sit one on top of the other. The bottom vertebra sits on top of the sacrum, which is really another five vertebrae that have fused together. The sacrum forms the back part of the pelvis. The top vertebra is specially modified to allow the skull to sit on it, and swivel in all directions.

When looked at from behind, the vertebrae should form a straight line. From the side though, the bones of the back are aligned in several smooth curves. The back curves in at the waist, out over the back of the chest, and in again at the neck. This careful alignment of bones is maintained by ligaments (which are stout bands of fibrous tissue) and muscles, that run along the length of the back. Between each vertebra is a cushion of cartilaginous material known as the disc. This has a semi-fluid centre (like a jelly-filled balloon) and absorbs the shocks the body receives in walking, running and jumping.

The **spinal cord** runs through holes in the centre of each vertebra. This cord is an extension of the brain, and passes through every vertebra from the skull to waist level. Between each vertebra, the spinal cord sends out nerves that supply that section of the body. Nerves run out from the neck to supply the arms, and from the lower vertebrae to supply the legs.

The **sacrum**, that big bone at the bottom of the spine, is attached to the pelvis by a complex network of ligaments positioned just under the dimples that many people have on either side of their back, just above their buttocks.

Back pain is the most common symptom complained of
by people in every part of the world.

BACK PAIN

Back pain may occur when the intricate arrangement of bones, ligaments, discs, muscles and nerves that makes up the back becomes strained, torn, broken, stretched or otherwise disrupted.

The most common cause of back pain is ligamentous and muscular **damage** from incorrect lifting. Lifting and twisting simultaneously is particularly dangerous. A poor posture can also add to muscular and ligamentous strain.

BACK PAIN

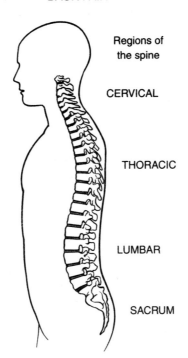

Regions of
the spine

CERVICAL

THORACIC

LUMBAR

SACRUM

FEMALE PELVIS

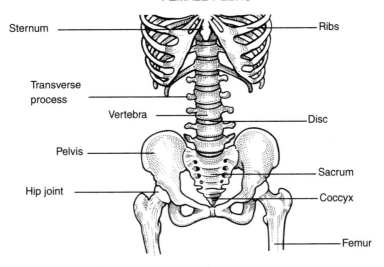

Sternum

Ribs

Transverse
process

Vertebra

Disc

Pelvis

Sacrum

Hip joint

Coccyx

Femur

In older people, arthritis may be the cause, when the smooth joints between the vertebrae become roughened and damaged by age and long years of use. This is **osteoarthritis**, but **rheumatoid arthritis**, which normally affects the hands and feet, may also affect the back.

A slight shift in the **position** of one vertebra on another, or inflammation of the surrounding tissues, may put pressure on a nerve, causing sciatica (leg pain) or localised back pain.

Direct **injuries** may fracture or dislocate the bones in the back, causing the spinal cord to be pinched, and paralysis of the body below that point.

There are discs of rubbery material between each vertebra that act as shock absorbers and allow movement between the discs. These intervertebral discs may be damaged by a sudden injury, gradual deterioration with age or many years of heavy work. A **damaged disc** may bulge (slipped disc) and press on a nerve as it leaves the spinal cord, to cause pain in both the back and down the course of that nerve. Discitis is an inflammation of the disc that causes local pain without pressing directly on a nerve.

A slipped disc is really a hernia of a disc, when part
of the disc wall weakens and allows the disc to bulge
in one direction and pinch a nerve.

Fibromyositis occurs in large muscles that have been overused and damaged repeatedly by heavy work or exercise. Scattered muscle cells are replaced by fibrous scar tissue to disrupt the structure of the muscle and cause a deep ache that worsens with use.

Osteoporosis is a thinning of the bones that occurs mainly in women after the menopause, due to a lack of calcium in the bones. It may result in bones breaking easily anywhere in the body, but particularly in the back where the weak vertebrae may collapse and cause pain.

Hormonal changes during **pregnancy** cause the ligaments throughout the body to slacken, and when this occurs in the back the vertebrae can shift slightly to cause considerable pain.

Menstrual **period pain** is a common cause of lower back pain, particularly in younger women who have not been pregnant.

Kidney stones may irritate the kidney to cause a dull ache on one side of the back, but if the stone starts moving down the ureter from the kidney to the bladder, excruciating pain will be felt running from the loin to the groin.

A **peptic ulcer** in the stomach is caused by the concentrated hydrochloric acid in the stomach penetrating the protective mucus that normally lines the organ, and eating into the stomach wall. Severe pain in the belly or back that is eased by eating, but worse after eating, is common.

Psychological and psychiatric conditions, including anxiety and depression, may cause muscle spasms and inappropriate perception of minor aches and pains that are magnified into a significant problem.

Cancer from one part of the body to another is called metastatic carcinoma, and the back is one site where these spreading cancers may settle to cause pain.

OTHER POSSIBLE CAUSES OF BACK PAIN MAY INCLUDE:

- scoliosis (a sideways curvature of the spine)

- posterior facet syndrome (small joints at back of vertebra are inflamed)

- Paget disease (in which the bones enlarge and soften in the back, legs and skull)

- Scheurmann's disease (an inflammation of the vertebrae in the centre of the back that is common in teenagers)

- hip disorders (e.g. osteoarthritis, poor circulation) may be felt as a pain in the back

- diffuse idiopathic spinal hyperostosis (excess bone deposited on spines on vertebrae)

- ankylosing spondylitis (a long-term inflammation of the small joints between the vertebrae in the back).

Back pain may also be due to diseases as diverse as kidney infections and menopause through to poor blood supply and a peptic ulcer.

Back pain does not necessarily come from the back. Many diseases of the organs in the chest and belly may cause back pain. Conversely, quite severe damage to the back may cause pain anywhere from the belly to the big toe, without any pain being actually felt in the back.

A woman's organs of reproduction are a common source of back pain. Infections of the Fallopian tubes (salpingitis) or uterus (pelvic inflammatory disease) may be felt in the back, as may endometriosis, a twisted ovarian cyst, and a prolapsed uterus (uterus slips down into the vagina).

There are many less common causes of back pain not covered in this list.

TREATMENT
Treatment will depend on the cause.

FOR PAIN ARISING FROM THE BACK ITSELF, TREATMENT MAY INVOLVE ONE OR MORE OF:

- rest and time with gentle mobilisation and correct posture

- physiotherapy and exercise regimes, with or without manipulation

- analgesics such as paracetamol or codeine

- anti-inflammatory medications. There are more than a dozen of these ranging from ibuprofen and indomethacin to diclofenac and rofecoxib.

- muscle relaxants such as diazepam to ease muscle spasm

- support belts

- potent steroid anti-inflammatory tablets or injections

- strong pain killers such as tramadol or (rarely and short-term) narcotics

- injections into the back of anti-inflammatories, steroids or disc-shrinking medications

- surgery of numerous types (always a last resort).

CURIOSITY

The 'dowager's hump' that many older women develop on the upper part of their back in old age is due to vertebrae in the upper back weakened by osteoporosis crumbling at their front edge and becoming wedge-shaped rather than square.

BAD BREATH

B ad breath is known in medical circles as halitosis. It, and its social implications, may be a major problem to an individual. Look after yourself, your family, friends, work mates and subsequently your career and social life by ensuring any bad breath you may have is adequately investigated and treated.

The way to fix the problem is to find out the cause and deal with that.

Most people who have it, don't know they have it.

CAUSES

The addictive habit of **smoking** is often to blame. Smoking causes the tongue to become deprived of its normal lubrication, and it becomes hairy and coated. This in turn traps microscopic food particles that decay in the crevasses of the tongue, causing the offensive odours.

Dental health is the other major factor involved. The gums may become very slightly detached from the teeth, forming tiny pockets in which food may become trapped. This is called periodontal disease, and the breakdown of saliva, food, bacteria and other foreign bodies in these pockets causes the production of rotten egg gas (hydrogen sulphide).

Sinusitis and other infections of the nose (e.g. rhinitis), throat (e.g. tonsillitis) and lungs (e.g. bronchitis, pneumonia) can cause bad breath because of the infected saliva and pus present in the airways. Damaged and scarred lungs will become infected more readily, or may have a constant low level of infection present in them (e.g. bronchiectasis, emphysema).

Fad diets that have excess protein and not enough carbohydrates are another cause, because the breakdown products of proteins are highly volatile acids that are expelled in the breath.

Alcoholics often have halitosis because the alcohol alters the balance of micro-organisms that normally live in the gut, causing an increase in the number of odour-producing bacteria.

OTHER CAUSES OF BAD BREATH MAY INCLUDE:

- liver failure

- hepatitis

- poorly controlled diabetes

- some types of cancer

- dehydration

- some drugs e.g. those used to treat angina, certain tranquillisers, lithium (used in psychiatry), griseofulvin (for fungal infections), penicillamine (for rheumatoid arthritis) and fluid tablets (diuretics).

TREATMENT
Treatment involves dealing with the cause if possible.
As a last resort, antiseptic mouthwashes and odour fighting gums and soluble strips can be used to disguise the bad breath.
   If you have a friend or colleague who appears blithely unaware of their problem, a quiet appropriate word, or even an anonymous note, is usually appreciated so that the one affected can deal with the problem and make more friends.

CURIOSITY
A nineteenth century Jewish book on child rearing tells parents that they can tell if their teenage children masturbate because they will develop bad breath. There is nothing to substantiate this curious advice.

BODY ODOUR

Bromhidrosis is the medical term for an unpleasant body odour, and in the same way as bad breath, it is important to look after yourself and control any body odour, in order to prevent social, work and family problems.

What is an unpleasant body odour to one person may actually be quite attractive to others. This is particularly the case in body odours due to spicy foods, as some of the spice may be excreted in the sweat.

People with body odour problems may not be aware that they have a problem, so a quiet word to them from a friend, or even a carefully worded anonymous note, may make them aware, so that they can seek a solution.

These people may also have problems in their personal, social, school and work life which may result in loss of friends, school bullying, failing to be promoted and missing social events.

CAUSES

The body produces two very different types of **sweat**.

About 2.5 million eccrine glands produce sweat all over the body in order to assist in regulating excessive body heat by evaporation, but apocrine glands produce a very different, oilier form of sweat in the armpits, groin and around the nipples, which contains the sexually attractive pheromones.

Increased sweating obviously occurs with exercise and in hot weather, but it may also increase with **stress**, and people who are suffering from long-term or persistent stress may develop a noticeable body odour that disappears when the stress goes away.

The **hormonal** changes associated with puberty, pregnancy and menopause may also cause a temporary increase in sweating.

Neither form of sweat has any significant smell, but the apocrine sweat is a good breeding ground for bacteria, and it is the breakdown of the oily apocrine sweat by bacteria which produces most body odour.

Some people have a slightly beery smell, despite not consuming large quantities of this intoxicant. In this case a **fungal** (yeast) infection may be responsible for the odour.

Diabetics whose sugar levels are poorly controlled may have an acetone-like (nail polish remover) smell about them. This is a serious sign, and they should be told of the problem and urged to seek immediate medical advice.

Rarely, an ammonia smell may be a sign of severe liver disease.

Zinc supplements in the diet may help some forms of body odour, as it increases the level of zinc in sweat and discourages bacterial growth.

MANAGEMENT

Body odour can obviously be controlled by regular **bathing**, particularly after vigorous exercise, but sometimes this is insufficient. Antiseptic soaps that reduce the number of bacteria on the skin is the next step.

Commercial **antiperspirants** and deodorants containing aluminium or zinc compounds that reduce sweating are the obvious next step. An antiperspirant blocks the pores in the skin and prevents the sweat leaving the skin, while deodorants allow sweat to escape but destroy bacteria or mask smells. Unfortunately, some people find that even these are inadequate.

Cotton clothing breathes better than synthetics, and is less likely to cause the accumulation of sweat and therefore odours. Cotton underwear should always be worn. Laundering clothes regularly, and using an antibacterial additive to the wash may also be helpful.

Hydrogen peroxide can be used to wash the skin in the armpit and groin, but ensure that there are no cuts (it will sting) and avoid the vagina.

In a small number of cases it is necessary for doctors to prescribe special **antibiotics**, either as a solution or tablet, that reduce the load of bacteria on the skin. These cannot be used long-term, only intermittently.

CURIOSITY

Pheromones found in the sweat from the armpits and groin are sexually attractive to the opposite sex, and change in a woman at different stages of her menstrual cycle. They are not perceived as odours, but can still subtly act to arouse.

BREASTS

Women should always look after themselves by looking after their breasts, as they can be both a source of pride and pleasure, as well as embarrassment and discomfort, let alone disease, if not carefully looked after.

DESCRIPTION

Understanding the structure and function of her breasts will enable a woman to look after them more effectively.

ANATOMY AND FUNCTION

Also known as the **mammary glands**, the breasts are glands that develop on the chest wall of women at puberty. Some women have breasts that are higher or lower on the chest, but when kneeling on all fours so the breast is hanging down, the nipple is usually over the fourth to sixth rib on each side. Some women have round breasts, while others have a more tubular shape. The size, shape and position of the breast is determined genetically, so women are likely to have similar-shaped and sized breasts to that of their mother and maternal and paternal grandmothers.

The primary **function** of breasts is to produce milk to feed babies, but they also have a very important role to play as secondary sexual characteristics and thereby to attract a suitable male partner.

The milk glands are arranged into 15 to 20 groups (lobes), each of which drains separately through ducts in the nipple. The amount of milk producing glandular tissue is similar in all breasts, regardless of their size. Larger breasts merely have more fat in them.

During pregnancy the glandular tissue increases to enlarge the breasts, and make them tender at times. The same phenomenon occurs to a minor extent just before a period in many women due to the increased level of oestrogen (sex hormone produced by the ovaries) in the bloodstream.

The breast also contains fibrous tissue to give it some support. The stretching of these fibres causes the breast to sag after breast feeding and with age.

A man's nipples react the same way as a woman's to stimulation.

When stimulated by suckling, muscles in the nipple contract to harden and enlarge it so that the baby can grip and suck on it. A similar response occurs with sexual activity, cold or emotional excitement.

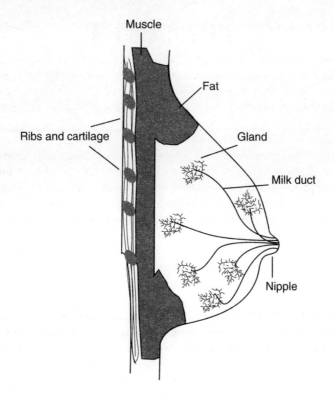

NIPPLE

The nipple is located at the apex of the breast and over the space between the fourth and fifth ribs in men.

In both sexes it is an **erogenous** area in that stimulation of the nipple is sexually stimulating, but in men it serves no other purpose. The nipple contains numerous small muscles that contract to make the nipple erect when stimulated by suckling, plucking, cold or anxiety. These muscles are more numerous in women as the nipple is considerably larger.

The nipple is surrounded by pigmented skin called the **areola**, which enlarges at puberty, and may darken further (chloasma) after pregnancy or hormonal medication use (e.g. contraceptive pill). The areola contains sebaceous (oil) glands that give it a bumpy appearance, particularly around its edge.

BREAST DEVELOPMENT

Breasts are normally a female characteristic, developing at puberty in the early teenage years, but any human, of any age or either sex, is able to develop breasts if given the sex hormone oestrogen. Those **men** who have decided to change their apparent sex, and those who wish to be transvestites, may take oestrogen in order to develop breasts, but there are a number of medical conditions that can also cause gynaecomastia (abnormal breast enlargement).

Boys with breasts? Not at all impossible, either by design or development.

Some **boys** going through puberty find that they are developing small lumps of tissue behind their nipples. This is caused by an imbalance in the sex hormones during this delicate stage of development. Most settle in a few months or a year, but a small number continue to develop excessive amounts of breast tissue and require an operation to remove it.

In men the menopause (**andropause**) occurs in the seventies, while in women it occurs in the late forties and early fifties. As testosterone levels drop in elderly men, the small amount of oestrogen that is present in the system of all men may no longer be suppressed by the testosterone, and start stimulating breast tissue development.

Women taking **oestrogen** as a hormone replacement therapy after the menopause, or on the oral contraceptive pill, may notice an increase in their breast size.

Obesity is an often overlooked cause for breast enlargement in both sexes, as fat may deposit in the breast area more easily than in the surrounding chest tissue.

Other causes of breast enlargement include **liver failure** (oestrogen normally produced by a man or woman may not be broken down and removed from the body at the normal rate), cancer or tumours of the testicle may prevent the normal production of testosterone, or in some cases (e.g. teratoma) may start to produce oestrogen instead, Klinefelter syndrome (only affects males who have additional X chromosomes matched with a single Y chromosome), Addison's disease (adrenal glands do not produce sufficient quantities of vital hormones), and a rare form of lung cancer (oat cell carcinoma) will affect sex hormone balance and cause breast enlargement in both sexes.

SYMPTOMS
Women can experience many different problems with their breasts from lumps to pain.

CRACKED NIPPLE
A common complaint, especially in breast feeding first-time mothers, is a cracked nipple. It usually starts a few days after the baby starts feeding and can be excruciatingly painful. Preparing the nipples for breast feeding (e.g. massaging in lanolin) should lessen the likelihood of this problem. If a crack does appear, soothing creams are available from chemists or doctors to settle the problem, and often the baby will have to be fed from the other breast for a few days until the worst of the discomfort passes.

NIPPLE ITCH
Itchy nipples are a relatively common problem. Women with small breasts may go without a bra and their nipples are irritated by clothing moving across them, or a loose fitting bra may constantly move across the nipple irritating it. Other causes include synthetic materials in a bra, **allergies** to soaps, perfumes and washing

powders, and fungal infections such as thrush (common in breast feeding mothers).

Treatments include lanolin and other skin moisturisers, anti-itch creams, anti-fungal creams if thrush is present, or prescribed mild steroid creams. Padding a bra may help small breasted women, and an adhesive dressing over the nipple can give quick relief.

NIPPLE DISCHARGE

The nipple of the breast will obviously discharge milk in a woman who is breast feeding, and will often leak milk between feeds, particularly when the breast is engorged with milk some hours after a feed. At other times a discharge will indicate some medical problem.

'Witch's milk' is a normal discharge from the nipple in many babies.

Sex **hormone imbalances** are the most common cause of abnormal nipple discharges. At almost any time during pregnancy, but particularly late in pregnancy, the higher levels of hormones in the body may stimulate premature breast milk production.

Hormones in the oral **contraceptive pill**, or hormone replacement therapy after the menopause, may overstimulate breast tissue to cause a discharge if the dose is too high.

The **pituitary gland** under the brain sends signals to the ovaries to increase or decrease sex hormone (oestrogen) production. A tumour or cancer of the pituitary gland or ovaries may result in excessive hormone levels and breast milk production.

Newborn **infants** of both sexes sometimes produce 'witch's milk', which is a discharge from the nipples in the first few days of life due to high levels of sex hormone passing over to the child from the mother through the placenta during birth. It is a harmless condition that settles quickly.

Other causes of an abnormal nipple discharge include breast cancer that involves the milk ducts (brown or blood stained discharge), kidney failure (may prevent the excretion of the normal amount of oestrogen and the levels of hormone increase), under- or over-active thyroid gland (hypothyroidism and hyperthyroidism), Cushing syndrome (over-production of steroids, or taking large doses of cortisone) and excessive stimulation of a woman's nipples for a prolonged period of time may result in a reflex which increases oestrogen levels and results in milk production.

Some non-hormonal **medications** may increase sex hormone production as a side effect. Examples include methyldopa and reserpine (used for serious high blood pressure) and tricyclic antidepressants.

BREAST PAIN

Any direct **injury** or blow to the breast may cause bruising and pain.

Many women experience painful tender breasts for a few days before each menstrual **period**. If this becomes a significant problem, medications are available to ease the discomfort.

In early **pregnancy**, one of the first signs of the pregnancy, other than missing a menstrual period, may be unusually sore and enlarged breasts.

The hormonal disturbances of the **menopause** may over-stimulate breast tissue to cause varying soreness. In the same way, excess oestrogen in hormone replacement therapy or the contraceptive pill will have the same effect.

Infections in the breast (mastitis), particularly during breast feeding, will cause hard, tender, painful, red lumps. If left untreated, an abscess may develop in the breast tissue.

Breast **cancer** may present as a painful lump in the breast, but sometimes there may be a firm painful area behind the nipple, with virtually no lump that can be felt. Large breasted women may not be able to feel a cancerous lump, but may experience pain on pressing on the affected area.

BREAST LUMPS

Breast lumps probably arouse more concern among women than any other condition. This is because of the fear of cancer in an organ that is so significantly associated with femininity and sexuality.

It is important to understand that there are many other causes of lumps in the breast, so if a lump develops, particularly in a young woman, the chances are that it is NOT a cancer. Fewer than one breast lump in ten seen by a doctor proves to be malignant.

There are no 'ifs', no 'buts' and no 'maybes': all breast lumps must be checked by a doctor if they persist beyond the next menstrual period.

If a lump is found, a general practitioner may arrange for an X-ray mammogram, ultrasound scan of the breast or a needle biopsy. These tests show the inside structure of the breast and can sometimes differentiate between **cysts**, cancers and fibrous lumps. If all the features of the examination and investigations in a young woman indicate that the lump is benign, it is safe to watch the lump, with regular checks by a doctor, because many disappear after a few months.

In an older woman, or if the lump persists, it should be removed by a small operation. In the majority of cases this is the only treatment necessary, and the scar should be almost invisible. If the lump is found to be cancerous, a more extensive operation may be necessary.

The earlier a **cancer** is diagnosed, the better the chance of cure, so surgeons have good reason for advising removal of a lump which appears to be benign, rather than waiting until an obvious cancer appears.

Infections in the breast (mastitis), particularly during breast feeding, will cause hard, tender, painful, red lumps. Blocked milk ducts during breast feeding might also be felt as a lump. If not cleared rapidly, mastitis is a possibility.

Other causes of breast lumps include cysts, over-stimulation of the breast by hormones (e.g. hormone replacement therapy, contraceptive pill, pregnancy), collections of fibrous tissue (fibroadenoma), mammary dysplasia and lumps of scar tissue in damaged fat caused by an injury to the breast.

INVESTIGATIONS
The breasts and their disorders may be investigated in many different ways.

BREAST EXAMINATION
It is commonly advised that women are taught **breast self-examination** by a doctor, and perform this easy procedure every month. Women who are menstruating should do this after their period has just finished.

The first step is inspecting the breasts in a mirror, with the arms at the sides and then raised above the head. Women should get to know the shape and size of their breasts, and note any changes that occur.

The next step is to lie down, and with one hand behind the head, examine the opposite breast with the free hand. This should be done by resting the hand flat on the chest below the breast, and then creeping the fingers up over the breast by one finger breadth at a time. Do this twice, once over the inside half of the breast, and then over the outside half. Check under the nipple with the finger tips and finally check the arm pit for lumps. Repeat the procedure on the other breast.

If the truth be told, more breast lumps are found by male
partners than by women self-examining.

Mammogram
A mammogram is an **X-ray** of the breast using a special technique to reveal the structure of the breast. It is one of the most significant diagnostic tools available for the detection of breast cancer.

A mammogram may be ordered to investigate a lump that has been found during a physical examination of the breasts, either by the patient herself, or by her doctor. However, women are being urged to have routine mammograms since it is the only reliable method of detecting cancer at the earliest possible stage, even before a lump can be felt. Unfortunately they are not 100 per cent reliable, and a mammogram should always be preceded or followed by a breast examination by a doctor.

Cancer cells are denser than ordinary cells and are impenetrable to certain X-rays. A tumour will therefore appear as a white patch on the mammogram picture. Mammography can sometimes detect the difference between benign and malignant tumours.

The rate of breast cancer rises markedly in women above 50, and regular mammograms are recommended for all women over this age, generally once every two years. Women younger than this should have regular mammograms if there is a high risk of developing breast cancer. Studies carried out in various parts of the world estimate that the death rate from breast cancer is reduced by up to 70 per cent in screened women.

Mammograms should be routinely performed every
two years in every woman over 50.

To have a mammogram, the woman will strip to the waist and sit or stand in front of a small table, leaning in such a way that her breast is resting on the table, where it will be placed in various positions and photographed by the X-ray machine. The breasts will be compressed to reduce the distance the X-rays must pass through them, and to reduce distortion caused by the curvature of the breast surface. The technique is especially valuable in the examination of large breasts, because the contrast is greater. However, a trained radiologist will detect any abnormalities in even the smallest breasts.

Having a mammogram is painless, although some women find the compression of their breasts uncomfortable. For routine mammograms, it is better to make the appointment in the first two weeks of the menstrual cycle when the breasts are not swollen and tender because of normal hormonal changes.

Modern mammography equipment delivers very little radiation and so is considered **safe**. Nevertheless, even small amounts of radiation increase the likelihood of getting cancer to a degree, and this needs to be taken into account when deciding on the frequency of routine tests. The older a woman gets, the less she is at risk from radiation, so those for whom a mammogram is of most value are at least risk from exposure to radiation.

If an abnormality is detected, it may be further investigated by an ultrasound and biopsy.

ULTRASOUND

Ultrasound is based on the fact that high-frequency **sound waves** bounce off tissues of different density at different rates. For example, bone reflects back nearly all sound waves that hit it, whereas fluids allow the waves to pass through. Sound waves are bounced off the organ being investigated, and the reflected waves are translated into a picture so the doctor can see what they mean.

Ultrasound machines produce a moving image from which selected still photographs are taken. Part of the patient's body is coated with oil, and a small pen-like probe that contains the sound recorder and microphone is placed on the skin. Once the area has been scanned, the instrument is moved a few centimetres and another scan is taken, and so on, until the entire area under investigation has been covered.

Breast ultrasounds, unlike a mammogram, require no
breast compression and cause no discomfort.

Almost any part of the body can be examined by ultrasound, with the exception of the head because the sound waves cannot penetrate bone. Because of the ribs, it is also difficult to see into the chest.

The breasts can be carefully checked for cysts, fibrous lumps or cancer by ultrasound, as the cancer cells reflect sound in a different way from normal cells. Ultrasound is also frequently used to guide a needle towards its destination in a biopsy.

Unlike X-rays, sound waves have no effect on the tissues exposed to them, so ultrasound is completely safe. It can be repeated as often as required without concern.

DISEASES

The various diseases affecting the breasts can vary from the mildly annoying to the very serious.

MASTITIS

Mastitis is an **infection** of the breast tissue, almost invariably in a breast feeding woman. It usually occurs if one of the many lobes in the breast does not adequately empty its milk, and may spread from a sore, cracked nipple. Women nursing for the first time are more frequently affected.

The breast becomes painful, very tender, red and sore, and the woman may become feverish, and quite unwell. Antibiotic tablets such as penicillin or a cephalosporin usually cure the infection rapidly and the woman can continue breast feeding, but if an abscess forms, an operation to drain away the accumulated pus is necessary.

In recurrent cases, bromocriptine may be used to stop or reduce breast milk production.

MAMMARY DYSPLASIA

Mammary dysplasia is also known as chronic cystic mastitis and **fibrocystic disease** of the breast. It is a common cause of breast lumps and cysts, and breast discomfort in middle-aged women, and is caused by overactivity of the ovaries in producing too much oestrogen. It is often an inherited characteristic.

Affected women develop multiple, tender, painful, small **lumps** in the breasts that vary in size and severity with the monthly hormonal cycle. They are usually worse just before a menstrual period. Large cysts may form permanently in the breast, and persistent pain and discomfort may significantly affect the woman's lifestyle.

Mammography (breast X-ray) and ultrasound may be used initially, but in most cases needle or surgical biopsy is necessary to confirm the diagnosis.

Initially a firm bra should be worn day and night. Individual cysts may be drained through a needle when they become too large or uncomfortable.

Medical treatment involves using drugs such as the contraceptive pill to regulate the menstrual cycle, nonsteroidal anti-inflammatories, danazol and progestogens. Avoiding caffeine helps some patients. The condition often persists until menopause, when it naturally subsides.

FIBROADENOMA

A fibroadenoma of the breast is a common **benign** growth of the breast, often affecting young women. The cause is usually unknown, but it may be the result of an injury to the breast. It is possible to feel one or more round, firm (but not hard) lumps within the breast tissue that are hard to catch hold of and tend to slide out from between the fingers when squeezed (thus sometimes known as a breast mouse) and are therefore not attached to surrounding tissue. They are not usually tender or painful.

A 'breast mouse' is a fibroadenoma that slips from between the fingers when squeezed and unlike a cancer, is not attached to surrounding tissue.

Mammography (breast X-ray) and ultrasound may be used initially, but in most cases a needle biopsy is necessary to confirm the diagnosis. If the diagnosis is confirmed to be benign, they may be left untreated, but if there is any doubt, they should be surgically removed. They persist long-term if not removed.

BREAST CANCER

Breast cancer (mammary carcinoma is the technical name) is an all too common cancer that affects one in every 11 women at some time in her life.

The absolute **cause** is unknown but it is more common in women who have a close relative (mother, sister, daughter) with the disease, in women who have not had a pregnancy, have not breast fed, have had a first pregnancy after 35 years, in white women, those who have had uterine cancer, and in higher socio-economic groups. On the other hand, women who start their periods late and those who have an early menopause have a lower incidence of breast cancer. About two per cent of all breast cancers occur in men as they have a tiny amount of breast tissue present just under the nipple.

The vast majority of breast lumps are not breast cancer,
but they might be. If you find a lump, always check it out.

The **symptoms** are a hard, fixed, tender lump in the breast. The nipple skin itself can become cancerous (Paget's disease of the nipple) causing a thick, firm, rubbery feeling to the nipple. There are many other causes of lumps in the breast and less than one in ten breast lumps examined by a doctor is cancerous.

The **diagnosis** of breast cancer is confirmed by an X-ray mammogram, ultrasound scan of the breast and needle biopsy.

The most common form of **treatment** is a lumpectomy in which only the cancer itself is removed, but if it is too large for this procedure a simple mastectomy, in which only the breast is removed, may be performed, leaving a cosmetically acceptable scar and scope for later plastic reconstruction of the breast. Often the lymph nodes under the arm will be removed at the same time. A course of radiotherapy and/or chemotherapy (drugs) may also be given.

A radical mastectomy in which the breast, underlying muscle and all the lymph nodes in the armpit and other nearby areas are all removed is done rarely, and only for very advanced cancer.

Up to two-thirds of all patients with breast cancer can be cured. In early cases the cure rate rises to over 90 per cent. In advanced cases the cancer may spread to nearby lymph nodes, the lungs and bones.

PAGET'S DISEASE OF THE NIPPLE

Paget's disease of the nipple (**nipple cancer**) is an uncommon type of cancer that starts in the milk ducts of the nipple, and may spread rapidly along these ducts, deep into the breast. The cause is unknown, but it is uncommon, occurring in only one in every 100 breast cancers.

There are often very few **symptoms** until the cancer is well-advanced, and no lump is felt. Symptoms include itching and irritation of the nipple, a thickening of the nipple and in advanced cases an ulcer may form. The cancer may spread to breast tissue and nearby lymph nodes. The diagnosis is confirmed by biopsy of the nipple.

Surgery to remove the nipple and the affected part of the breast is performed, followed by radiotherapy and chemotherapy when necessary. The more advanced the cancer when first treated, the poorer the survival rate.

BREAST FEEDING

LACTATION

Breast feeding is technically known as lactation.

After birth, a woman's breasts automatically start to produce milk to feed the baby. The admonition 'breast is best' features prominently on cans of infant formula and on advertising for breast milk substitutes in many third-world countries, and there is little doubt that it is true. Because of poverty, poor hygiene and poorly prepared formula, bottle-feeding should be actively discouraged in disadvantaged areas.

Breast milk is very cheap, very convenient and requires no preparation.

Breast feeding protects the baby from some childhood infections, and stimulation of the breast also helps the mother by a reflex that causes the uterus to contract to its pre-pregnant size more rapidly.

Babies don't consume much food for the first three or four days of life. Nevertheless, they are usually put to the breast shortly after birth.

For the first few days the breasts produce **colostrum**, a very watery, sweet milk, which is specifically designed to nourish the newborn. It contains antibodies from the mother which help prevent infections. Breast feeding may be started immediately after birth in the labour ward. All babies are born with a sucking reflex, and will turn towards the side on which their cheek is stroked. Moving the baby's cheek gently against the nipple will cause most babies to turn towards the nipple and start sucking. Suckling at this early stage gives comfort to both mother and child. In the next few days, relatively frequent feeds should be the rule to give stimulation to the breast and build up the milk supply. The breast milk slowly becomes thicker and heavier over the next week, naturally compensating for the infant's increasing demands.

After the first week, the **frequency** of feeding should be determined by the mother and child's needs, and not laid down by any arbitrary authority. Each will work out what is best for them, with the number of feeds varying between five and ten a day.

Like other beings, babies feed better if they are in a relaxed comfortable environment, with a relaxed comfortable mother. A baby who is upset will not be able to concentrate on feeding, and if the mother is tense and anxious, the baby will sense this and react, and she will not be able to produce the 'letdown reflex' which allows the milk to flow. The milk supply is a natural supply-and-demand system. If the baby drinks a lot, the breasts will manufacture more milk in response to the vigourous stimulation. Mothers of twins can produce enough milk to feed both babies because of this mechanism.

Breast milk is very sweet to taste.

While milk is being produced, a woman's reproductive hormones are suppressed and she may not have any **periods**. This varies greatly from woman to woman, and some have regular periods while feeding, some have irregular bleeds, and most have none. Breast feeding is sometimes relied upon as a form of contraception, but this is not safe. The chances of pregnancy are only reduced, not eliminated. The mini contraceptive pill, condoms, and the intrauterine device can all be used during breast feeding to prevent pregnancy.

It is important for the mother to have a nourishing **diet** throughout pregnancy and lactation. The mother's daily protein intake should be increased, and extra fresh fruit and vegetables should be eaten. Extra iron can be obtained from egg yolk, dark green vegetables (e.g. spinach), as well as from red meat and liver. Extra fluid is also needed.

INVERTED NIPPLE
Some women have flat or inverted nipples. The nipple is also inverted if it retreats when the woman tries to express milk by hand. If a woman intends to breast feed, the doctor will examine the breasts during an antenatal visit, and if the nipples are flat or inverted, a nipple shield may be worn to correct the problem. The shield fits over the nipple drawing it out gently, making it protrude enough for the baby to feed. Stimulating the nipple by rolling it between finger and thumb, and exposing the breasts to fresh air (but not direct sunlight) may also help.

BREAST ENGORGEMENT
One of the most common breast feeding problems is engorgement, which is not only uncomfortable but may lead to difficulty in feeding and to infection. If the breasts are swollen and overfilled with milk, **expressing** the excess milk usually relieves the discomfort. This can be done by hand under a shower or into a container, or with the assistance of a breast pump. At other times, expressed milk may be kept and given to the baby by a carer while the mother is out or at work. Breast feeding need not tie the mother to the home.

Engorged breasts can be eased by cold lettuce leaves, as the cooling effect is pleasant and they are the right shape to tuck inside a bra.

The infant may find it difficult to suckle on an overfilled breast, so expressing a little milk before the feed may be helpful. A well fitted, supportive bra is essential for the mother's comfort. Mild analgesics such as aspirin may be necessary, particularly before feeds, so that the feeding itself is less painful. Heat, in the form of a warm cloth or hot shower, will help with the expression of milk and with releasing milk from blocked areas of the breast.

Engorgement usually settles down after a few days or a week, but if the problem persists, fluid tablets can be used to reduce the amount of total fluid in the body and make it more difficult for the body to produce milk. In severe cases, partial suppression of the milk supply may be necessary.

INADEQUATE BREAST MILK

If the milk supply appears to be inadequate, increasing the **frequency** of feeds will increase the breast stimulation, and the reflex between the breast and the pituitary gland under the brain is also stimulated. This gland then increases the supply of hormones that cause the production of milk. Sometimes, medications that stimulate the pituitary gland can be used to increase milk production, or even induce milk production in mothers who adopt a baby.

A mother who is tense and **anxious** about her new baby may have trouble breast feeding. The mother should be allowed plenty of time for feeding and relaxation so that she becomes more relaxed and never feels rushed. A lack of privacy can sometimes be a hindrance to successful breast feeding. Lots of reassurance, support from family, and advice from doctors, health centre nurses or associations that support nursing mothers can help her through this difficult time.

The best way to determine if the baby is receiving adequate milk is regular **weighing** at a child welfare clinic or doctor's surgery. Provided the weight is steadily increasing, there is no need for concern. If the weight gain is very slight, or static, and increasing the frequency of feeds fails to improve the breast milk supply, then as a last resort supplementation of the breast feeds may be required. It is best to offer the breast first, and once they appear to be empty of milk, a bottle of suitable formula can be given to finish the feed.

INABILITY TO BREAST FEED

Unfortunately, for a variety of reasons, not all mothers are capable of breast feeding. Those who can't should not feel guilty, but should accept that this is a problem that can occur through no fault of theirs, and be grateful that there are excellent feeding formulas available for their child.

The most common **reason** for breast feeding failure is emotional or physical stress. The harder the woman tries to succeed, the more she fails. Being relaxed with the baby, the concept of breast feeding, and the physical and emotional surroundings is vital.

There are other reasons for being unable to breast feed. A mother who has a significant illness, be it an infection, dietary problems, cancer or any other form of debilitation, is not going to be as successful at breast feeding as a woman who is in perfect health. In less developed areas of the world, malnutrition may be a factor, but even in developed countries, a fad diet may lack vital nutrients and have an adverse effect. Rarely, damage to the pituitary gland under the brain may be responsible.

Cosmetic Procedures

If a woman is having physical or social problems with her breasts, she may wish to have them altered by an appropriate form of cosmetic surgery. If performed for the right reasons, this may have a significant impact upon the quality of her life.

BREAST ENLARGEMENT

Women desiring breast enlargement (**augmentation**) fall into three broad groups. Those who were born with small breasts, those who have suffered a sagging or shrinkage of the breasts after breast feeding or with age, and those who have had a breast removed because of cancer (breast reconstruction). Provided the patient is healthy, will benefit from the procedure, and is willing to have the operation there are no other criteria to be met.

The **operation** involves a two or three day stay in hospital. Techniques vary from one surgeon to another, but normally a small cut is made under each breast, and through this a plastic bag of silicone or saline gel (a prosthesis) is inserted to increase the size and improve the shape of the breast.

Often a small tube is left behind in the wound to drain off excess fluids that may accumulate. Bandages are tightly bound around the chest and breasts for a few days.

Larger breasts do not necessarily mean a better sex life.

The patient should rest for a week to ten days after the operation before returning to normal duties. The stitches are taken out in two stages about one and two weeks after the operation. After six weeks the breasts should feel and look completely natural, and the tiny scar will be hidden under the breast fold when standing.

Complications are unusual, but include excess bleeding and infection. The most common postoperative problem is breast capsule contraction. This occurs months after the procedure and is caused by the body laying down too much fibrous tissue around the implant, which results in the breast feeling firmer than normal.

There has never been any link demonstrated between this operation and the development of breast cancer, the woman can still breast feed after the operation, and can still check herself routinely for breast lumps.

An attractive bust may improve a woman's self-image and esteem, but the operation should not be done for the wrong reasons.

*There are no creams or lotions that will alter breast size,
no matter what they say in the advertisement.*

BREAST REDUCTION

Women with very large breasts can find them to be both uncomfortable and embarrassing. They develop fungal and heat rashes under the breast, and tired shoulder and back muscles from supporting them. They can get in the way when performing some tasks, and may make the woman look fatter than she is. Many women gain enormous benefit by having a breast reduction operation performed, and find that the sooner such a procedure is undertaken, the better.

There are a number of different ways of reducing breast size, but in the most common **operation**, a slice of tissue and fat is removed from the underside of the breast, so that the resulting scar is in the fold under the breast, and barely noticeable. If nothing further is done, the nipple would be left pointing at the floor instead of straight ahead, so a further vertical cut must be made, to allow the nipple to be moved further up the smaller breast. The resultant vertical scar is below the nipple on an area of the breast that is rarely exposed to public view.

BREAST REDUCTION OPERATION

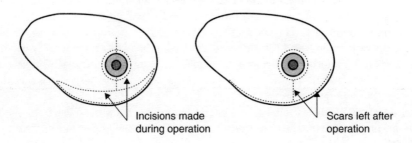

Incisions made
during operation

Scars left after
operation

After the operation, the woman will feel much more comfortable, she will still be able to breast feed, and no one except her most intimate friends need ever know.

BREASTS' DIFFERENT SIZES

Most women have slight differences in the sizes of their breasts, in the same way that most of us have one foot or hand a fraction larger than the other. All humans (male and female) have a tiny nodule of breast tissue present behind the nipple from birth.

At puberty, the oestrogens in women stimulate this tissue to grow into a breast. The degree of stimulation, the size of the original nodule, and (most importantly) hereditary tendencies will determine your breast size. In some women the breast tissue on one side does not react as much to the stimulating hormones as the other side.

Some women are born with no nodule of breast tissue behind one nipple, and therefore there is nothing there for the hormones to stimulate at puberty.

There is no magical medication, cream or diet that will correct uneven breasts, but plastic surgery has been known to improve a woman's self-image and appearance dramatically.

CURIOSITY
Women who have soft ear wax have a much higher risk of breast cancer than those with hard ear wax.

BREATHLESSNESS

U nexplained breathlessness is often a sign of significant disease, so look after yourself and find out the cause sooner rather than later.

CAUSES

If you run up stairs, become emotionally excited or upset, or **exercise** in any way, you will become short of breath, but the better your state of fitness, the longer it takes. Pain, anxiety, fright, hysteria and a high fever of any cause may cause rapid breathing, which is a bit different to breathlessness.

Most medically significant causes of **dyspnoea** (shortness of breath) can be related to the lungs, the throat (mouth, pharynx, larynx) and the heart.

Common **lung causes** include asthma (a temporary narrowing of the tubes through which air flows into and out of the lungs), any significant infection of the lungs (e.g. bronchitis, pneumonia, bronchiolitis), chronic obstructive airways diseases (e.g. chronic bronchitis, emphysema, bronchiectasis), cystic fibrosis (a birth defect of lung function) and a pneumothorax (air escapes from the lung into the chest cavity).

Less common lung causes of dyspnoea include lung collapse because of a chest injury, a blood clot in one of the major arteries within the lungs (pulmonary embolism), fluid accumulation within the pleura that surrounds the lung (pleural effusion), the rupture of an artery in the lung, asbestosis or silicosis, carbon monoxide poisoning, infantile respiratory distress syndrome (hyaline membrane disease) and sarcoidosis.

Throat causes for shortness of breath include croup (a viral infection of the throat in children), severe postnasal drip that may clog the throat and make breathing difficult, and an abscess, polyp or tumour in the throat or on the vocal cords that may affect breathing.

The **heart** may also be responsible, with conditions such as congestive cardiac failure (a damaged heart is unable to beat effectively enough to clear blood out of the lungs and pump it out to the rest of the body), a heart attack (myocardial infarct) or damaged valves in the heart (particularly a narrowed mitral valve).

OTHER LESS COMMON POSSIBLE CAUSES FOR BREATHLESSNESS
INCLUDE:

- gross obesity (may restrict the muscles available to move the chest and lungs)

- stroke (cerebrovascular accident)

- reflux oesophagitis

- severe scoliosis (abnormal back curvature)

- overactive thyroid gland

- nerve and muscle disorders that affect muscle contraction

- imbalances in the vital electrolytes (sodium, potassium, chloride) in blood due to kidney disease, abnormal diet, medications or injury that may affect the function of both lungs and heart.

STRIDOR

Difficulty in breathing (stridor) is subtly different to breathlessness. Patients with stridor may actually whistle as they try to draw breath, and it is far more common in children than adults.

Many different bacterial and viral infections of the throat may cause stridor, including laryngitis (infection of vocal cords), diphtheria (now mainly prevented by vaccination), glandular fever (infectious mononucleosis), tracheitis (infection of windpipe) and most significantly, croup.

Croup is a viral infection of the throat in children which causes swelling of the tissues in the throat that results in a seal-like barking cough, difficulty when breathing in, and excessive chest movement with breathing, in a child under five years of age.

A particularly sinister cause in small children is the inhalation of a **foreign body** (e.g. peanut, plastic block) into the windpipe (trachea) or larynx where it causes a partial obstruction of the airway.

A growth, polyp, cyst, tumour, haemorrhage (bleed) or abscess in the throat may also be responsible.

HYPERVENTILATION

Hyperventilation is the term used by doctors for rapid breathing, usually at a rate above 35 breaths per minute in an adult. Rapid shallow breathing may alter the balance of carbon dioxide and oxygen in the lungs, and thus the blood. The blood becomes more alkaline, and irritates small muscles, particularly in the hands, which go into spasm. This is known as **tetany** (totally different to a tetanus infection) and patients have fingers and sometimes wrist, forearms and feet, which are pointed in a firm spasm. Hormonal and calcium imbalances in the blood may also cause tetany. Breathing into a paper bag for a few minutes increases the level of carbon dioxide in the lungs, slows the breathing and eases the spasm.

*Breathing into a paper bag works far better than a plastic one for
hyperventilation, as it does not collapse as completely.*

Obviously, **exercise** will cause rapid breathing, but so will pain, anxiety, fright,
hysteria and a high fever of any cause.

Most bacterial and viral **infections** cause a fever, and therefore might be responsible for hyperventilation, but infections of the lungs and throat are more likely to
be responsible.

Other common **causes** of hyperventilation include a blood clot in one of the major
arteries within the lungs (pulmonary embolus), pneumothorax (occurs if air escapes
from the lung into the chest cavity), and a stroke (cerebrovascular accident).

An uncommon cause is Rett syndrome (an inherited condition of girls that
causes episodes of hyperventilation, seizures, subnormal mentality, constipation
and repetitive hand movements).

Some medications (e.g. adrenaline, pseudoephedrine – used for runny noses)
may cause rapid breathing as a side effect.

WHEEZE

A wheeze occurs when a person has **difficulty breathing out**. They can usually get
some air into the lungs, but then have to force the air out, creating a harsh rasping
wheeze. The cause of a wheeze is usually a disease of the lungs or airways.

Asthma is a temporary narrowing of the tubes (bronchi) through which air flows
into and out of the lungs. This narrowing is caused by a spasm in the tiny muscles
which surround the bronchi. The problem is further aggravated by the excess
production of phlegm in the lungs and swelling of the lung tissue through inflammation. The narrowing of the airways causes shortness of breath and wheezing.
Asthmatics usually find they cannot breathe out easily because, as they try to
exhale, the lung collapses further and the small amount of space left in the airways
is obliterated. Asthmatic symptoms also include coughing, particularly in children,
and tightness and discomfort in the chest.

*Asthma, eczema and hay fever are really all the same disease
(atopy) but occurring in different organs.*

An inhaled **foreign body** (e.g. peanut, small plastic block, poorly chewed food) is
a serious and potentially life threatening cause of a wheeze. The Heimlich manoeuvre (standing behind an adult patient and suddenly squeezing their chest to expel
the foreign body) may need to be applied by a person who has studied first aid in
order to clear the airway before an ambulance or doctor can reach the victim. If the
object cannot be expelled, and the patient loses consciousness and stops trying to
breathe, apply mouth-to-mouth resuscitation to force air past the obstruction.

OTHER CAUSES OF A WHEEZE MAY INCLUDE:

- anaphylaxis (severe, life-threatening reaction to an allergy-causing substance)

- congestive cardiac failure (damaged heart that is unable to beat effectively
  enough to clear blood out of the lungs)

- emphysema

- bronchitis (infection of the bronchi that carry air within the lungs)

- bronchiolitis (lung infection of children under two years of age).

- bronchiectasis (bronchi are damaged, scarred and permanently overdilated)

- reflux oesophagitis (stomach acid is inhaled)

- lung cancer

- cystic fibrosis (genetic defect of mucus glands)

- under-active parathyroid glands (hypoparathyroidism)

- carcinoid syndrome (rare tumour in the intestine).

CURIOSITY
The internal oxygen-absorbing surface area of an adult lung is equivalent to that of a tennis court.

BURNS

In order to look after yourself and your family, it is important to know the first aid steps in dealing with a burn.

EXPLANATION

A burn is damage to body tissues by excess heat. A burn can be caused by fire, contact with something hot, boiling water or steam (scald), electricity, the sun, or excess friction. They are classified according to three degrees of severity.

- First degree refers to burns where the skin has reddened, such as in sunburn.

- Second degree burns are where the superficial layers of skin are damaged, such as in a blister from hot coffee.

- Third degree burns are when the full thickness of the skin has been burnt away.

*Burns by open flames, boiling liquids and hot objects
are all treated in the same way.*

Burns are painful and distressing, and all but minor burns are serious and need medical attention. Third degree burns are sometimes less painful as the nerve endings will have been destroyed. Extensive burns may lead to fluid loss and shock, and the victim will need urgent help.

FIRST AID

THE FIRST AID TREATMENT OF BURNS INVOLVES THE
FOLLOWING STEPS:

- If necessary **put out the flames**. Hold a rug or blanket in front of you as you approach so that you will not get burnt yourself, and envelop the victim in it. Wrap it tightly around the victim to smother the flames and lower them to the ground. You can also use water to douse the flames but not if there is a likelihood of electrocution, and make sure you do not create scalding steam.

- Remove hot **clothing** if it will come off easily, but do NOT remove any fragments sticking to the skin because you may remove the skin with it.

- **Cool** the burnt area with cold water. If the victim is comfortably able to move and the burn is easily accessible, e.g. on an arm, hold the burn in a bucket of cold water or cold running water for at least 20 minutes. If not, gently apply cold water compresses.

- Do NOT prick or break any **blisters** and do not apply any lotions, ointments, or oily dressings as they will have to be removed later, which will be painful and damaging.

- **Cover** the burnt area with a clean (sterile if possible) non-stick dressing. If not available, use a wet cloth.

- **Bandage** the burnt area lightly – a torn up sheet is ideal. If the burns are on the face, cut holes for the eyes, mouth and nose.

- Allow the victim to **rest** in a comfortable position, if possible using pillows for support.

- **Raise** injured limbs to reduce swelling and fluid loss. If the face is burnt, try to keep the victim sitting up.

- Give frequent sips of **water** to replace lost fluids – but NOT alcohol.

- Watch for signs of **shock** and treat if necessary.

- Give mouth-to-mouth **resuscitation** or cardiopulmonary resuscitation if required.

Putting butter on a burn is a bad idea – use cold water instead.

TREATMENT
Once under medical care, second degree burns are treated with antibiotic creams or other dressings. Third degree burns usually require skin grafts unless very small.

Extensive second and third degree burns may be life threatening because of the loss of body fluids through the burn area and the absorption of large amounts of toxic waste products into the blood that can cause kidney and liver failure.

Once in a hospital burns unit, a patient can be kept alive on a ventilator and fluids can be replaced through drips into a vein. Antiseptic paints, creams, amniotic sac membrane (recovered from the placenta of mothers who have just delivered a baby) or pig skin may be used to protect wounds after the burnt tissue has been cleaned or cut away (surgical debridement). Pressure may be applied in various ways to reduce scarring.

Skin taken from unburned areas of the body is grafted to areas that have been totally destroyed in a late stage of treatment. Tissue cultures of the patient's own skin cells, or those of a donor, are used in severe cases to replace missing skin.

Rehabilitation from a severe burn takes months or years, and may involve plastic surgery to correct contractures (tight scars) or improve appearance. Physiotherapists, occupational therapists, and even speech pathologists (for inhaled hot gas burns) may all play a part.

CURIOSITY
Patients who die from severe burns tend to do so from dehydration through loss of fluid through the burnt skin that can no longer hold water in the body.

BURPING

urping is normal, but excessive burping may not be, so look after yourself by using antacids initially, but if these are not effective, seek medical advice. Burping is bringing up air or gas from the stomach into the mouth. That air has to get in to the stomach in the first place to be burped, and in the vast majority of cases, it gets in by being swallowed.

People who **eat quickly** tend to swallow air with their food. If a person is nervous, before an exam or interview etc., they may swallow more often as a sign of anxiety and take in extra air. Drinking fizzy liquids, such as lemonade or beer, will also take gas in to the stomach. If small amounts of gas are swallowed, it will move on into the gut to be absorbed or passed through the anus as flatus. Otherwise excess gas tries to escape by going up and out through the mouth.

This is not as easy as it seems because there is a muscular valve at the top of the stomach that stops the food and acid in the stomach from running back up the oesophagus (gullet) into the mouth when bending or lying down. Only when sufficient pressure builds up, or the person can relax the muscular valve themselves, can the air escape, causing the often unexpected and embarrassing explosion. When the gas escapes, it may take small amounts of acid and food with it, causing heartburn or nausea at the same time.

Champagne is a notorious cause of burping.

A change in **diet** can be the answer to persistent burping. An increase in fibre in the diet and a decrease in processed foods will help the situation, but all of us over-indulge or eat inappropriate combinations of foods at different times, and suffer the consequences of stomach pain, belching, nausea and flatus (farts).

A **hiatus hernia** occurs when part of the stomach pushes up through the diaphragm (the sheet of muscle that separates the chest and abdominal cavities) into the chest. The muscle ring that prevents stomach acid from coming back up into the oesophagus then fails to work effectively, allowing reflux oesophagitis to occur very easily.

The excess amounts of acid present in the stomach of patients with a **peptic ulcer** may also damage the muscle ring at the lower end of the oesophagus, and increase the amount of burping.

A wide range of **medications** to relieve excess stomach gas are available. The simpler ones available without prescription from chemists contain substances such as simethicone (which breaks up the bubbles of gas), peppermint oil and charcoal. Simethicone can also be used to relieve wind in babies. If these do not work, doctors can prescribe drugs to prevent the gut spasms, and reduce the production of gas.

CURIOSITY

Burping partly fermented gas from food in the stomach may be a cause of bad breath.

CANCER

L ook after yourself by ensuring that any suspicion of cancer is assessed quickly and appropriately, and be aware of your family history so that any cancer tendency can be investigated regularly.

EXPLANATION

Cancer, the crab of astrology, is so named because the ancients could see the abnormal cancer cells clawing their way into the normal tissue, destroying everything in their path. Doctors now understand a great deal about cancer, but do not fully understand what starts the process. Although the specific cause of cancer is unknown in many cases, sun exposure, a low-fibre diet and smoking are well-known precipitating factors.

Cancer (malignancy or neoplasm) **occurs** when otherwise normal cells start multiplying at an excessive rate, and the cells made by the rapid process of reproduction are abnormal in shape, size and function. Although they may have some slight resemblance to the cells around them, cancer cells cannot perform the correct work of that type of cell, and they prevent the normal cells around them from working properly, thus enabling the cancerous cells to spread.

To try and avoid cancer, don't smoke, don't be promiscuous, eat sensibly, avoid excessive sun exposure and choose your parents carefully.

Cancer is not just one disease process – dozens of different **types** of cancer occur in different parts of the body, and each type causes different problems and responds differently to treatment. Several different types of cancer can be found in the lungs, for example. There are, however, two main groups of cancers according to the type of tissue affected:

- Sarcomas are tumours originating in connective tissue (bone, cartilage, muscle and fibre).

- Carcinomas are tumours originating in the epithelial cells (tissue comprising the external and internal linings of the body).

SIGNS

THE EARLY **SIGNS** OF CANCER ARE:

- a lump or thickening anywhere in the body

- sores that will not heal

65

- unusual bleeding or discharge

- change in bowel or bladder habits

- persistent cough or hoarseness

- change in a wart or mole

- indigestion or difficulty in swallowing

- loss of weight for no apparent reason.

INVESTIGATION
Investigation of a cancer depends upon the organ involved and may include blood tests, urine tests, sputum tests, faeces tests, X-rays, endoscopy, radioactive scans, ultrasound scans, microscopic examinations and magnetic resonance imaging.

TREATMENT
Over half of all cancers can be **cured**, and that excludes the skin cancers that rarely cause death. The cure rate is far higher in those who present early to a doctor, because the less the cancer has spread, the easier it is to treat.

Treatment may involve surgery to remove the growth, drugs that are attracted to and destroy abnormal cells, irradiation of the tumour with high-powered X-rays, specifically developed vaccines or combinations of these methods.

SURGERY
The surgical treatment of cancer is merely the cutting away of as much of the cancerous tissue as possible. It is now common, if possible, to use chemotherapy first to reduce the size of the cancer before surgery. In other cases, radiotherapy and chemotherapy are used after the surgery once wounds have healed. The area to be removed, and the effectiveness of the surgery, varies dramatically from one form of cancer to another.

CHEMOTHERAPY
The **cytotoxics** and **antineoplastics** form a large, diverse group of drugs that are used to destroy cancer cells within the body in a process known as chemotherapy. 'Cyto' means cell, so 'cytotoxic' means toxic (harmful) to cells, while antineoplastic means 'against cancer'.

These drugs can be given by tablet or injection, and different drugs are used to attack different types of cancer. Unfortunately they are not all as specific in attacking cancer cells as we would wish, and normal cells may also be attacked and destroyed. The balance between giving enough of the drug to kill the cancer cells and not enough to kill too many normal cells is a very fine one.

The effectiveness of cytotoxic drugs varies dramatically from one patient to another and one disease to another. Some forms of cancer are very susceptible to cytotoxic drugs (e.g. acute leukaemias), while others are resistant.

Side effects are very common, and again variable. Nausea, vomiting, diarrhoea, muscle pain, loss of hair, weight loss, fatigue and headaches are just a few of the many complications possible. Patients taking this type of medication will be closely monitored by their doctors through regular blood tests and clinic visits. Long-term treatment for many months is usually required, and other medications may be added to control the side effects.

Examples of medications used to treat cancer include bleomycin, carmustine, chlorambucil, cisplatin, cytarabine, daunorubicin, etoposide, fosfestrol, goserelin, mercaptopurine, methotrexate and tamoxifen, but there are many more, and new ones become available almost every month. They should never be used in pregnancy, and may aggravate liver disease and infections.

Cortisone and other steroids cause euphoria (false happiness) when given as an injection into a vein, and have been misused to 'cure' cancer patients.

RADIOTHERAPY

Radiotherapy had its beginnings when Marie Curie, the discoverer of **nuclear radiation**, noted the effect the radiation had upon her hands, and theorised on the possibility of these invisible rays being used to destroy unwanted tissue. Radiotherapy is the treatment of cancer with various forms of ionising radiation. Different types of radiation may be used for different degrees of penetration into the tissue. The time of exposure also varies, depending upon the depth and sensitivity of the cancer. Some cancers are known to be very susceptible to irradiation, while others are quite resistant.

Once a patient is diagnosed as having a tumour that is sensitive to radiotherapy, they will be referred to one of the special clinics attached to major hospitals that have the facilities to apply radiotherapy. There the patient is assessed, the location of the cancer is determined, and special marks will be applied to the patient's skin to allow the beam of radiation to be accurately directed at the cancer.

The patient is firmly secured to a stretcher so that no movement of the area affected by cancer is possible. Then following the plotted guide lines on the skin, the radiation machine is rotated around the patient to give the maximum possible dose of irradiation to the cancer, while avoiding damage to the skin and other vital internal organs.

Depending on the site of the cancer, it may be attacked from only a few directions, or every imaginable direction that is safe. The aim is to destroy the cancer cells and allow the body's natural defence mechanisms and waste clearance cells do the rest of the work.

In other situations, a small amount of radioactive material may be briefly implanted into the cancer within the body, to destroy the surrounding malignant cells.

IMMUNOTHERAPY

Immunotherapy is the enhancement of the body's natural immunity as a method of preventing, or (more recently) of treating disease. Immunisation against a wide range of diseases such as polio, influenza, measles, typhoid, mumps, etc., is a well known role of this area of medicine.

The new role of immunotherapy is in treating cancer, and specifically engineered antibodies are now being used to destroy some types of cancer cells. **Antibodies** are normally produced by the body as a reaction to an invading organism. Antibodies against the measles virus are produced by an attack of measles in order to destroy the invading virus, and these antibodies remain for the rest of the patients life to prevent a further attack of measles.

With genetic engineering techniques that have been developed within the last decade, specific antibodies have already been designed to detect certain types of cancer, and their use experimentally to treat these cancers is under way.

Cancer cells from the patient are cultured artificially, and a **vaccine** to destroy these cells is developed. This vaccine is then given to the patient, quite often with very good results. Unfortunately this process is very time consuming, technically difficult and expensive, and a vaccine must be developed specifically for each patient. Leukaemias, melanomas and lymphomas (lymph gland cancers) are the main areas of success to date.

Immunotherapy is a new science, and medical practitioners are only just beginning to grasp its complexity and potential. Almost certainly immunotherapy will be as significant in the future as the first antibiotics were in 1940.

Women smokers have an increased risk of cancer of the cervix.

CANCER TYPES

THE MOST COMMON TYPES OF NON-SKIN CANCER ARE:

CANCER	INCIDENCE PER 100,000 PEOPLE
Prostate	142
Breast	137
Lung	67
Colon and rectum	54
Bladder	21
Lymphatic system (lymphomas)	20
Ovary	16
Melanoma	15
Kidney	11
Leukaemia (white blood cells)	11
Pancreas	10
Cervix	9
Stomach	7
Thyroid	7
Brain	6
Testes	5
Oesophagus	4.9
Liver	4.8
Larynx	4.3

Tongue	2.5
Vulva	2.5
Gums	1.6
Small intestine	1.6
Tonsils	1.4
Throat	1.4
Anus	1.3
Salivary glands	1.2
Bones and joints	0.9
Pleura (membrane around lung)	0.9
Lip	0.9
Uterus	0.8
Mouth	0.8
Vagina	0.8
Nose	0.7
Penis	0.7
Eye	0.7
Thymus	0.6
Ureter	0.6
Peritoneum (abdomen lining)	0.5

PROSTATE CANCER

Prostatic or prostate cancer describes any one of several different types of cancer of the prostate gland, depending on which cells in the gland become cancerous. The cause is unknown, but those who have sex infrequently may be more susceptible. It is rare before 50 years of age, but up to 20 per cent of all men over 60 may have an **enlargement** of the prostate. The percentage of these men whose enlargement is due to cancer steadily increases with age, with virtually every male over 90 years of age having some degree of prostate cancer.

This is a very **slow-growing** cancer that may give no symptoms until many years after it has developed. Symptoms usually start with difficulty in passing urine and difficulty in starting the urinary stream. In advanced stages there may be spread of cancer to the bones of the pelvis and back.

Specific blood tests can detect most cases, but it is often diagnosed by feeling the gland using a gloved finger in the back passage. Ultrasound scans and biopsy of the gland may also be performed.

It is treated with a combination of surgery, drugs and irradiation. Early stages may not be treated in the very elderly, because it is unlikely to cause trouble in their lifetime.

Brachytherapy is a process in which tiny radioactive particles are injected into the prostate to create radiation which destroys the cancer.

Orchidectomy (removal of the testes) is sometimes performed to remove all testosterone from the man's body, as this stimulates growth of the cancer.

If the cancer is localised to the gland itself, the five-year **survival** rate is over 90 per cent. With local spread, the survival rate drops to about 70 per cent, but with spread to the bone, only 30 per cent of patients survive five years.

The rarest type of cancer is the almost completely unknown cancer that effects the epididymis, the sperm collecting tubes around the testes.

BREAST CANCER

Breast cancer is covered under the BREAST section in this book.

LUNG CANCER

The terms lung cancer, bronchial carcinoma and bronchogenic carcinoma describe any of several different types of cancer affecting lung tissue. The **incidence** of this type of cancer is steadily increasing, particularly in women, and it is the most common form of internal cancer.

Smoking causes 90 per cent of all lung cancers, but this effect of smoking is usually delayed until the patient is 55 or older. Other causes of lung cancer include asbestos dust, irradiation and chrome dust.

There are several different types of lung cancer, depending on the cells within the lung that are affected. The common types are:

- **Squamous cell** carcinoma is a relatively common form, in which symptoms usually occur early, but the cancer doubles in size every three months on average, and spreads early to lymph nodes.

- **Oat cell** (small cell) carcinomas are far more serious, double in size every month on average, spread rapidly to other parts of the body, and are almost impossible to cure.

- **Adenocarcinomas** and large cell carcinomas develop at the edge of the lung, have few symptoms, are not easily detected, double in size every three to six months, but spread early to distant parts of the body.

- **Secondary** cancers are the spread of cancer from other parts of the body to the lungs. These are common, but they are not caused by smoking, and their treatment involves the treatment of the original cancer as well as that in the lung.

Many other rarer types of lung cancer are known.

In future decades, lung cancer may become a disease affecting more women than men, as more young women now smoke than young men.

The early warning **signs** are weight loss, a persistent cough, a change in the normal type of cough, coughing blood and worsening breathlessness. Later symptoms include loss of appetite, chest pain, hoarseness and enlarged tender lymph nodes in the armpit. Spread of the cancer to other organs is the next stage, most commonly to bone and the brain, and blockage of the veins draining the head and arms (superior vena cava syndrome).

One quarter of patients have no symptoms when the diagnosis is made, often by a routine chest X-ray, so smokers should consider having a routine chest X-ray every few years.

The cancer is **diagnosed** by chest X-rays, CT scans, sputum examination, and a biopsy of the tumour using a bronchoscope (tube into the lung) if possible.

Prevention is always better than cure, and that means stop smoking. Even in heavy smokers, after five years of non-smoking, the risk of developing lung cancer will reduce to near normal.

Treatment involves major surgery, irradiation, and potent drugs, depending on the type of cancer present. Radiation may be used to shrink the original tumour, but is primarily used to treat cancers that have spread to other organs.

Fewer than 20 per cent of all patients with lung cancer survive more than five years from diagnosis. Those with small cell (oat cell) carcinoma usually die within a year, while those with squamous cell carcinoma tend to live longer than average.

BOWEL CANCER

Colorectal cancer is cancer of the large bowel, which forms the last two metres of the intestine.

The absolute **cause** is unknown, but a low fibre and high fat diet may be a factor and there is a definite family tendency. It is more common in men, and most develop in the last 10cm of the gut. Finding polyps on a routine colonoscopy or CT scan, ulcerative colitis and chronic bowel infections are also risk factors. Any polyps found are always removed to prevent them from becoming cancerous.

Screening for colorectal cancer can be done by performing a colonoscopy every five years over the age of 50 in all those at high risk, and by testing the faeces on at least three occasions for the presence of blood on all those who wish to have the test.

Symptoms include alteration in normal bowel habits, passing blood with the faeces, weight loss, colicky pains in the abdomen and constant tiredness. A large cancer can be felt as a hard lump in the abdomen. If left untreated, a gut obstruction, or perforation which allows faeces to leak into the abdomen and causes peritonitis, will occur.

A colonoscopy and/or barium enema X-ray will confirm the diagnosis. Blood tests may show anaemia due to the constant slow leaking of blood from the cancer. People with a bad family history can have a faeces sample tested for blood.

Treatment involves major surgery to remove the cancer, the bowel for some distance above and below the cancer, and the surrounding lymph nodes. Up to three per cent of patients may die during or immediately after surgery. Chemotherapy (drugs) and radiotherapy may also be used. Regular examinations of the colon are then required lifelong to detect any recurrence.

If the cancer has not spread away from the large intestine, two out of three patients will survive for more than five years, and are probably cured as most recurrences occur within four years. If the cancer has spread, the survival rate drops steadily, depending on the degree of spread.

COLORECTAL CANCERS ARE STAGED BY THE DUKES SYSTEM THUS:

Stage A: Cancer limited to lining of gut – over 95 per cent cured.

Stage B1:   Cancer extends into muscle surrounding gut – about 85 per cent cured.

Stage B2:   Cancer extends through full thickness of gut wall – about 80 per cent cured.

Stage C: Cancer has spread to surrounding lymph nodes in the pelvis – cure rates vary from 35 per cent to 60 per cent.

Stage D: Cancer has spread to distant organs (e.g. liver, lung) – less than ten per cent cured.

Cancers closer to the anus are more difficult to treat and more likely to result in a colostomy.

George Papanicolou (as in the Pap Smear Test) was a Greek/American physician (b. 1883) who developed a staining process to detect cancer cells in bodily secretions.

CANCER OF THE CERVIX

Cancer of the cervix involves the part of the **uterus** (womb) which opens into the top of the vagina. It is one of the more common forms of female cancer, and more common in women who have multiple sexual partners, women who are smokers, and much more common in women who have been infected with the human papilloma virus which causes genital warts.

There may be no **symptoms** for several years after the cancer is present, then abnormal vaginal bleeding, foul discharge, pain and/or bleeding on intercourse, and discomfort in the lower abdomen may occur.

The cancer may be detected at an early stage by a **Pap smear** test. If a Pap smear result is suspicious, the cervix will be more closely examined through a microscope that looks into the vagina (a colposcope). Biopsy of a suspicious area can then confirm the diagnosis.

It is easily treated in early stages by burning away the cancerous area with diathermy or laser, or a cone-shaped area of tissue may be excised. These forms of treatment do not interfere with the woman's ability to become pregnant, or function normally in her sexual responses. Only if the cancer is advanced is a hysterectomy required or radiation therapy used. If left untreated the cancer may spread to the lymph nodes in the pelvis, the uterus, ureters and other organs.

Ninety-nine per cent of early stage cancer is **cured**, 65 per cent of cases with medium stage survive, but only five per cent of those with spread outside the pelvis are alive after five years. Regular Pap smears can therefore save lives.

MELANOMA

Melanoma is covered under the SKIN CANCER section in this book.

CURIOSITY

Bruising around the belly button (Cullen's sign) may indicate conditions as varied as a ruptured ectopic pregnancy and cancer of the pancreas.

Extract from an 1830 medical text book:
'To obtain recovery in cases of cancer, aconite (a potent poison) is recommended for persons of sanguine temperament; arsenic is better for bilious or melancholic temperament; and graphite for those of lean habit'.

CHECK UP

L ook after yourself by having regular check ups by your general practitioner, the doctor who should know you and your family, on a regular basis. Don't swap practices for different problems, as your medical records will become fragmented, leading to a deterioration in the overall quality of your care. Doctor swapping is a health hazard.

The 'annual check up' has been a much used phrase in literature and conversation, but is it necessary? How often should it be done? What should be done?

It is probably not necessary for everyone to have a full check up every year, but they should be done on a regular basis, and the older you are, the more frequently they need to be performed.

FREQUENCY

It is reasonable to have one thorough medical examination at about 30 years of age. If nothing abnormal is found, and you are otherwise in good health, no further check should be needed until you are 40. From then until 55 a five yearly check up would be advisable, and after the late fifties, they should gradually become more frequent until they become an annual event by 70 years of age.

Women need more frequent check ups than this for their Pap smear tests. These should be done every 24 to 36 months from the early twenties until old age. Women should also check their breasts themselves every month, and report any abnormalities to their doctor immediately. Breast X-rays (mammograms) are recommended in women, starting in their late forties.

Many 'executive health checks' are of more benefit to the doctor's wallet than the patient's health.

WHAT TO CHECK

The most important part of any check up is what you tell the doctor. At the beginning of the consultation the doctor will ask 20 or 30 wide ranging questions. The answers to these will lead the doctor to ask more detailed questions about some areas of your health, and will enable the correct tests and investigations (if any) to be ordered.

Hopefully, your answers will not cause any concern to the doctor, and they will be able to undertake a physical examination of your throat, nose, ears, eyes, chest and abdomen.

Your **smoking** habits, **weight**, **diet**, **alcohol** intake and **exercise** levels will all be assessed, and appropriate advice will be given when necessary.

A **blood pressure** reading will be made using an inflatable cuff around the upper part of the arm. Control of high blood pressure, which may start relatively early in life, will do more to reduce the incidence of heart disease than any other factor.

Most doctors routinely order a **cholesterol** and **triglyceride** blood test at the first check up, but if this is satisfactory, it does not need to be repeated for some years. It is necessary to fast for 12 hours and go without alcohol for 72 hours before this test to reach an accurate reading.

Any suspicious **spots** or moles on your skin will be checked during the examination to ensure that they are not malignant.

Some doctors recommend **faeces testing** for blood to detect early bowel problems, but the cost and inconvenience of this test related to its effectiveness is still a matter of controversy in medical circles.

No matter how fit, healthy, full of life and vigour you feel,
no one is bullet-proof from disease and illness.

Unless there are indications from the examination so far, it is not necessary for any further investigations to be performed. Routine chest X-rays are now frowned upon by the National Health and Medical Research Council, and a cardiograph (ECG) is only indicated if there is a likelihood of heart disease.

More important than any routine check up is the early presentation to a doctor when any symptoms or changes to your body occur. Far too many patients leave it too long to see a doctor after they notice a swelling, change in bowel habits, unusual pain or other problem.

It is far better to be reassured today that your problem is of no concern, than to be told after several weeks that you have left it too late for effective treatment.

CURIOSITY

Abnormal may be normal. If a wide enough range of blood tests are performed, statistically ten per cent of them will be abnormal, as the quoted normal range is that which is found in 90 per cent of the population. The top and bottom five per cent are considered to be outside the normal range, regardless of whether any disease is present.

CHEST PAIN

I n looking after yourself, always have chest pain checked by a doctor. A crushing pressure-like chest pain is a medical emergency requiring immediate ambulance attention.

EXPLANATION

A pain in the chest is a very distressing symptom, as patients are often concerned that it may be serious, and rightly so. Because chest pains might be caused by a life-threatening condition involving the heart or lungs, medical help should be sought rapidly unless there is an obvious cause.

Other organs that may cause chest pain include the oesophagus, breast bone, ribs, aorta (main artery of the body), thymus gland, lymph nodes, smaller arteries, veins or nerves, as well as the structures around the area such as the muscles, ligaments, skin, breasts or the vertebrae in the back.

The nature of the pain (sharp, ache, dull, pressure), whether it is constant or intermittent, if it is affected by eating, exercising, coughing or taking a deep breath, if it starts in one area then moves to another, what tends to make the pain better or worse, and the presence of associated symptoms such as vomiting, cough, shortness of breath, loss of appetite, fever and pain on swallowing may enable the doctor to make a definitive diagnosis.

INVESTIGATIONS

Investigations to further aid a doctor may include blood tests, X-rays (but these show only bones, and not soft tissue), CT scans (computerised cross sectional X-rays which show some soft tissues), electrocardiographs (ECG – read the electrical activity of the heart), lung function tests (blowing into various machines), endoscopy (passing a flexible telescope tube in through the mouth and down the oesophagus or into the lungs), and as a last resort, surgery.

ECGs were first performed on volunteers who knelt with hands and feet in buckets of water which acted as electrodes on the skin.

CAUSES

COMMON CAUSES OF CHEST PAIN INCLUDE:

- An **injury** to the chest that causes bruising, fractured ribs, muscle or ligamentous tears, may cause pain in varying parts of the chest that is usually worsened by any movement.

- Viral **infections** frequently cause generalised muscle inflammation, resulting in aches and pains in varying muscle bundles, including those in the chest and back.

- **Arthritis** of the vertebrae in the back may cause pinching of nerves and pain not only in the back, but running around the sides of the chest to the front as well. Changes in position often vary this pain.

- A **heart attack** (myocardial infarct) occurs when one of the small arteries supplying the heart muscle becomes blocked by a piece of clot or debris from a cholesterol plaque. Pain may occur in any part of the chest, neck, jaw or arms (left more than right), but the usual sites for pain are the left chest, lower front of neck, central chest and front of left shoulder. It is usually described as a crushing pressure or severe ache rather than a sharp pain. It is not affected by movement, eating or coughing, and does not usually vary in intensity. If in doubt, see a doctor now!

- **Angina** is a pressure-like, squeezing pain or tightness in the chest, usually central, that starts suddenly, often during exercise, and settles with rest.

- **Pneumonia** is a bacterial infection of the tiny air bubbles (alveoli) that form the major part of the lung and enable oxygen to cross into the bloodstream. The symptoms include fever, cough and chest pains.

- **Pleurisy** causes severe localised pain that is worse with breathing, coughing or any movement of the chest.

- The stomach contains concentrated hydrochloric acid, and is protected from this by a thick lining of mucus. If the acid comes back up into the unprotected oesophagus (**reflux oesophagitis**), intense burning may be felt behind the breast bone, as well as a bitter taste, shortness of breath and burping.

- A **hiatus hernia** may cause burning pain behind the breast bone, burping and an acid taste at the back of the tongue.

- **Tietze syndrome**, which is a painful, tender swelling of one or more of the carti-lages that join the end of each rib to the side of the breast bone.

- A **blood clot** (pulmonary embolus) in one of the major arteries within the lungs (pulmonary thrombosis) will cause severe damage to that section of lung beyond the clot, leading to its collapse, pain and shortness of breath.

A blood clot in the deeper calf veins of the lower leg may cause a subsequent blood clot in the lungs which is characterised by chest pain and shortness of breath.

If an **aneurysm** on the aorta enlarges, leaks or bursts, pain may be felt in this area that varies from an ache to severe pain, depending on the degree of damage.

LESS COMMON CAUSES OF CHEST PAIN INCLUDE:

- pneumothorax (air in the chest outside the lung)

- a foreign body (e.g. food, small toy) caught in the oesophagus or a bronchus

- shingles (viral infection of a nerve)

- bronchiectasis (lung damage)

- myocarditis (infection of the heart muscle)

- abnormalities of the heart structure that may be present at birth (e.g. Fallot's tetralogy)

- severe anaemia

- failure of the major valves in the heart (particularly the mitral valve between the left ventricle and atrium)

- cancer in the lymph nodes within the chest

- cardiac neuroses (excessive concern about heart disease)

- slipping rib syndrome

- Bornholm disease (pleurodynia – chest wall inflammation)

- cholecystitis (inflammation or infection of the gall bladder)

- peptic ulcer

- back pain (pinched nerve from arthritis between the vertebrae).

CURIOSITY

Extract from an 1821 medical guide book for lay people:

'Love, though at first but a moral malady, very frequently gives rise to pains in the chest and organic diseases of the heart and lungs'.

CHOKING

L ook after yourself, your family and friends, by knowing how to deal with a sudden episode of choking.

Choking occurs when a foreign body gets stuck in the airway so that breathing is obstructed. When choking occurs, the victim may have a violent fit of coughing and the face and neck will become deep red, turning to purple. They will make a superhuman effort to breathe, and if unsuccessful will claw the air and clutch at the throat before turning blue in the face and collapsing.

Often the object will be dislodged by the coughing. If not, try to remove it with your finger – but be extremely careful not to push it down further. If that is unsuccessful, two or three sharp blows between the shoulder blades may clear it. Make sure the person is in a position in which the object can fall out easily – e.g. an adult should sit and lean forward. If the victim is lying down, turn them gently to one side.

MANAGEMENT

If this fails, there are several ways in which you may proceed:

1. The **Heimlich manoeuvre** is a method of relieving a person who is choking on inhaled food or other object.

   Place your arms around the victim's chest from behind, with your clenched fists over the breast bone. As suddenly and as hard as you can, push on the breast bone and squeeze the chest.

   The procedure may need to be repeated several times, but there is a risk of breaking ribs, particularly if the victim is smaller than the helper.

   The Heimlich manoeuvre is named after the American surgeon, Henry Heimlich (b. 1920).

2. Lie the patient in the **coma position** on their side on the floor, give several sharp blows between the shoulder blades, and then if necessary, give several firm quick pushes on the side of the chest wall below the arm pit.

3. Place the victim on a table so that they are **hanging** over the edge from the waist up, with the top of their head on the floor. Try the chest compression again so that it is aided by gravity.

If all these measures fail and the victim is unconscious, lie them on their back and tilt the head backwards to maximise the airway. Sit astride the victim and place the heel of your hand on the upper abdomen just above the navel. Cover it with the heel of your other hand. Give a sharp downward and forward thrust towards the victim's head. Give up to four thrusts if necessary. If the victim does not splutter and start breathing, start mouth-to-mouth **resuscitation**.

As the victim starts breathing normally, place them in the lateral or coma position and get medical help. It is especially important to tell the doctor if chest compression has been used, so that the internal organs can be checked.

If all efforts to dislodge the object fail, you will have to blow air past it by using mouth-to-mouth resuscitation until medical help is obtained.

If you have a **child** who is choking, sit down and lie the child face down across your lap, with the head low. Give two or three blows between the shoulder blades with the heel of your hand. If this is unsuccessful, administer chest compression.

A **baby** can be held upside down in your arms while you slap it between the shoulder blades or administer chest compression.

CURIOSITY

A morbid fear of choking is called pnigerophobia by doctors.

CHOLESTEROL

D o you know your cholesterol level? Is it satisfactory? If not, look after yourself and see your general practitioner to have an accurate test performed by an accredited laboratory.

EXPLANATION

A yellow/white fatty substance called cholesterol is responsible for a large proportion of the heart attacks, strokes, circulatory problems and kidney disease in the Western world. Yet cholesterol is **essential** for the normal functioning of the human body. It is responsible for cementing cells together, is a major constituent of bile, and is the basic building block for sex hormones. Only in excess (when the patient is said to have hypercholesterolaemia) is it harmful.

About 70 per cent of the body's cholesterol is actually **manufactured** in the liver, and only 30 per cent is obtained through the diet. If too much cholesterol is carried around in the blood stream, it may be deposited in gradually increasing amounts inside the arteries. Slowly, the affected artery narrows, until the flow of blood is sufficiently obstructed to cause the area supplied by that artery to suffer. If that area is the heart, a heart attack will result; if it is the brain, a stroke will occur. This deposition of fat is known as **arteriosclerosis**, or hardening of the arteries.

LEVELS

The level of cholesterol in the body is determined by **inherited** traits and **diet**. The people most affected by high levels of cholesterol are overweight middle-aged men. Women, and some normal weight people may be affected too, but not as frequently.

It has been proved that if cholesterol levels are within normal limits, the risk of heart attack is greatly reduced. It is therefore important for anyone who feels they may be at risk, and everyone at 40 years of age, to have a blood test to determine their cholesterol level. For this test to be accurate, it is necessary to fast for 12 hours (usually overnight), and avoid alcohol for 72 hours before the blood sample is taken.

If the cholesterol level is below **4.5 mmol/L**, there is no need for concern. If it is above 5.0 mmol/L, the doctor will probably order tests to find out what types of cholesterol are present. Lower levels of cholesterol are of concern in patients who have diabetes or a history of heart attack or stroke, smokers and patients with some other diseases. Levels should also be lower in young people than old, and males than females.

TYPES

There are two main **subgroups** of cholesterol – high density (which protect you from heart attacks and strokes) and low density (which are bad for you). The ratio between these two types of cholesterol will determine the treatment (if any) that is required.

Xanthomata are a complication of excess cholesterol. Small, fatty, yellow lumps appear on the skin around the eyes, and on the knees, elbows and buttocks. They may be destroyed by cautery (burning) or removed surgically.

If the patient is found to be in the high risk group, there are several measures they can take to bring the levels back to normal. The first step is to stop smoking, limit alcohol intake, take more exercise and lose weight if obese. If these measures are insufficient, doctors will recommend a diet that is low in fat and cholesterol. On this, many people return to within normal cholesterol levels after a month or two.

TREATMENT

The first step in treatment is always a trial of diet, and only if this fails is medication considered.

DIET

A low cholesterol diet has the following rules:

| FOODS ALLOWED | Vegetables, chicken breast, cereals, margarine, fruit and nuts, dark chocolate, fish, olive oil, lean meat, pasta, skim milk, wine and beer. |
| FOODS TO AVOID | Sausages, hamburgers, pies, mince, chicken skin and legs, pizza, offal (liver, kidneys, tripe), roast meats (particularly surface), game meat, lamb chops, calamari, prawns, milk chocolate, eggs and egg products, oysters, and all dairy products (cream, milk, butter, yoghurt, cheese, custard). |

MEDICATIONS

Despite a strict diet, there are still some people who cannot keep their cholesterol levels under control. They will require further lifelong medical management by the regular use of **medications** (hypolipidaemics) that are designed to lower the level of fat in the blood. These are prescribed by a doctor only when necessary.

Once the fatty deposits of cholesterol are deposited inside the arteries, they remain there permanently. There are new drugs that may partially remove these deposits over many years, and surgical techniques are available to clean out clogged arteries, but diet has little effect at this late stage. As in all diseases, prevention is much better than cure.

The drugs used to lower cholesterol are **hypolipidaemics**. The term 'hypo' means low (as opposed to 'hyper', meaning high), lipids are fats, and the term 'aemia' refers to the blood (compare 'anaemia' – lack of blood), so a hypolipidaemic is a drug that lowers fat in the blood. The fats include both cholesterol and triglycerides. A combination of diet and drugs are used to control excess levels of fat in the bloodstream.

Fat-lowering hypolipidaemics include tablets in the newer statins subclass which are generally more convenient, effective and have fewer side effects than the older medications such as clofibrate and probucol (tablets), colestipol and cholestyramine (powders to mix with water) which are taken after meals to remove fats from the blood. These older medications can be useful additive treatment to the statins and in some diabetics and obese patients, but they interact with a number of other medications that may be essential for the patient's well-being.

Medication does not cure excess cholesterol, merely controls it,
and must be continued lifelong or the problem will rapidly recur.

The drugs in the **statins** class include atorvastatin (Lipitor), cerivastatin (Lipobay), fluvastatin (Lescol, Vastin), pravastatin (Pravachol) and simvastatin (Lipex, Zocor). Side effects may include constipation, diarrhoea, excess wind, nausea and headache. They should not be used in pregnancy or severe liver disease. Regular blood tests are necessary to check liver function and fat levels.

Cholestyramine (Questran) is an old-fashioned medication used to reduce blood cholesterol, the itch of liver failure, and in some other intestinal diseases. Side effects may include constipation, belly discomfort, excess wind, heartburn and a rash. It must be used with care in pregnancy, and not in gall bladder disease. The powder must always be mixed with water, and not swallowed dry.

Clofibrate (Atromid S) is another older style medication that reduces both blood cholesterol and triglyceride levels. Side effects may include nausea, vomiting and diarrhoea. Must be used with care in pregnancy, and not in patients with liver failure.

Colestipol (Colestid) is a hypolipidaemic used in difficult cases. Its most common side effect is constipation. It must not be used in patients with diabetes or thyroid disease. The powder must always be mixed with water, and not swallowed dry.

Gemfibrizol (Jezil, Lopid) also reduces both blood cholesterol and triglyceride levels. Side effects may include heartburn, belly pains, nausea and diarrhoea. It must be used with caution in pregnancy, and may reduce fertility.

Nicotinic acid is one of the oldest medications used to reduce blood cholesterol and triglycerides, and it also aids poor circulation. Side effects may include a rash, itch, nervousness, heart changes and stomach upsets. It must be used with care in pregnancy, and not in patients with a peptic ulcer or a recent heart attack.

Probucol (Lurselle) is reserved for patients with severe high blood cholesterol level. Side effects may include diarrhoea, nausea, excess wind and belly pains. It must be used with care in pregnancy, and not in patients with a recent heart attack or heart disease.

Fenofibrate is a less commonly used medication in this class.

ARTERIOSCLEROSIS

Arteriosclerosis, or **hardening of the arteries**, is a degeneration of the arteries in the body, making them hard and inelastic. It is usually associated with atherosclerosis, which is the the excessive deposition of hard fatty plaques and nodules within the artery and its wall.

It usually occurs in the elderly, and those who have a high blood level of cholesterol, but may also be caused and aggravated by high blood pressure. Hard fatty deposits form at points of turbulence within a major artery (e.g. the junction of two arteries, or a bend in the artery) to narrow the artery and gradually restrict the flow of blood to the tissues beyond.

Symptoms depend on which arteries are affected. An affected artery is less able to cope with pressure changes and more likely to rupture, causing a leak of blood, sometimes into vital structures such as the brain. If a neck artery (carotid artery) is involved, patients cannot cope with sudden changes in position (e.g. getting out of bed) without becoming dizzy or light-headed. If the leg arteries are involved, the leg muscles become painful, particularly when climbing slopes or stairs (claudication). If heart arteries are involved, angina occurs. If arteries to the brain are involved, the patient may develop a multitude of bizarre symptoms, become light headed, dizzy, confused, or black out, as the brain does not receive sufficient blood to operate correctly.

The heart is very badly designed. Most organs have multiple arteries supplying each area, but in the heart there is only one artery for each area, so if a blood clot blocks an artery there are always serious consequences.

An embolism occurs when a piece of the hard fat within the artery breaks away and travels with the blood along the arteries to a point which is too narrow for it to pass. This causes no problem in most parts of the body, but if the blockage is in the heart or brain, a heart attack or stroke will occur.

Arteriosclerosis is **diagnosed** by doppler flow (ultrasound) studies on the movement of blood through arteries, and by angiograms (artery X-rays) in which an X-ray visible dye is injected to outline an artery. Cholesterol levels can be checked by a fasting blood test.

The condition is better **prevented** than treated, by keeping cholesterol levels and blood pressure within normal limits. Narrowed arteries can be opened slightly with medications that relax the muscles in the artery walls, or that ease the passage of blood cells through the narrowing, but in advanced cases, surgery is necessary.

THERE ARE THREE TYPES OF **SURGERY** POSSIBLE:

- bypass grafts use tubes of synthetic material, or arteries or veins from elsewhere in the body, to bypass the blocked area.

- endarterectomy involves opening the blocked artery and cleaning out the fatty deposits.

- balloon angioplasty is used to dilate blocked arteries by passing a fine tube, with a deflated balloon at the end, along an artery and into the narrowed segment where the balloon is inflated, forcing open the blockage. Sometimes a stent (tube shaped metal grid) is left behind to keep the artery open.

Medication can help many cases, and surgery can be extremely successful in curing the condition.

CURIOSITY

Droplets of cholesterol are produced in the cells lining the small intestine and found circulating in the blood where they are called chylomicrons.

COLONOSCOPY

Those who have abnormal bowel symptoms, or a family history of bowel cancer, should look after themselves by having a colonoscopy regularly from age 50 onwards.

ANATOMY

The **colon** is the major part of the large intestine and consists of a large loop that circuits the belly. Dividing the ileum of the small intestine from the colon is a muscular valve which opens to let food into the colon but otherwise remains closed to prevent the food passing back into the small intestine.

The colon starts at the caecum and passes up through the abdomen as the ascending colon. When it reaches just below the liver, it makes a sharp turn and travels across the abdomen to the left side near the spleen as the transverse colon. It then makes a sharp downwards turn and becomes the descending colon. This extends down the left side of the abdomen to the pelvis. At the bottom of the descending colon is an S-bend, called the sigmoid colon, which empties into the rectum.

LARGE INTESTINE

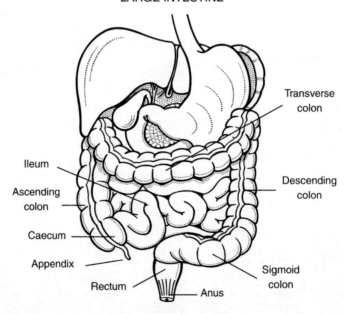

Food that is not digested in the small intestine passes into the colon. Here most of the water content is extracted to be reabsorbed into the bloodstream, and the remaining semisolid waste passes into the rectum to be stored until it is eliminated from the body through the anus.

At 65mm, the large intestine is nearly twice the diameter of the small intestine, and is 1.5 to 2m in length from caecum to anus.

A redundant colon is one that is too long and has too many twists and turns, usually in the sigmoid area. A full colonoscopy may be impossible in a redundant colon.

PROCEDURE

A colonoscopy is an examination of the large bowel or colon using a **colonoscope**, which is a flexible tube which combines the features of magnification and illumination. It is two metres long and enables the doctor to view the entire colon.

For the lower third of the colon, an instrument called a **sigmoidoscope** may be used, which is rigid but shorter than the colonoscope and enables an examination of the bowel for polyps, tumours and other diseases. The instrument used for seeing inside the rectum and anus is called a **proctoscope**.

Before having a colonoscopy, the patient will be given a laxative or an enema and then be instructed to drink only clear fluids for the day before the test is performed. A solution must also be drunk in the day before the test to thoroughly cleanse the bowel. It is unusual to feel any discomfort during the procedure as an effective sedative is given. The examination takes about an hour, and any polyps found will be removed during the procedure.

As with any procedure, there are **risks**. Perforation of the bowel may occur in about one in every 2000 procedures, and this will require an open operation to close the hole. Bleeding into the bowel, particularly after the removal of a polyp, is another rare complication. Even in the best circumstances, about five per cent of cancers present will be missed. One in every 16 000 patients die from the complications of a colonoscopy.

VIRTUAL COLONOSCOPY

Virtual colonoscopy uses a sophisticated spiral **CT X-ray** or MRI (magnetic resonance imaging) scanner, to obtain a three dimensional X-ray picture of the colon that will usually detect polyps and tumours over 10mm in diameter. Unlike a normal colonoscopy, it is a non-invasive procedure, but still involves the same degree of bowel preparation with special diets, laxatives and enemas to clean out the gut before the procedure.

This investigation is currently too expensive to allow its widespread use, but is appropriate in some circumstances. Unlike conventional colonoscopy, any polyp detected cannot be removed, and a further procedure is necessary.

CURIOSITY
From the teeth to the anus, the digestive tract is about ten metres long. Using gastroscopes doctors can examine the top two metres, and colonoscopes examine the bottom two metres, but the middle six metres of small intestine often remains a mystery with difficult-to-diagnose diseases.

COMMON COLD

T he best way to look after yourself with a cold is to take rest, more rest, and yet more rest, until completely better.

EXPLANATION

A common cold is a **viral** infection of the upper respiratory tract. One or more of several hundred different rhinoviruses may be responsible. A cold is a distinct entity from influenza, which is caused by a different group of viruses.

The viral infection causes the lining of the nose, sinuses and throat to become red, sore and swollen; and phlegm and mucus are produced in great quantities to give a stuffy head, sore throat and runny nose to their victim. A secondary bacterial infection may cause pharyngitis or sinusitis.

The toxins (poisons) created by the body destroying the viruses circulate around in the blood stream to cause the fever and muscular aches that are also associated with a cold. While the patient is suffering, the body is busy producing the appropriate antibodies to fight the infection. Once the number of antibodies produced is adequate to destroy most of the viruses, the symptoms of the disease disappear.

Colds spread from one person to another in droplets of moisture in the breath, in a cough or in a sneeze. Once inhaled, the virus settles in the nose or throat and starts multiplying rapidly. Crowds, confined spaces (e.g. buses, aircraft) and air conditioners that recycle air are renowned for spreading the virus.

Most adults have a cold every year or two, usually in winter. Children, because they have not been exposed to these viruses before and so have no immunity to them, may have ten or more infections a year.

MANAGEMENT

No cure or prevention is possible. The symptoms can be eased by aspirin or paracetamol for headache and fever, and medications for the cough, sore throat, runny nose and blocked sinuses. The more the patient rests, the faster the infection will go away. Many vitamin and herbal remedies are touted as cures or preventatives, but when subjected to detailed trials, none can be proved to be successful.

Colds usually last about a week, but some people have a briefer course, while in others the first cold may lower their defences so that they can catch another one, and then another, causing cold symptoms to last for many weeks.

The technical term used by doctors for a common cold is coryza.

VIRUSES

A virus is an infective agent smaller than a bacteria, is not a cell, is unable to be seen using a light microscope, has no internal metabolic processes, and is unable to replicate without the use of a living cell.

Viruses are unimaginably small, and millions could exist on this full stop. They can be found anywhere in the environment – in the body, or in a drop of sweat, in saliva, or the skin of the family dog.

Every virus in the body is under constant attack by the body's defence system. Every minute, millions more viruses enter the body through the mouth or nose. As they enter, the defence system uses its special cells and protein particles (**antibodies**) to repel the attack.

Sometimes the defences are overwhelmed for a short time by the rapidly multiplying viruses. When this happens, the patient may feel off-colour for a day or two. If the virus numbers manage to totally defeat the defenders, a full-blown viral infection will develop. Viruses can cause diseases as diverse as measles, hepatitis, cold sores, chickenpox, glandular fever, AIDS and the common cold.

Virus particles are so small that they cannot be seen by even the most powerful light microscope, and special electron microscopes have to be used. They are neither animal nor plant, but particles that are so basic that they are classified into a group of their own. They are not alive in any sense that we understand, but are overgrown molecules that are intent on reproducing themselves at the expense of any host that happens along.

Because they are not truly alive, they cannot be killed, and so antibiotics that are effective against the much larger living cells known as bacteria have no effect on viruses. Other than for a limited number of viruses that cause genital herpes, shingles and cold sores, doctors have no cure for virus infections.

PREVENTION

Doctors can **vaccinate** against some viral diseases, such as measles and influenza, to prevent them; but others such as the common cold cannot be prevented.

Viral infections can best be avoided by a good, well-balanced diet, reasonable exercise, avoiding stress, avoiding extremes of temperature, and avoiding those who already have the infection.

CURIOSITY

Viruses function with about ten genes, while bacteria are far more complex organisms requiring over 1000 genes. A bacteria can be, and frequently is, infected with a virus. A bacteria can therefore catch a cold, albeit with very different symptoms to those experienced by humans.

CONSTIPATION

L ook after your bowels and look after yourself. Some wits argue that the anus controls the rest of the body, because if it fails to work properly, the rest of the body suffers.

We have all experienced the strain and discomfort of constipation at some stage of our lives as a result of changes in diet, dehydration or reduced activity, but if it persists, a specific cause should be sought so that long-term complications do not occur.

Normal bowel activity can vary from two or three times a day to two or three times a week, or even once a week in some individuals. Constipation increases with age and is far more common in the elderly than the young.

To be medically significant, constipation must cause discomfort in the abdomen, pain around the anus, bleeding, tears (both pronunciations of the word are appropriate), piles or another problem.

Passing faeces twice a week is just as normal as three times a day,
provided neither habit causes discomfort.

Hard dry motions are usually due to inadequate fluid intake, eating too much junk food with too little fibre, or lack of exercise. They may also be due to repeatedly ignoring signals to pass a motion and allowing the bowel to become distended, which reduces the urge to eliminate and the problem becomes self-perpetuating.

The major **complications** of persistent constipation are piles (bleeding under the skin caused by over stretching of the anus and straining), anal tears (fissures) and megacolon (an overdilated lower end of gut that cannot contract properly). All these problems can worsen constipation as well as being a result of the problem, as patients with piles and tears are reluctant to pass motions because of pain, while megacolon prevents normal lower bowel contraction to move faeces along.

CAUSES

There are many different **causes** of significant constipation.

Bedridden patients often find they become constipated due to the lack of activity and body movement. Even a healthy person who becomes less active because of a broken leg or bad dose of the flu may suffer the same effects.

Changes in **diet**, particularly if more protein and less fibre is suddenly eaten, and lack of fluid (dehydration) will both cause the faeces to harden and dry.

In the last three months of **pregnancy**, many women find that constipation becomes a problem as the growing baby puts pressure on the bowel.

A **prolapse** of the bowel occurs when it bulges forward into a woman's vagina, or slides out through the anus due to weakening of the support structures with pregnancy or age. Straining to pass a motion only worsens the prolapse without moving the faeces.

Many different **medications** can have constipation as a side effect. Examples include codeine, narcotics (e.g. morphine), antacids, anticonvulsants (for epilepsy and fits), antidepressants, diuretics (fluid tablets) and iron.

LESS COMMON CAUSES OF CONSTIPATION MAY INCLUDE:

- hypothyroidism (underactive thyroid gland)

- tumours or cancers of the last part of the large intestine

- irritable bowel syndrome (abnormal bowel spasms)

- depression

- neuroses and psychiatric disturbances

- Hirschsprung disease (birth defect of bowel nerve supply)

- diabetes mellitus

- persistent high levels of calcium in the blood stream (hypercalcaemia) from kidney or parathyroid gland disease

- abnormal balances of sodium, potassium or chloride in the blood.

Extensive **investigations** (e.g. colonoscopy, barium enema X-ray) may be necessary to determine cause in persistent cases.

TREATMENT

Treatment of constipation should be aimed at treating the underlying cause if possible. **Dietary** methods are the next choice, and only if neither is possible should laxatives or other medications be used. Patients should change their diet by avoiding white bread, pastries, biscuits, sweets and chocolates, and adding plenty of fluids and fibre-containing foods such as cereals, vegetables and fruit. If necessary, fibre supplements may be used. Pear and prune juice, and rhubarb stew may be very effective.

Laxatives are the next step, but dependence can develop rapidly. They vary in effectiveness and strength, but the weakest ones (e.g. paraffin, other oils, senna and cascara) should be tried first. As a last resort, enemas may be used to clear out the lower gut.

The prognosis of constipation depends on the cause, but the condition can usually be well managed by appropriate treatment.

Long-term unrelieved constipation may result in megacolon.

MEGACOLON

A megacolon is a massive **distension** of the descending and sigmoid colon, the last parts of the large intestine.

Long-term constipation and retention of faeces stretches the large bowel, or it may be a complication of ulcerative colitis, associated with some psychiatric and low intellect disorders, a symptom of an underactive thyroid gland (hypothyroidism), due to excessive use of narcotics, or a birth defect (Hirschsprung disease).

The symptoms of megacolon include severe constipation, sometimes associated with lower abdominal pain and a watery diarrhoea as liquid faeces flows around the blockage. Rarely the bowel may rupture causing life threatening peritonitis.

Doctors then treat any underlying disease, remove faeces build up, recommend a special high fibre diet, and advise the careful use of laxatives. Surgery in the form of a colostomy (opening bowel onto skin) is a last resort, but it is often a persistent condition that requires constant and repeated treatment.

The anus has been described by some pundits as one of the smartest parts of the body, because what other structure could let gas out below while retaining solids and liquids above?

ANUS

The anus consists of a narrow fleshy tube surrounded by a muscular ring that relaxes when faeces or wind is passed, but remains firmly closed at all other times. It connects the storage area for faeces (the rectum) with the outside of the body, is about 3cm long, and can dilate to about 2cm without discomfort.

A ring of veins around the anus may be damaged to form piles, and the anal canal can tear if over-stretched.

CURIOSITY

Excessive modesty is a very frequently cause of constipation in Japanese women.

CONTRACEPTION

T he use of an appropriate form of contraception by you or your partner is vital in looking after both yourselves and your relationship.

TYPES

Attempts to find some way of having sex without producing babies have a long history.

Documents from Mesopotamia, 4000 years ago, record that a plug of dung was placed in the woman's vagina to stop conception. In Cleopatra's Egypt, small gold trinkets were inserted into the uterus of the courtesans as a form of early intra-uterine contraceptive device. At the same time, camel herders pushed pebbles into the wombs of the female camels so that they would not get pregnant on long caravan treks.

More recently, in the eighteenth century in France, the renowned philanderer Casanova used a thin pig's bladder as an early condom or 'French letter'. Prior to this there were similar devices made from leather or gut.

Finding a safe, effective and reliable contraceptive has proved a difficult task.

Today, a very wide range of safe and effective contraceptives are available. They include:

- contraceptive pill

- morning after pill

- medroxyprogesterone injection

- implants

- spermicides

- condom

- female condom

- diaphragm

- cervical cap

- contraceptive sponge

- intrauterine devices

- natural family planning

- tubal ligation

- vasectomy

CONTRACEPTIVE PILL

The development of the oral contraceptive pill by American scientist Gregory Pincus and Dr John Rock in 1959, and its widespread release in 1962, revolutionised the lives of modern women, and changed society as a whole forever. For the first time, there was an effective, safe, reliable, easy to use, reversible contraceptive that did not interfere with lovemaking and had no aesthetic drawbacks.

The oral contraceptive pill is the **safest** and most effective form of reversible contraception. There are many different dosage forms and strengths, so that most women can find one that meets their needs. The main types are the monophasic (constant dose) two-hormone pill, the biphasic (two phase) and triphasic (three phase) hormone pills in which the hormone doses vary during the month, and the one hormone mini-pill.

The first contraceptive pills released were 30 times stronger than modern low-dose pills.

The pill has several positive **benefits** besides almost perfect prevention of pregnancy. It regulates irregular periods, reduces menstrual pain and premenstrual tension, may increase the size of the breasts, reduces the severity of acne in some women, and libido (the desire for sex) is often increased. It even reduces the incidence of some types of cancer.

Two different hormones control the menstrual cycle. At the time of ovulation, the levels of one hormone drops and the other rises, triggering the egg's release from the ovary. When the hormones revert to their previous level two weeks later, the lining of the uterus (womb) is no longer able to survive and breaks away, giving the woman a period.

The pill maintains a more constant hormone level, and thus prevents the release of the egg. In fact, it mimics the hormonal balance that is present during pregnancy, so the side effects of the pill are also those of pregnancy. The body, being fooled into thinking it is pregnant by the different hormone levels, does not allow further eggs to be released from the ovaries.

With the triphasic pills, the level of both hormones rises at the normal time of ovulation, and then drops slightly thereafter to give a more natural hormonal cycle to the woman, while still preventing the release of an egg.

The **hormones** commonly used in contraceptive pills include ethinyloestradiol, levonorgestrel, norethisterone, gestodene, and mestranol. Another less commonly used hormone is ethynodiol diacetate. There are some specialised types of contraceptive pills which have added benefits such as the improvement of acne when the hormones cytoperone and ethinyloestradiol (Diane) are combined.

When the pill is stopped (or the sugar pills started) at the end of the month, the sudden drop in hormone levels cause a hormone withdrawal bleed (period) to start. If the woman stops taking the pill, her normal cycle should resume very quickly (sometimes immediately) and she is able to become pregnant.

If taken correctly, the pill is very effective as a contraceptive. But **missing a pill**, or suffering from diarrhoea or vomiting can have a very pregnant result. Some antibiotics can also interfere with the pill. If any of these things occur, continue to take the pill but use another method of contraception until at least seven active pills (not the sugar ones taken when you have your period) have been taken.

In its early days there were some questions raised about the wisdom of **long-term** reliance on the pill, but a woman on today's pill is taking a hormone dose that is less than four per cent the strength of the original. It is much safer to take the contraceptive pill for many years than it is to have one pregnancy, and that is the realistic basis on which to judge the safety of any contraceptive.

A few women do have unwanted **side effects** from the contraceptive pill. These can include headaches, break-through bleeding, nausea, breast tenderness, increased appetite and mood changes. If these problems occur, they can be assessed by a doctor, and a pill containing a different balance of hormones can be prescribed. Rarely, a serious complication, such as a blood clot in a vein, may occur.

Tetracycline antibiotics, commonly used for acne, may interfere with the liver absorption of oral contraceptives to the extent that they may loose their contraceptive effect.

Although the contraceptive pill is very safe, there are some women who **should not use** it. Those who have had blood clots, severe liver disease, strokes or bad migraines must not take the pill. Heavy smokers, obese women and those with diabetes must be observed closely, and probably should not use the pill after 35 years of age.

There is no need these days to take a **break** from the pill every year or so. This may have been the case in earlier years, but is no longer necessary. It is possible (and safe) to take the active pills of a monophasic (constant dose) contraceptive pill without a break for three months or more, then have a one week break when a period will occur. This way the woman will only have four periods a year, but some women have break-through bleeds when attempting this.

In its most commonly used forms, the pill is a combination of the hormones oestrogen and progesterone. There is also a 'mini-pill', which contains only a progestogen hormone and is suitable for some women, including breast feeding mothers, who cannot take the combined pill. The mini-pill is less reliable than the combined pill and is more likely to give rise to irregular bleeding, but serious side effects are much less common. It is vital to take it at the same time each day.

The effects of the pill are readily **reversible**. If a woman decides to become pregnant, she could find herself in that state in as little as two weeks after ceasing the pill, with no adverse effects on the mother or child.

MORNING AFTER PILL

The morning after pill is a short course of a high dose of sex hormones (often an oral contraceptive) which must be taken within 72 hours of sexual intercourse. Two doses are taken twelve hours apart and they are often given with a second medication to prevent vomiting, which is the most common side effect.

MEDROXYPROGESTERONE INJECTIONS

Medroxyprogesterone (**Depo-Provera**) injections are a means of contraception in which a synthetic form of the female sex hormone progesterone is injected, causing the ovaries to stop producing eggs. One injection lasts for 12 weeks or more, depending on the dose given.

IMPLANTS

It is possible to have an small rod-shaped, hormone-containing implant (commercially called **Implanon**) inserted into the flesh on the inside of the upper arm. This gives almost 100% protection against pregnancy for three years. In most women, their periods cease for this time, but in some, irregular bleeding leads to the implant being removed. It is essential for the implant to be removed after the three year period to prevent ectopic pregnancies.

SPERMICIDES

Spermicides are creams, foams, gels and tablets which act to kill sperm on contact. A spermicide must be inserted no more than 20 minutes **before** intercourse and a new application must be used before each ejaculation. Generally the use of spermicides is advised with a diaphragm or condom.

Contraceptive risk must be measured against the significant
risk of not using a contraceptive, i.e. the risk of childbirth.

CONDOM

The condom is the simplest barrier method of artificial contraception. A condom is a thin rubber **sheath** which is placed on the penis before penetration. When the man ejaculates, the sperm are held in the rubber tip.

FEMALE CONDOM

There is also a female version of the condom, which is a thin rubber or plastic pouch that is inserted into the vagina before sex and contains the penis and ejaculated sperm when used.

DIAPHRAGM

The diaphragm for women works on a similar principle as the condom, in that it provides a physical barrier to the sperm meeting the egg. A diaphragm is a **rubber dome** with a flexible spring rim. It is inserted into the vagina before intercourse, so that it covers the cervix. It is best used with a spermicidal cream or jelly to kill any sperm that manage to wriggle around the edges.

CERVICAL CAP

Like the diaphragm, the cervical cap is a barrier method of contraception, but it is much smaller because it fits tightly over the cervix, rather than filling the vagina. The cap must be fitted very carefully and should be used with spermicides.

The most effective form of contraception is abstinence.

CONTRACEPTIVE SPONGE

A contraceptive sponge is impregnated with spermicide and is inserted into the vagina so that it expands to cover the cervix. Like a diaphragm, it is inserted **before** intercourse but is disposable and thrown away after use.

INTRAUTERINE DEVICE

The IUD is a piece of plastic, shaped like a T, which may be covered by a thin coil of copper wire or may be impregnated with a hormone (**Mirena**). It is inserted by a doctor through the vagina and cervix to sit inside the uterus (womb). The device can remain in place for three to five years before its needs to be changed.

NATURAL FAMILY PLANNING

Natural family planning is a form of **periodic abstinence** from sex (not having sex at those times of the month when a woman is fertile). The trick is knowing just what are the safe and not so safe times. Obviously, it is essential for both sexual partners in this situation to co-operate fully in the contraceptive process. The man must be as aware of the woman's cycle as she is herself. For this reason alone, this method of contraception does not suit all couples.

A woman can only become pregnant for a short period each month, a few days either side of ovulation. Because sperm can live for up to five days in the woman after ejaculation, and because the woman is fertile for two or three days after ovulation every month, sex must be avoided for seven to eight days during every cycle.

There are many different ways of calculating the fertile time of the month. The most common is a simple mathematical **calculation**, as a woman usually ovulates 14 days before her next period starts. If the woman has a regular 28 day cycle, she should not have sex from days 9 to 16 of her cycle (where day one is the first day of the period) in order to avoid pregnancy. If her cycle varies significantly, other clues to ovulation must be observed.

*Natural family planning is relatively effective, but accidents
do occur and have very pregnant consequences.*

Changes in body **temperature** can give a guide to ovulation, as the temperature first dips, then rises about half a degree centigrade at the time of ovulation. Changes in vaginal secretions also occur just before ovulation, and these can be noted on a glass slide. Breast tenderness and lower abdominal pain may be other relevant signs in some women. The **Billing's method** of contraception is a combination of the above factors.

Many people practise this form of contraception successfully for several years, but it is notoriously **unreliable**. The failure rate depends a great deal on the couple's commitment to follow the rules strictly, and the woman's own ability to note her own bodily changes. The percentage of women falling pregnant in one year while using natural family planning has varied from five per cent to 25 per cent in different clinical studies.

Natural family planning can be used in combination with other forms of contraception, such as condoms, spermicidal foam or diaphragms, which are used at the time of the month when pregnancy may occur. No couple should undertake this form of contraception without consulting a doctor who understands, and is prepared to teach, natural family planning.

TUBAL LIGATION

A tubal ligation (having the tubes tied, clipped or blocked) is an **operation** that usually renders a woman permanently unable to have children. As a contraceptive it is almost 100 per cent effective, but as with all surgical procedures, failures may occur, and women should be aware of this when they have the procedure.

VASECTOMY

A vasectomy is **procedure** in which the vas deferens (sperm tubes) of a man are cut and tied or clipped in order to prevent him from fathering children. It is a simpler operation than the sterilisation (tubal ligation) of a woman. It should be considered to be a permanent procedure at the time it is performed, but there is always a small risk that the cut sperm tubes may spontaneously reconnect at a later time, making the man fertile again.

Coitus interruptus, or withdrawal of the penis
before ejaculation, is not a method of contraception,
but a form of Russian roulette.

CONTRACEPTIVE FALLACIES

Many people believe that if a woman is **breast feeding** she cannot get pregnant. It is true that breast feeding stops ovulation in some women for some time. However, it is not a reliable or predictable method. Of women who breast feed and have intercourse without contraception, 40 per cent become pregnant.

Young girls often think that they can't get pregnant the '**first time**'. They can and frequently do. Pregnancy depends on whether your body has released an egg, not on the number of times you have had intercourse. You can get pregnant on the first time or the tenth time or the hundredth time or any other time.

Another fallacy is 'I've had sex before and nothing happened, so I'm probably **sterile**'. Very few women are sterile and the chances of you being one of them are slim. You are far more likely to have been lucky and your luck is probably running out.

'I'm too **young** to get pregnant'. If you have started your periods, you are not too young. You can even get pregnant before you have your first period – because the period comes after the egg has been released.

So-called **astrological** birth control is said to work in much the same way as the natural family planning method and dictates that you will avoid pregnancy if you abstain from intercourse during your sun-moon phase – the same phase that existed on the day that you were born. According to some astrologers, women release eggs twice each month, one in mid-cycle and once during the sun-moon phase. There is no scientific basis for this belief, and for a young girl who adopts it when embarking on a sexual relationship it is likely to prove futile nonsense.

OTHER OLD WIVES TALES SAY THAT A GIRL WON'T GET PREGNANT IF SHE:

- sneezes before or after having sex

- holds her breath when the boy reaches climax

- jumps up and down after intercourse so that the boy's sperm flows back out

- douches after intercourse so that the sperm is washed away

- has sex during her period.

None of these are true. Any girl or boy who is old enough to have sex is old enough not to lie to themselves with such nonsensical stories, but to find out about proper contraception and how to use it.

CURIOSITY

Quote from Marie Stopes, promoter of planned parenthood, 1921:

'The penile sheath (condom) is to be condemned, for it prevents the absorption of seminal juices by the woman through the wall of her vagina. These seminal juices are essential for the good health of the woman'.

COUGH

Look after yourself by treating a cough appropriately, initially with medications from a chemist, but if it persists, see a doctor before you drive your family and work mates, as well as yourself, crazy with your persistent hacking.

A cough is one of the most common conditions presenting to doctors, and the causes can vary from the totally innocuous to the deadly serious. A cough may be dry or moist, hard, productive, painful, associated with a wheeze, persistent or intermittent, and the phlegm produced may be clear, yellow, brown, green or blood-stained, and all these characteristics and more assist the doctor in making a diagnosis.

CAUSES

Many causes come from the throat and lungs (respiratory tract), but anything from heart failure to thyroid gland disease may cause a cough.

Any bacterial or viral **infection** (e.g. common cold, influenza) of the respiratory tract, from the nose to the lungs, may cause a cough. In the nose, excess phlegm production with a common cold may not only cause the nose to run, but phlegm may run back into the throat (a postnasal drip) to irritate this and stimulate a cough. An infection in the sinuses will cause a similar effect. The throat itself may be inflamed with minimal phlegm, but irritated to produce a hard dry cough. In the lungs, infections can cause inflammation of the major air tubes (bronchi) to cause bronchitis, or pus may accumulate in the tiny bubbles (alveoli) from which oxygen is absorbed into the blood to cause pneumonia.

Smoking is the most common cause of a persistent cough. 'Smoker's cough' typically occurs on waking, eases after half an hour or so, then flares after each cigarette during the day, and worsens again as temperatures drop at night.

Allergy reactions in the nose (hay fever) and throat can create copious amounts of clear phlegm that pour down the back of the throat, as well as out the front of the nose.

Coughing can be used as a subtle form of communication, from the polite cough to attract attention, to the carefully timed coughs used to cheat on the British television program 'Who Wants to be a Millionaire'.

Asthma is a temporary narrowing of the tubes through which air flows into and out of the lungs (the bronchi). Symptoms may include shortness of breath, wheezing, difficulty in breathing out easily, coughing (particularly in children) and a tightness and discomfort in the chest.

OTHER **LUNG DISEASES** THAT MAY CAUSE A COUGH INCLUDE:

- emphysema (over dilated damaged lungs)

- bronchiectasis (chronic lung infection and damage)

- pleurisy (inflammation of the membrane around the lungs)

- inhaled foreign body such as a peanut

- lung cancer (bronchial carcinoma)

- pulmonary embolism (blood clot in an artery supplying the lung)

- smoke inhalation

- near drowning

- toxic gases (e.g. exhaust fumes)

- hyper-reactive airways disease (a condition similar to asthma in which there is wheezing, cough and shortness of breath)

- whooping cough (pertussis)

- tuberculosis (TB)

- cystic fibrosis (birth defect of lung and bowel function)

- Q fever (caught from cattle)

- brucellosis (also caught from infected cattle)

- psittacosis (caught from birds)

- Legionnaire's disease (severe bacterial infection)

- sarcoidosis (cancer-like illness)

- anthrax

- abscess in the lung.

CONDITIONS OUTSIDE THE LUNGS WHICH MAY CAUSE A COUGH
INCLUDE:

- congestive heart failure

- reflux oesophagitis

- a foreign body in an ear (e.g. hard wax, peanut) in a child may cause a reflex cough even though the lung itself is not infected

- psychogenic (the patient coughs repeatedly to attract attention, then sub-consciously develops a habit of coughing constantly)

- aortic aneurysm (dilated artery that puts pressure on the trachea)

- damage to the valves (e.g. mitral valve) between the chambers of the heart

- pericarditis (inflammation of the membrane around the heart)

- goitre (enlarged thyroid gland puts pressure on the larynx).

Many **medications**, but particularly those used for heart failure and high blood pressure (ACE inhibitors), may have a cough as a side effect.

> *Coughing at the moment an injection is given*
> *significantly reduces the pain of an injection.*

COUGHING BLOOD
A cough that produces blood-stained mucus is much more significant than any other form of coughing.

Any **prolonged coughing** bout can result in the coughing up of blood, or blood-stained phlegm (haemoptysis), caused by damage to the pharynx (throat), larynx (voice box), trachea (main airway) or bronchi (smaller airways) in the lungs. As a result, bronchitis, pneumonia and many other infections that cause a cough may cause the problem. The occasional coughing up of blood under these circum-stances is usually of no significance, but when the coughing of blood, particularly when not mixed with much phlegm, becomes a regular occurrence, assessment by a doctor is essential.

A **bleeding nose** will not only lose blood out through the nostrils, but some will run down the back of the nose into the throat, from where it may be coughed up. If the bleeding comes from a polyp, tumour or cancer at the back of the nose, nearly all the bleeding will be back into the throat.

An **injury** to the chest, such as a fractured rib that pierces the lung, or a crush injury that damages the lung (e.g. car accident), will cause bleeding into the airways and haemoptysis.

Bronchiectasis occurs if the tubes within the lung that carry air (the bronchi) are damaged, scarred and permanently overdilated. The damage can be present from birth in diseases such as cystic fibrosis, or be caused in childhood by immune deficiencies. Bronchiectasis may develop in adult life due to recurrent attacks of pneumonia or to the inhalation of toxic gases (e.g. smoking). Patients have a constant cough that brings up large amounts of foul phlegm, and they may cough up blood, become anaemic, lose weight, have chest pains and develop frequent attacks of pneumonia and other lung infections that are triggered by minor stress, a cold or flu.

Lung cancer (bronchial carcinoma) is usually a result of smoking. The early warning signs are weight loss, a persistent cough, a change in the normal type of cough, coughing blood and worsening breathlessness.

A **blood clot** in one of the major arteries within the lungs (pulmonary thrombosis) will cause severe damage to that section of lung beyond the clot, leading to its collapse, coughing, pain and shortness of breath.

Tuberculosis (TB) causes a productive cough, haemoptysis, night sweats, loss of appetite, fever, weight loss and generalised tiredness.

Tumours, polyps, cancer or ulceration of the pharynx, larynx, trachea or other airways can cause bleeding that irritates the airway or lung to trigger coughing.

The medical term for the coughing of blood is haemoptysis.
It is a very significant symptom.

LESS COMMON CAUSES OF COUGHING UP BLOOD INCLUDE:

- an inhaled foreign body (e.g. peanut)

- damage to the valves (e.g. mitral valve) between the chambers of the heart which may lead to back pressure into the lungs leading to a build up of blood in the lungs which can leak into the airways to irritate them and cause a cough which brings up blood-tinged phlegm

- an abnormality in the blood clotting mechanism (e.g. a lack of platelets in the blood, haemophilia)

- cystic fibrosis

- an abscess in the lungs

- rare tropical diseases (e.g. hookworm, ascariasis)

- inflammation from smoke inhalation, near drowning, toxic gases (e.g. exhaust fumes) or other irritants.

COUGH MEDICINES

Antitussives are the mixtures, lozenges or tablets that stop coughing. They act by directly soothing the inflamed throat, decreasing the sensitivity of the part of the brain that triggers the spasm of coughing, decreasing the amount of phlegm in the throat, anaesthetising the throat, reducing inflammation, reducing pain, and by almost any combination of these methods. There are dozens of different cough mixtures (antitussives). They differ from expectorants, which are designed to increase coughing but make the coughing more effective so that phlegm can be cleared from the lungs and throat.

It is far better to treat the cause of a cough
(if possible) than to use cough suppressants.

Codeine is one of the most common ingredients of cough mixtures and acts as a suppressor of the brain's cough centre and as a painkiller. It is a mild narcotic, and its main side effect is constipation. There are a number of related drugs (e.g. pholcodine, dihydrocodeine, dextromethorphan) which act in a similar way.

Most antitussives are available without prescription and have minimal side effects. Many have an alcohol base and also contain mild narcotics or antihistamines, so care must be taken with driving and operating machinery.

Other cough suppressants may include guaiphenesin, senega, camphor and thymol. Antihistamines, decongestants, mucolytics and analgesics are often combined with these ingredients.

The only potent antitussive that requires a prescription is hydrocodone, which may have drowsiness and blurred vision as side effects, and is addictive.

CURIOSITY

Extracts from an 1830 medical text book:

'Pleurisy has as its common consequence a violent cough. The physician must without loss of time take away ten ounces of blood and cause a vomit with 80 grains of ipecocanna (sic)'.

'Cigarettes give immediate relief in cases of Hay Fever, Chronic Bronchitis, Influenza, Cough and Shortness of Breath, and their daily use affects a complete cure'.

CUTS

K nowing how to give first aid for a significant cut, and knowing when to obtain further treatment, is important in looking after yourself and those around you.

A **laceration** is merely any cut or tear that penetrates through the skin.

FIRST AID

THERE ARE THREE ESSENTIALS IN DEALING WITH ANY CUT:

- stop the bleeding

- prevent infection

- repair the wound.

No matter how large the wound, the best way to stop bleeding is to **apply pressure** directly over the injury. Tourniquets should not be used unless there is direct bleeding from a large artery. A piece of clean cloth several layers thick (e.g. a clean folded handkerchief) is the best and usually most convenient dressing. Tissues tend to disintegrate and contaminate the wound.

The cloth should be applied over the bleeding area and held there firmly by the person giving first aid or by the victim. If it is likely to be some time before further treatment can be given, the dressing can be held in place by a firm bandage, provided it is not so tight as to cause pain or restrict the supply of blood to the parts of the body beyond the bandage.

If an arm or a leg is involved, that part of the body should be elevated above the level of the heart. Unless the wound is minor, the patient should lie down to avoid fainting or shock.

Doctors always like to know what has caused a cut so that they can determine if a tetanus injection and/or antibiotics are necessary.

Provided medical attention is readily available, no other first aid is necessary, as the doctor will ensure the cleanliness of the wound and its repair. If there is likely to be a significant delay before a doctor can be seen, it is advisable to clean any dirt out of the wound with a diluted antiseptic, or clean water if no antiseptic is available. Do not use harsh antiseptics such as hydrogen peroxide. Ensure that bleeding has stopped first, and do not disturb any clots that may have formed.

Minor cuts will heal without suturing, provided the edges of the wound are not gaping. If the edges do not lie comfortably together, if a joint surface is involved, if the wound continues to bleed, or if the scar may be cosmetically disfiguring, then it is essential to have the cut correctly repaired by taping or sutures.

Although it will sting, a dirty wound that is likely to become
infected may be cleaned with any alcoholic spirit (e.g. whisky, gin)
if medical attention is likely to be delayed.

SUTURING

Sutures are threads used to close a wound anywhere in the body, be it caused by an injury or operation, or in the skin or an internal organ. The **thread** of the suture can be made from silk, linen, gut, nylon, or any one of innumerable other synthetics. Some are designed to remain permanently, while others must be removed after healing has occurred, or will dissolve and disappear after a predetermined time.

Almost invariably the thread is bonded almost seamlessly with a steel needle which will vary in shape and size depending on its intended use. Needles used in the skin are usually diamond shaped in cross section, while those used on internal tissues are usually round in cross section.

If a cut (laceration) is being sutured, a local anaesthetic will usually be given into the tissue around the wound by injection. After this there should be no pain felt, although there may be sensations of pulling or pressure.

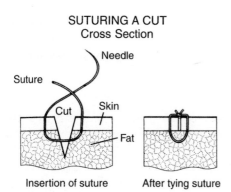

SUTURING A CUT
Cross Section

Needle

Suture

Cut   Skin

Fat

Insertion of suture   After tying suture

The doctor inserts the needle through the skin to one side of the cut, curls it around under the skin, and brings it out through the skin on the other side, then pulls on the two ends of the thread to bring the wound edges together, and ties the ends firmly so that it is kept closed.

Usually sutures must be removed from the skin, and the timing will depend on the site and size of the wound. A small cut on the face may have sutures removed in four or five days, while a large deep cut on the thigh may need the support of the sutures for two weeks or more.

The **removal** of sutures is a painless procedure, with only a pulling sensation, but if their removal is delayed beyond the ideal time, the healing process may bury the sutures making removal more difficult. Sutures must be removed in a way that prevents any infection entering the healing wound as the thread is pulled through.

CURIOSITY
A wound caused by an animal or human bite is often left unsutured as they are very prone to infection, which is less likely to happen if the edges are left apart.

DEPRESSION

It is essential to look after your mental health as well as your medical health. Everyone should realise that it is really an artificial divide that separates the two types of health, as many mental conditions, including depression, can have a biochemical cause and their management is no different to that of high blood pressure, gout or diabetes. Look after yourself, and if your family or friends comment that you may be suffering from a low mood or personality change, seek professional help.

DEFINITION
Depression is also known as an affective disorder, melancholia, hypothymia or a nervous breakdown. It is a medical condition, not just a state of mind, that affects 30 per cent of people at some time in their life. Patients are not able to pull themselves together and overcome the depression without medical aid, although a determination to improve the situation certainly helps the outcome.

Depression may be a symptom (having a bad day and feeling sad), personality type (inherited with the genes), reaction (depressed because of loss of job, death in family etc.) or a disease (depression due to chemical imbalances in the brain). It is usually a mixture of several of these.

TYPES
There are two main types of depression, endogenous and reactive, with very different causes.

> *Depression is a disease like diabetes. Diabetes is due to low levels of insulin in the blood, depression to low levels of serotonin in the brain.*

ENDOGENOUS DEPRESSION
Endogenous depression has **no obvious reason** for the constant unhappiness, and patients slowly become sadder and sadder, more irritable, unable to sleep, lose appetite and weight, and feel there is no purpose in living. They may feel unnecessarily guilty, have a very poor opinion of themselves, feel life is hopeless and find it difficult to think or concentrate. After several months they usually improve, but sometimes it can take years. It is due to an imbalance of the chemicals (neurotransmitters) that normally occur in the brain to control mood. The neurotransmitters include serotonin, noradrenaline and dopamine. If too little of any one is produced, the patient becomes depressed – if too much, the patient may become manic.

Endogenous depression can be further subdivided, depending on the combination of neurotransmitters that are too low. The subtypes are:

Type	Neurotransmitter level too low	Characteristics
Non-melancholic depression	Serotonin	Obsession, panic, compulsions, anxiety
Non-psychotic melancholia	Serotonin, noradrenaline	+ lack of energy, tired
Psychotic melancholia	Serotonin, noradrenaline, dopamine	+ unmotivated, no pleasures, lack of concentration, no insight.

Patients with endogenous depression are not able to pull themselves together and overcome the depression without medical aid, but doctors can alter the abnormal chemical balance by giving antidepressant medications. When they do start to improve, some patients with depression go too far the other way and become over-happy or manic. These patients are said to be manic depressive, have bipolar personality (generally severe swings of mood) or cyclothymic disorder (milder mood changes).

There are no diagnostic blood tests or brain scans to prove the presence of endogenous depression, and the final diagnosis depends on the clinical acumen of the doctor.

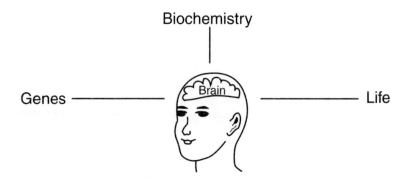

DEPRESSION
Factors causing the condition

REACTIVE DEPRESSION
Reactive depression is the sadness that occurs after a death in the family, loss of a job, a marriage break-up or other disaster. Patients are depressed for a **definite reason**, and, with time, will often be able to cope with the situation, although some patients do require medical help.

OTHER TYPES

There are many other causes of depression that overlap between the two types above or that have totally independent causes.

The **elderly** often become depressed because they are confused, ill, unable to sleep as well as they would like, in discomfort, have no pleasure in life and can see no future. A change in attitude, environment and a bit of medication may often change their outlook dramatically.

The **hormonal** changes associated with menopause often trigger significant clinical depression. The varying hormone levels may cause wide variations in mood that can be corrected by hormone replacement therapy.

Many women find that the normal sex hormone variations during the month will also cause mood changes, with depression and irritability being particularly common just before a menstrual period (**premenstrual tension** – PMT).

Many other **diseases** may have depression as a component, but doctors must be careful to differentiate between depression caused by the disease process itself, and depression in the patient because they are upset at having the disease.

There is no identifiable cause for most cases of depression.

POSSIBLE **MEDICAL CAUSES** FOR DEPRESSION MAY INCLUDE:

- tumour, cyst, abscess, cancer or infection of the brain

- stroke (cerebrovascular accident)

- hypothyroidism (a lack of thyroxine)

- Parkinson disease (degeneration of part of brain that co-ordinates muscle movement)

- serious viral infections (e.g. AIDS, hepatitis, influenza, glandular fever)

- pernicious anaemia

- systemic lupus erythematosus (an autoimmune disease)

- multiple sclerosis (a nerve disease that affects nerves randomly and intermittently)

- abnormalities in the levels of potassium, sodium, bicarbonate and chloride (electrolytes) in the blood due to kidney or other diseases.

A number of **medications**, including cortisone, methyldopa (used for high blood pressure), beta blockers (used for heart disease) and various hormones (including the contraceptive pill) may have depression as a side effect.

There are many rarer medical causes of depression.

POSTNATAL DEPRESSION

Postnatal (or postpartum) depression is a spontaneous form of depression that occurs in some women just before, or soon after childbirth, and is a response to the effect on the brain of sudden changes in hormone levels.

The woman experiences constant unhappiness for which there is no reason. They are unable to sleep, lose appetite and weight, and feel there is no purpose in living. They may feel unnecessarily guilty, have a very poor opinion of themselves, feel life is hopeless, find it difficult to think or concentrate, worry excessively about their infant or neglect the child. Rarely it may lead to attempted or actual suicide. It is diagnosed after careful psychiatric assessment.

Medications are prescribed to control the production of depressing chemicals in the brain (e.g. fluvoxamine, moclobemide, nefazodone, paroxetine, venlafaxine) while hospitalised or given intensive home support. Shock therapy (electroconvulsive therapy – ECT) may be used as a last resort. Virtually all cases settle with support and medication in a few weeks.

SEASONAL AFFECTIVE DISORDER

Seasonal affective disorder is a special form of depression that is a common condition in far northern climates where there may be daylight for only two or three hours a day during winter. The cause is an inappropriate regulation of time by the body's internal clock, which is controlled by the hormone melatonin produced in the pineal gland at the front of the brain.

Patients become irritable and depressed, and suicide may occur in severe cases.

It is difficult to manage, but living in very bright light for part of the day, antidepressant medications, or taking melatonin may help.

Patients with depression need to be constantly reassured
that the problem is not in any way their fault, and that
with time, medication and patience, it can be successfully treated.

TREATMENTS

PSYCHOLOGISTS

Psychologists are not medical doctors but have undertaken a course of training to obtain a Master of Arts degree in psychology from a university. Many further their studies to earn postgraduate degrees and doctorates (PhD). Psychologists deal with behavioural, social and emotional problems (e.g. marriage counselling, dealing with badly behaved children, coping with stress). They can also help many patients cope with depression, particularly reactive and postpartum depression, and are often involved in a team approach to the problem.

MEDICATIONS

Numerous **medications** (antidepressants) that control the production or activity of the depressing chemicals in the brain are available to treat depression, but most antidepressant drugs work slowly over several weeks. Hospitalisation in order to use high doses of drugs or other treatments, and to protect the patient from the possibility of suicide, is sometimes necessary when the disease is first diagnosed. The other form of treatment used is shock therapy (electroconvulsive therapy – ECT), which is a safe and often very effective method of giving relief to patients with severe chronic depression.

Untreated depression may lead to attempted or actual suicide, which can be seen as a desperate plea for help.

Antidepressants are used to control depression. Depression caused by a biochemical imbalance in the brain requires appropriate medication to correct it before a tragedy occurs. There are many sub-classes of antidepressants including SSRI, RIMA, SNRI, tricyclics and MAOI.

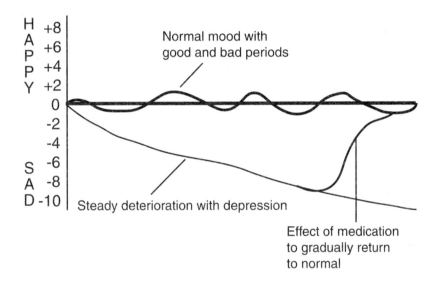

SSRI
Selective serotonin reuptake inhibitors (SSRI) is a class of antidepressants that has received a great deal of publicity because of the extraordinary efficacy of one of its members – fluoxetine (Prozac). Introduced in 1992, this group has revolutionised the management of depression and anxiety because of its speed of action, safety and minimal side effects, and they are now the most widely used antidepressants. Other drugs in this class include paroxetine (Aropax), sertraline (Zoloft), escitalopram (Lexapro) and citalopram (Cipramil). Side effects may include nausea, drowsiness, sweating, tremor, a dry mouth and impotence.

RIMA
Reversible inhibitors of mono amine oxidase (RIMA) antidepressants are a class of very safe antidepressants introduced in the early 1990s. The only one generally available is moclobemide (Aurorix). Side effects may include disturbed sleep and dizziness.

SNRI
Serotonin and noradrenaline reuptake inhibitors (SNRI) is a class of antidepressants that was introduced in 1996 and is normally used in resistant cases of depression. Venlafaxine (Efexor) is the most common drug in this class. Side effects may include dizziness, drowsiness and a dry mouth.

Antidepressants are very effective, but they are slow to work, and as a result they are not addictive. No addict wants to take a pill that gives them a high several weeks later.

TRICYCLICS
Tricyclic antidepressants were the most widely used drugs in this class until the introduction of SSRI, and are still very effective in treating most cases, but they are slow to act, taking two to four weeks to reach full effectiveness. They also cause some sedation, and so are normally taken at night. Other side effects may include a dry mouth, tremor, dizziness, constipation, rapid heart rate, blurred vision and excess sweating. Examples include amitriptyline (Tryptanol), clomipramine (Anafranil), dothiepin (Prothiaden), doxepin (Sinequan), imipramine (Tofranil), nortriptyline (Allegron) and trimipramine (Surmontil). Mianserin (Tolvon) is a variant on the tricyclic theme that tends to be safer in patients with heart problems.

MAOI
Monoamine oxidase inhibitors (MAOI) are potent antidepressants that are only used in severe and chronic cases of depression. They are slow to become effective, and their effects may persist for a couple of weeks after they are stopped. They do not cause drowsiness, but they interact violently with many other drugs and some foods, including soy sauce, cheese, red wine and pickled foods. Any patient on MAOI should be given a list of foods and drugs they must avoid by their doctor. This list must be observed carefully, or serious side effects may occur. Other side effects may include dizziness, constipation, dry mouth, drowsiness and nausea. MAOI should not be taken at the same time as tricyclic antidepressants, and only with extreme care by epileptic patients. If taken correctly, they can dramatically improve a depressed patient's life. Examples include phenelzine (Nardil) and tranylcypromine (Parnate).

MIRTAZAPINE
Another newer antidepressants is mirtazapine (Avanza, Remeron). Its use at present tends to be restricted to more severe depression that cannot be controlled by other classes of medication. It interacts with alcohol and benzodiazepines (e.g. Valium) and may cause increased appetite, weight gain, dizziness and headaches.

ELECTROCONVULSIVE THERAPY
Electroconvulsive therapy (ECT, shock treatment) has been used successfully by psychiatrists since the 1930s to treat severe depression and other mental disease, but it has been subjected to much media criticism and vilification by consumer

groups in the past few decades. The adverse reactions to shock treatment come mainly from a misunderstanding of the procedure and what it can and cannot achieve.

A patient about to undergo ECT is thoroughly examined, and an electro-encephalogram (EEG), and X-rays of the back and neck may be performed. The patient will be stopped from eating or drinking for eight hours before the treatment.

Despite its bad press, shock treatment can be very effective and life-saving in severely depressed patients.

For the procedure, the patient is usually taken to a specially equipped room or operating theatre. They will be asked to empty their bladder. Electrodes are attached to the temples, and then a brief general anaesthetic is administered. During this anaesthetic, which lasts only a couple of minutes, an electric current is passed through the brain. This electric current causes the patient to have an epileptic-like seizure that lasts five to 15 seconds, but because the patient is anaes-thetised, the actual body and muscle movement is only slight or non-existent, and the patient has no pain or discomfort. The patient recovers rapidly from the anaes-thetic, is confused for about an hour, may have lost any memory of events in the few hours before the shock treatment was given, and may suffer a dull headache for a day or two. There are no other side effects, and normal activity can be resumed an hour or so after the procedure.

The ECT is repeated up to three or four times a week for eight to 12 or more treatments. Occasionally, more intensive programs of shock treatment are carried out under strictly monitored conditions. Up to 70 per cent of patients with severe depression are significantly improved by ECT, and overall it is more effective than medication in these patients.

Depression is not a diagnosis that patients should fear, as medication and coun-selling by a general practitioner, psychologist or psychiatrist will cure or control the vast majority of cases.

CURIOSITY

Depression is not a new disease. In the nineteenth century, women with a 'delicate constitution' were often depressed and they secluded themselves from society for months on end. In the first half of the twentieth century the expression 'nervous breakdown' was the favoured term.

DIABETES

The term diabetes is derived from the Greek word for syphon and indicates that water goes through the person with the disease.

Everyone over 40 should look after themselves by having blood checks every few years to check for diabetes, and consult a doctor if they develop characteristic symptoms. A good diet, not being overweight, and regular exercise will delay the onset of diabetes.

DEFINITIONS

There are three totally distinct medical conditions called diabetes, and all have the symptoms of excessive thirst and the frequent passing of urine. It was not possible for doctors to differentiate between the three forms of diabetes until the end of the nineteenth century, so the name of diabetes has stuck with all of them because of their similar symptoms.

Diabetes mellitus type one (juvenile diabetes or insulin dependent diabetes mellitus) develops in children and young adults due to a lack of insulin production by the pancreas.

Diabetes mellitus type two (maturity onset diabetes or non-insulin dependent diabetes mellitus) is the most common form and develops in middle-aged and elderly people as the cells in their body develop resistance to insulin.

Diabetes insipidus is a rare disease caused by a disorder of the pituitary gland.

A sudden increase in thirst and frequency of passing urine
are the classical symptoms of all types of diabetes.

Insulin disorders are involved in both forms of diabetes mellitus.

Glucose is used as fuel by every cell in the body. When glucose is eaten, it is absorbed into the blood from the small intestine. Once it reaches a cell, it must cross the fine membrane that forms its outer skin. This is normally impermeable to all substances, but insulin has the ability to combine with glucose and transport it across the membrane from the blood into the interior of the cell. Insulin is made by cells in the Islets of Langerhan in the pancreas, which sits in the centre of the abdomen.

DIABETES MELLITUS TYPE ONE

Diabetes mellitus type one is also known as insulin dependent diabetes mellitus (IDDM) or juvenile diabetes, and causes excessive levels of glucose in the blood.

SYMPTOMS

Only ten per cent of diabetes suffer from this form of diabetes mellitus which is caused by a lack of insulin production by the Langerhan cells in the pancreas, which lies across the centre of the abdomen. Most people develop this type as a child or in early adult life.

Symptoms include excessive tiredness, thirst, excess passing of urine, weight loss despite a large food intake, itchy rashes, recurrent vaginal thrush infections, pins and needles and blurred vision. Patients become steadily weaker because their muscles and other organs cannot work properly.

The diagnosis can be confirmed by blood and urine glucose levels and a glucose tolerance test (GTT).

By measuring the amount of glucose in certain blood cells, the average blood glucose level over the past three months can also be determined. The level of insulin can also be measured in blood.

Daily self-testing is advisable to ensure that disease control is adequate. Both blood and urine tests for glucose are available, but the blood tests are far superior.

MANAGEMENT

Diet is an essential part of treatment because the amount of glucose eaten is not normally constant, and diabetics lack the means of adjusting the amount of glucose in their blood with insulin. The diet must restrict the number of kilojoules (calories) being eaten, and sugar in all its forms should be eaten only with great caution.

Fat should not account for more than a third of the total calories, and cholesterol intake should be restricted. Protein should be obtained more from poultry and fish than red meats. Carbohydrates other than sugar can be consumed freely. Grains and cereals with a high fibre content should be the main part of the diet. Artificial sweeteners such as aspartame (NutraSweet) can be used to flavour food and drinks.

Fat cells can react abnormally to insulin very easily, and so overweight diabetics must lose weight. Exercise is encouraged on a regular daily basis. Patients should carry glucose sweets with them at all times to use if their blood sugar levels drop too low.

The simplest diet rule for diabetics is no sugar, minimal fat.

When first diagnosed, patients are often quite ill, and most are hospitalised for a few days to stabilise their condition. **Insulin** injections must be given regularly several times a day for the rest of their life. Initially derived from pigs and cattle, human insulin has now been produced by genetic engineering techniques.

Insulin cannot be taken by mouth as it is destroyed by acid in the stomach, but can be injected into any part of the body covered by loose skin, although the same site should not be used repeatedly. The newer pen-style delivery systems enable diabetics to easily dial the required dose and inject as necessary with minimal inconvenience. There are many different types of insulin that vary in their speed of onset and duration of action.

COMPLICATIONS

The complications of type one diabetes mellitus include an increased risk of both bacterial and fungal skin and vaginal **infections**, the premature development of **cataracts** in the eye, microscopic haemorrhages and exudates that destroy the **retina** at the back of the eye, damage to the **kidneys** that prevents them from filtering blood effectively, poor **circulation** to the extremities (hands and feet) that may cause chronic ulcers and even gangrene to the feet, the development of brown skin spots on the shins, and sensory **nerve damage** (diabetic neuropathy) that alters the patient's perception of vibration, pain and temperature.

Until the isolation of insulin in the 1920s, most patients with type one diabetes died within a year or two of diagnosis.

There are also complications associated with treatment such as a '**hypo**' in which too much insulin is given, excess exercise undertaken or not enough food is eaten, and blood glucose levels drop (hypoglycaemia) to an unacceptably low level. The patient becomes light-headed, sweats, develops a rapid heart beat and tremor, becomes hungry, then nauseated before finally collapsing unconscious. Glucose drinks or sweets given before collapse can reverse the process, but after collapse, an injection of glucose is essential. In an emergency, a sugary syrup or honey introduced through the anus into the rectum may allow a diabetic to recover sufficiently to take further sugar by mouth.

Rarer complications of treatment are adverse reactions to pork or beef insulin, and damage to the fat under the skin if the same injection site is used too frequently. Diabetic **ketoacidosis** is the most severe complication, which results in significant biochemical imbalances in the blood (see below).

On the other hand, with the correct treatment and careful control, patients should live a near-normal life, with a near-normal life span.

DIABETES MELLITUS TYPE TWO

Diabetes mellitus type two is also known as maturity onset diabetes or non-insulin dependent diabetes mellitus (NIDDM).

SYMPTOMS

Nine out of ten of diabetics suffer from the maturity onset form of diabetes mellitus, which is far more common in **obese** patients. There is adequate insulin production, but cells throughout the body fail to respond to the insulin, so glucose cannot enter the cell.

The symptoms include excessive tiredness, thirst, excess passing of urine, visual problems, skin infections and sensory nerve problems. Many patients are totally without symptoms when the diagnosis is discovered on a routine blood or urine test.

Most people can avoid type two diabetes by avoiding obesity.

Blood and urine glucose levels are high in untreated or inadequately treated patients. A blood glucose tolerance test (GTT) is performed to confirm the diagnosis and determine its severity.

By measuring the amount of glucose in certain blood cells, the average blood glucose level over the past three months can also be determined.

Regular **blood testing** of glucose levels is also necessary, but normally on a weekly rather than daily basis. Urine tests are often inaccurate in the elderly, as their kidney function may be reduced to the point where glucose cannot enter the urine.

MANAGEMENT

Diet is an essential part of the management in the same way as in type one diabetes mellitus (above). Overweight diabetics must lose weight, and exercise is encouraged on a regular daily basis.

Education of patients with diabetes is very important, so that they understand what they can and cannot eat and drink. Older people who develop diabetes can often have the disease controlled by diet alone or a combination of tablets and diet.

Tablets (e.g. metformin, glimepride, tolbutamide, chlorpropamide, glibenclamide, glipizide) make the cell membrane respond to insulin again (see below). Weight loss is a vital part of treatment because if normal weight levels can be maintained, the disease may disappear.

Poorly controlled diabetes results in clogging of capillaries and damage everywhere in the body from the eyes to the toes.

COMPLICATIONS

The complications of type two diabetes mellitus are the same as those of type one (above), but tend to develop more slowly and less dramatically.

With the correct treatment and careful control, patients should live a near-normal life, with a near-normal life span.

DIABETES IN PREGNANCY

Pregnancy may trigger diabetes in a woman who was previously well but predisposed towards this disease. One of the reasons for regular antenatal visits to doctors and the urine tests taken at each visit is to detect diabetes at an early stage. If diabetes develops, the woman can be treated and controlled by regular injections of insulin. In some cases, the diabetes will disappear after the pregnancy, but it often recurs in later years.

A common cause for a very large baby is diabetes in the mother.

If the diabetes is not adequately controlled, serious **consequences** can result. In mild cases, the child may be born grossly overweight but otherwise be healthy. In more severe cases, the diabetes can cause a miscarriage, eclampsia (severe high blood pressure and fitting in the mother), malformations of the foetus, urinary and kidney infections, fungal infections (thrush) of the vagina, premature labour, difficult labour, breathing problems in the baby after birth, or death of the baby within the womb.

Diabetic women tend to have difficulty in falling pregnant, unless their diabetes is very well-controlled.

DIABETIC KETOACIDOSIS

Ketoacidosis is a severe complication or initial presentation of diabetes mellitus. It is due to a build-up of waste products and glucose in the bloodstream because of untreated or under-treated diabetes. Patients who are careless about their treatment, diet and self-testing may be affected. Almost invariably, it is the juvenile insulin dependent diabetics that develop this complication.

The **symptoms** include mental stupor, nausea, vomiting, shortness of breath and eventually coma. Blood sugar levels are very high and other blood and urine tests are abnormal.

Treatment involves the emergency injections of insulin, but urgent hospital treatment is necessary to control the situation adequately. If left untreated, death will occur due to kidney, heart or brain damage.

The prognosis is good with prompt medical care, but permanent organ damage may occur if treatment is delayed.

*Type one diabetes often presents dramatically with patients
in a coma, while type two has an insidious onset.*

INVESTIGATION

Both forms of diabetes are **diagnosed** in the same way, by directly measuring the level of glucose in the blood, and with a test on the response of the body to increased glucose in the diet (glucose tolerance test).

GLUCOSE

Blood sugar (glucose) tests are used to diagnose hyperglycaemia and hypoglycaemia (too much or too little sugar in the bloodstream) which may be associated with diabetes. Diabetics must **regularly measure** their blood glucose levels, and should aim to keep them at a fasting level below 8 mmol/L and above 3.5 mmol/L. A level over 10 is considered to be dangerous, and below 3.5 there is a risk of having a 'hypo' due to excessive medication lowering the level too much.

The level of glucose in the blood is controlled by insulin. Excess sugar in the body is converted to glycogen and stored in the liver. When glycogen stores are full, it is converted to fat for storage.

The level of glucose can be more accurately measured in a blood sample by a laboratory. Fasting for eight hours or more before the test is necessary. The normal range is 3.5 to 6 mmol/L (60 to 100 mg/100 mL in the US).

A **high** level of glucose in the blood may be due to diabetes mellitus (a level over 7.0 on a fasting test is diagnostic) and numerous other conditions such as infection, hyperthyroidism (over-active thyroid gland), hyperpituitarism (over-active pituitary gland in the brain), hyperadrenocorticism (over-active adrenal glands on the kidneys), liver disease, burns, steroid treatment and a recent meal.

A **low** level of glucose in the blood may be due to vomiting, diarrhoea, insulinoma (tumour of pancreas), excess insulin production, hypoadrenocorticism (adrenal gland under-activity), hypopituitarism (under-active pituitary gland in the brain), hypothyroidism (under-active thyroid gland), severe liver disease, hepatoma (liver cancer), alcoholism, after stomach surgery, unpreserved blood specimen and medications (e.g. insulin, laxatives, diabetes drugs, fluid tablets – diuretics).

Regular blood tests are essential lifelong after diabetes is diagnosed.

GLUCOSE TOLERANCE TEST

A blood glucose tolerance test (GTT) may be performed to **confirm** the diagnosis of diabetes mellitus. After fasting for 12 hours, a blood sample is taken, then a sweet drink is swallowed, and further blood samples are taken at regular intervals for two or three hours. The pattern of absorption and elimination of blood glucose is measured to confirm the diagnosis of diabetes mellitus. The blood sugar level should not exceed 8 mmol/L (140 mg/100 mL) after 30 minutes, and should return to normal within two hours. No sugar should appear in the urine.

Diabetic (and potential diabetic) patients do not produce adequate insulin to clear glucose from blood rapidly. The test may be affected by drugs such as fluid tablets (diuretics), steroids, lithium, phenytoin and phenothiazines.

GLYCOSYLATED HAEMOGLOBIN

The glycosylated haemoglobin (GHb or **HbA1c**) is a very important and regularly performed management test for diabetes of all types. It is a measure of the glucose in red blood cells. The normal range is five to eight per cent of haemoglobin as HbA1c.

A **high** level indicates above average normal glucose level (i.e. diabetes, poorly controlled diabetes, non-compliance with treatment). A falsely high reading can occur in uraemia (kidney failure) and beta thalassaemia (inherited blood disease), while a falsely low reading may be due to haemolytic anaemia (breakdown of red blood cells), blood loss.

Glucose reacts with, and attaches to, haemoglobin in red blood cells. This test is a measure of compliance and efficacy of treatment as the life cycle of a red blood cell is about 3 months. The test should not be used to change the treatment for diabetes unless there are two abnormal tests at least three months apart. The test is inaccurate in conditions of shortened red blood cell lifespan (e.g. haemolytic disease, blood loss).

TREATMENT

Hypoglycaemics are drugs that lower the level of sugar (glucose) in the bloodstream by allowing the sugar to cross the membrane surrounding a cell and to enter the interior of the cell. They are used mainly in the maturity onset (type two) form of diabetes mellitus.

Alteration to the dosage of all types of hypoglycaemics may be required with changes in exercise or diet, surgery or the occurrence of other illnesses, particularly if a fever is present. A doctor should be consulted immediately in these situations. As well as treatment with hypoglycaemics, all diabetics must remain on an appropriate diet for the rest of their lives. Regular blood tests and urine tests are essential for the adequate control of all forms of diabetes. Most patients now use small machines to test their own blood sugar.

HYPOGLYCAEMICS FALL INTO TWO MAIN GROUPS:

- Insulin, which is normally produced by the pancreas to transport sugar across the cell membrane, can only be given by injection, and is invariably required in type one diabetes which has its onset in children and young adults.

- Maturity onset (type two) diabetes has its onset in the middle-aged and elderly, and is normally treated by hypoglycaemic tablets and diet, but sometimes insulin is also required.

Modern diabetes tablets can sometimes be used just once a day.

HYPOGLYCAEMIC TABLETS

THE HYPOGLYCAEMIC TABLETS FALL INTO SEVERAL SUB-CLASSES:

BIGUANIDES

Biguanide hypoglycaemics tend to be used more in obese patients. Metformin (Diabex, Diaformin) is the only commonly used medication in this subclass. Side effects may include nausea and belly discomfort. It should not be used in pregnancy or alcoholics.

SULFONYLUREAS

The sulfonylureas are a class of drugs that come as tablets that are used only in maturity onset (type two) diabetes. Excessive use, or overdosage, can cause a 'hypo' attack as in insulin overuse. Examples include chlorpropamide (Diabinese), glimepride (Amaryl), glibenclamide (Daonil, Euglucon), gliclazide (Diamicron), glipizide (Minidiab) and tolbutamide (Rastinon). Side effects may include nausea, weakness and belly discomfort. They should not be used in pregnancy, thyroid disease, and severe liver or kidney diseases, and should not be combined with insulin.

ACARBOSE

Acarbose (Glucobay) is used in difficult to control mature onset diabetes. Side effects may include nausea and diarrhoea. It must be used with caution in pregnancy, and blood tests to check liver function must be performed regularly.

INSULIN

Insulin is a natural hormone produced by cells in the islets of Langerhan which are in the pancreas (an organ in the centre of the abdomen). It is essential for insulin to be present in the blood, because without it, cells cannot absorb glucose.

   The amount of insulin present in blood can be measured by sensitive tests. The blood specimen should be collected after a 15 hour fast and then during a glucose tolerance test.

Normal results are:
   Less than 19 mIU/L (less than 0.9 µg/L) fasting.
   50 to 130 mIU/L 1 hour after 75 g glucose.
   Less than 100 mIU/L 2 hours after 75 g glucose.

These results can be interpreted thus:
   Low level of insulin after glucose – Diabetes due to lack of insulin (type one diabetes), malnutrition.
   High level after glucose – Diabetes due to lack of tissue response to insulin (type two diabetes), insulinoma, Reaven syndrome, pregnancy.

Unfortunately, insulin is destroyed by the acid and digestive juices in the stomach and gut, and therefore cannot be given to diabetics in tablet form. It is currently only available as an **injection**, but experiments with an inhaled form are under way.

Insulin has been derived from the pancreas of cattle or pigs for the 60 years up to the early 1990s since it was originally identified and isolated by the Canadian doctors, Banting and Best. Because it was derived from animals, there were occasional reactions to the foreign animal protein present in the insulin. Since 1990, genetically engineered human insulin has almost totally replaced the animal insulin. The new form causes virtually no adverse reaction after injection.

Many diabetics inject their insulin through their clothing, and when they over-indulge, merely give themselves an extra shot.

There are many different **types** of insulin available. They vary in their speed of action (how quickly they work after injection) and their duration of action (how long they last after injection). Some can be given by doctors as an injection directly into the bloodstream in acutely ill patients, others are combinations of long and short-acting insulins that enable diabetics to have only one or two injections a day, rather than four or more of the short-acting types. Each diabetic will have trials of a number of these combinations to find the one best suited to them.

INSULIN TYPES

TYPE	ALTERNATE NAME	ONSET OF ACTION	PEAK ACTION	DURATION
Aspart		20–40 min	4 hours	6–10 hours
Biphasic	Neutral and isophane mix	30–60 min	4–12 hours	24 hours
Isophane		2–4 hours	4–12 hours	24 hours
Lente	Insulin zinc suspension (IZS)	3 hours	6–10 hours	24 hours
Lispro		15 minutes	1 hour	3.5–4.5 hours
Neutral		30–60 min	4 hours	6–10 hours
Ultralente	Crystalline insulin zinc susp. (CIZS)	4–6 hours	10–30 hours	24–36 hours

There are a number of ways of administering **insulin injections**, including the traditional syringe and needle, injecting guns, and a new type of calibrated tube that looks like a ball point pen and is just as easy to carry in a pocket or purse but injects very precise doses of insulin.

Insulin is almost always required in the juvenile (type one) form of diabetes, and occasionally in the maturity onset (type two) form.

Overuse of insulin, or a reduction in normal food intake or exercise, can lead to a sudden drop in blood glucose (hypoglycaemia) and collapse of the patient. Most diabetics are aware of the onset of a hypoglycaemia ('hypo') attack, and are prepared to deal with it by sucking a glucose sweet or swallowing a sweetened drink. Relatives and close friends should be made aware of symptoms of hypo-glycaemia and first aid requirements.

Insulin is safe to use in pregnancy, breast feeding and children. Pregnancy, illness, infections, change in diet, exercise and stress may cause a change in insulin requirements, so regular monitoring of blood sugar levels is essential.

Patients should vary the site of insulin injection and never inject into vein.

Many drugs **interact** with, or alter the requirements for, insulin. These include corticosteroids, thiazides, frusemide, ethacrynic acid, protamine, isoniazid, phenoth-iazines, salbutamol, phenytoin, anabolic steroids, ACE inhibitors, sulfonamides, oral contraceptives, thyroxine, MAOI, salicylates, beta blockers and the herbs ginseng and karela. Alcohol may increase the need for insulin.

Surprisingly, Corn Flakes have a high glycaemic index
(bad in diabetes), while fried sausages have a low GI.

GLYCAEMIC INDEX

The **glycaemic index** (GI) is a measure of how much a food affects the blood sugar level. This is very important for diabetics who need to keep their blood sugar level within specific limits. Diabetics can determine their diet by referring to the GI of foods they eat.

Different foods have different effects on the blood sugar level, and a GI level between 0 (no effect) and 100 (serious effect) has been given to most foods, and comprehensive lists of these are available from doctors, dieticians and diabetic educators.

DIABETES INSIPIDUS

Diabetes insipidus is an uncommon type of pituitary gland failure. This gland lies under the centre of the brain and controls all other glands in the body. The condition may be triggered by a head injury, or develop slowly over many months because of a brain infection, tumour or stroke. It occurs when the pituitary gland fails to produce the hormone vasopressin that controls the rate at which the kidney produces urine. Without this hormone, the kidney constantly produces large amounts of dilute urine.

Patients have a huge urine output, are constantly thirsty, lose weight, develop headaches and muscle pains, become easily dehydrated, and may have an irregular heart beat. The diagnosis can be confirmed by a series of ingenious blood and urine tests after exposing the patient to varying degrees of water intake.

It can be controlled by regular injections of **vasopressin** which last from one to three days. Milder cases can be treated with a nasal spray containing a synthetic form of vasopressin, but this only lasts for a few hours.

Although diabetes insipidus cannot be cured, it is usually well controlled. Some cases do settle spontaneously, but most patients require lifelong treatment.

CURIOSITY

Sir Frederick Grant Banting (1891–1941) was a Nobel prize winning Canadian physiologist who, in cooperation with then medical student Charles Best, first discovered in 1922 that a lack of insulin, produced in the pancreas, was responsible for diabetes. His discovery has saved the lives of millions of diabetics since then.

DIARRHOEA

Diarrhoea is the frequent and excessive discharge of watery fluid from the bowel. Diarrhoea is really a symptom of disease rather than a disease itself. Look after yourself by treating diarrhoea appropriately, and seeking medical advice if it persists.

Everyone experiences diarrhoea at some time. The ten metres of an adult human gut is very sensitive to irritants, and any irritation of the lower half, particularly the last two metres (the large intestine), will result in diarrhoea.

Diarrhoea may be considered by a patient to be the more frequent passing of motions that are softer than usual, but to be medically significant, the motions must be at least part liquid and be passed more than four times a day.

CAUSES

Diarrhoea can be caused by conditions of the intestine, or diseases outside the gut that alter the body's chemistry or other functions.

By far the most common cause of diarrhoea is a viral infection of the intestine (**viral gastroenteritis**). This infection is passed from one person to another by close contact or on the breath, and usually occurs in epidemics, often in springtime. The usual symptoms are six to twelve hours of vomiting followed by one to three days of diarrhoea, and painful gut spasms usually occur.

The rota virus and noro virus are the most common ones to cause viral gastroenteritis.

Food poisoning is due to bacteria, or a toxin produced by bacteria, being present in food. The diagnosis is most strongly suspected when a whole family or group of people is affected simultaneously. The symptoms and the severity of the attack will depend upon the bacteria causing the poisoning, the amount eaten, and the age and general health of the victim. Most attacks of food poisoning occur abruptly, within eight hours (and often one or two hours) of eating the contaminated food, but some types may take up to 24 hours to give symptoms. The patient suddenly starts vomiting, and has explosive diarrhoea associated with intermittent belly pain.

Bacterial gastroenteritis is usually more severe than the viral form, and includes infections by bacteria such as *Shigella*, *Salmonella typhi* (causes typhoid) and *Yersinia*. These are usually responsible for the 'Delhi belly' and 'Montezuma's

121

revenge' suffered by travellers to less developed countries. *Vibrio cholerae* is the bacteria responsible for cholera, the most severe of the bacterial gut infections.

Giardia lamblia is a microscopic animal that can easily enter the body and cause an infection (**giardiasis**) in the small intestine. It passes from one person to another by poor personal hygiene. The condition is far more common in children than adults, who may have no symptoms.

OTHER POSSIBLE INTESTINAL CAUSES OF DIARRHOEA MAY INCLUDE:

- irritable bowel syndrome (spasms of the large intestine with stress)

- diverticulitis (infected outpocketings of the large bowel)

- lactose intolerance (a reaction to the sugar in milk)

- appendicitis

- cancer of the rectum or colon (large intestine)

- food allergies (e.g. eggs, milk, chocolate, peanuts)

- ulcerative colitis (lining of the large intestine becomes ulcerated and bleeds)

- Crohn's disease (a thickening and inflammation of the small or large intestine)

- intussusception (an infolding of the gut on itself)

- surgery to shorten the intestine (prevents adequate absorption of fluids)

- regular anal sex (causes inflammation of the rectum)

- pseudomembranous colitis (severe, rare side effect of antibiotics)

- amoebiasis (an infestation of the gut with microscopic animals)

- blood clot in an artery supplying the bowel.

Strangely severe constipation may actually present as diarrhoea because liquid faeces from further up the bowel can seep around the outside of a large faecal mass in the rectum that is impossible to pass through the anus.

The diarrhoea from cholera may be so severe that
death occurs within hours of its onset.

CONDITIONS OUTSIDE THE INTESTINE MAY ALSO CAUSE DIARRHOEA. THESE MAY INCLUDE:

- psychological, physical or emotional stress, fear and anxiety (may cause involuntary spasms of the gut)

- psychiatric conditions (e.g. depression)

- excess thyroxine (hyperthyroidism)

- pernicious anaemia

- deficiencies of other essential vitamins (e.g. vitamin B3 in the disease pellagra)

- mineral deficiencies

- diabetes mellitus

- inflammation or infection of the organs in the pelvis around the rectum (e.g. bladder, vagina)

- abscess in the pelvis

- Addison's disease (failure of the adrenal glands on top of each kidney)

- cirrhosis (damage to the liver)

- septicaemia (bacterial infection of the blood)

- alcoholism

- AIDS

- toxic shock syndrome

- uraemia (kidney failure).

There are many **medications** that may have diarrhoea as a side effect. Examples include antibiotics (particularly penicillin), antacids, methyldopa (for high blood pressure), beta blockers (for heart disease), theophylline (for asthma and bronchitis), colchicine (for gout), digoxin (for heart disease) and quinine (for malaria). Overuse of laxatives will naturally result in diarrhoea.

There are dozens of other rare causes of diarrhoea.

Faeces may be examined to determine the cause, along with blood tests and sometimes colonoscopy and X-rays.

TREATMENT

Treatment involves determining and treating the cause if possible. Mild attacks are dealt with by diet and fluids, more serious ones require medication to slow the flow, and severe attacks may need fluids to be replaced by an intravenous drip.

Dehydration is the main complication, and the risk is much greater in children under five years of age.

In an emergency, a mixture containing a level teaspoon of salt and eight level teaspoons of sugar or glucose into a litre of boiled water may be given by mouth to treat dehydration.

ANTIDIARRHOEALS

Antidiarrhoeals are one of the most popular drug groups with patients. When you just have to go and go and go – and you want to stop – antidiarrhoeals are just the thing to help.

There are some types of diarrhoea that they are not suitable for, including those associated with jaundice (yellow skin), bacterial gut infections, and diarrhoea during pregnancy. Diarrhoea has a vast number of causes, and the exact treatment chosen will depend on that cause. Many types of diarrhoea require no medication but a correct diet.

The most commonly used antidiarrhoeals include diphenoxylate and atropine (**Lomotil**), kaolin (old fashioned and not particularly effective), **codeine** (also an analgesic – pain killer) and loperamide (**Imodium**).

CURIOSITY

Extract from Pugh's Almanac of 1900.

'In the seventy six great towns of England and Wales, there were during July, August and September of this year (1899), 14,306 infant deaths from diarrhoea'.

DIET

Eating the correct foods is one of the best, and most important ways in which you can look after yourself.

Humans are **omnivores** – they eat all types of food, both from vegetable and animal origin. In fact there are only two things that humans consume on a regular and normal basis that were not at some stage of their production alive as either an animal or plant (see last sentence of this entry for the answer to what these two things are).

The rules of a good diet revolve around the aphorism of 'all things in moderation'. A diet heavy in fat is harmful, but a totally fat-free diet is also harmful. Alcohol in small to medium quantities is beneficial, but in excess is harmful. Moderate drinkers actually live longer than teetotallers. Even water in excess can be harmful.

There is no 'best' food or 'best' diet, it is up to each individual to work out what is best for them by selecting appropriately from all food groups, including carbohydrates, proteins, fats and an appropriate amount of fibre.

Generally **fresh** foods are better (and often cheaper) than processed and packaged foods, as they contain a higher percentage of essential vitamins that may be degraded by processing. As a result, many manufacturers add back in vitamins at the end of the processing in order to replace those that have been lost. Often they claim that their product has been 'vitamin enriched' if they add in more vitamins than were originally present.

FOODS

All animals require food that is appropriate to their needs. The food requirements of humans can best be demonstrated by the food pyramid, which shows which foods are required and in what proportions.

A healthy diet contains adequate quantities of six groups of substances – proteins, carbohydrates, fats, fibre, vitamins, and minerals. The first three contain kilojoules (i.e. produce energy) and the second three do not. It is also essential to have a supply of safe drinking water, as a person can live for weeks without food, but only a few days without water.

GOOD DIET

A GOOD WELL BALANCED DIET SHOULD INCLUDE:

- **protein** from foods such as fish or other seafood, poultry, very lean meat, or eggs, dried peas, beans or lentils

HEALTHY FOOD PYRAMID

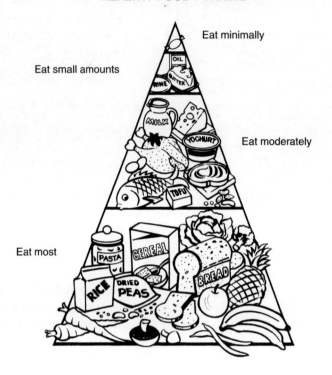

Eat minimally

Eat small amounts

Eat moderately

Eat most

- some salad and three or four **vegetables**, including at least one serve of a green leafy variety and one yellow variety such as carrots

- two or three pieces of **fruit**

- **cereal** or grains, such as rice

- **bread** (some dieticians recommend that this should be wholemeal or whole grain but others are content with white bread)

- some **dairy** products, preferably low-fat for most adults (women in particular should ensure that they get an adequate supply of milk, yoghurt or cheese to prevent the loss of calcium in their bones after menopause which causes osteoporosis).

CARBOHYDRATE

Carbohydrates are molecules that contain carbon, hydrogen and oxygen. They are the body's preferred source of **energy** as the process of digestion converts them into forms of sugar that the body can use easily. They should make up 50–60 per cent of the diet. Sugar, bread, pasta, potatoes and cereals are all rich in carbohydrates. Sugar, however, is not the best means of getting adequate carbohydrates as it has no minerals, vitamins or fibre, and is not always metabolised properly because it enters the bloodstream too quickly.

THERE ARE TWO TYPES OF CARBOHYDRATES:

- Simple carbohydrates are found in fruits, some vegetables, sugar and honey.

- Complex carbohydrates (starches) are found in potatoes, cereals, bread, rice and pasta.

When excess carbohydrates are consumed, they are converted into glycogen and stored in the liver and muscles as a form of energy store.

Foods low in carbohydrates include meats, poultry, eggs, fish, most shellfish (contain practically no carbohydrates) and salad vegetables (e.g. lettuce, arugula, mushrooms, cucumber, celery, alfalfa sprouts, bok choy, radishes, peppers), while fats like olive oil, butter, cheddar, mozzarella, Swiss and other cheeses have small amounts of carbohydrate.

Chocolate is an excellent food that keeps for years without preservatives due to its high content of antioxidants, and as a result is found in most survival kits.

FAT
The main function of fats is to provide energy, although minute amounts are used in growth and repair. Fats enable energy to be **stored** and play a role in insulation. Most fats come from animal products, although some are found in plant foods such as olives, peanuts and avocados. Excess fat is laid down in the body as fatty tissue and is the main cause of obesity.

Depending on chemical composition, fats are either saturated or unsaturated. Saturated fats are more likely to increase the amount of cholesterol in the body and therefore increase the risk of heart disease. Broadly speaking, animal fats, especially those in milk, butter, cheese and meat are highly saturated, and the fat in fish, chicken, turkey and vegetable products is unsaturated. Most of the fat in chicken and turkey is in the skin, which can be removed.

Cholesterol and **triglycerides** are types of fat that are found only in animal products such as meat, eggs and dairy products. These fats can also be manufactured by the body from other types of fat, and are essential in the body for the formation of many chemicals including sex hormones. The rate at which cholesterol and triglyceride are manufactured by the body is determined to a considerable extent by inheritance. Excess levels of these fats in the blood stream can cause hardening of the arteries, heart attacks and strokes.

*A side effect of excess fibre consumption is an
increase the production of intestinal gases.*

FIBRE
Fibre consists of thread-like strands of **cellulose** or cell products that are not normally digested by humans. Fibre is a part of most vegetables, cereals, nuts and fruit, and the insoluble parts that cannot be broken down by intestinal bacteria and digested, is passed out in the faeces.

Fibre food does not cause indigestion because it cannot be digested, and does not always look stringy. For example, peas and beans are high in fibre, cucumber is very low, and celery is in between. The average person should eat 40g of fibre a day.

A high-fibre diet is one way of overcoming obesity, since it makes the stomach feel full so one feels less hungry, but there are fewer kilojoules to be absorbed from the food into the body. Furthermore, the fibre residue in the bowel increases the size and wetness of the stools, and so eases defecation and prevents constipation. The downside may be an increase in flatulence (wind).

Diseases that **benefit** from a high-fibre diet include diverticulitis (small outpocketings of the large bowel), diabetes, gallstones, arteriosclerosis (hardening of the arteries), irritable bowel syndrome, cancer of the bowel, varicose veins, piles and hernias. The incidence of these diseases is significantly less in populations who eat high-fibre diets. Moderation, however, is important. A diet made up entirely of fibre-based foods would lack essential nutrients, fats, carbohydrates and vitamins.

PROTEIN

A protein is a complex molecule that forms the basis of all life, and is composed of two or more **amino acids**. Protein is essential in the diet for growth, repair and replacement of tissue. Animal products (meat, fish, eggs, cheese) provide much protein in a form able to be used by the body. Vegetable proteins exist in peas, beans and other legumes, as well as in grains (and thus bread). If more protein is eaten than the body needs it will provide extra energy, but if not used it will be converted to fat and stored.

Caffeine is a mild stimulant that acts on the body to increase alertness, increase the rate at which the body metabolises (burns) food, and increase urine production.

VEGETARIAN DIET

There are far more vegetarians in the world than meat eaters, simply because vegetables, grains and the like are easier to keep without refrigeration and are usually more readily available, but most people in the developed world for many generations have been enthusiastic consumers of meat. To a degree this is changing, for reasons including health, religion, environmental concerns and fashion.

There are three main types of vegetarian diet. The most common form is **lacto-ovo-vegetarianism** in which milk and eggs are consumed, but no flesh. Other vegetarians avoid red meat but eat fish, while a **vegan** diet excludes all animal products, i.e. not only meat and fish but also dairy produce and eggs.

There is no reason why a vegetarian diet cannot be as healthy as a diet containing meat, provided that protein is obtained from nuts, cereals or pulses (e.g. beans). Vegetarians also need to ensure they get adequate supplies of iron, zinc and calcium, which are found in good supply in meat and milk. Women in particular have double the iron needs of men and should take care to avoid iron deficiency. Women also seem to suffer more from loss of calcium. Generally an adequate supply of these minerals can be obtained from dairy products, but if these are not included in the diet, substitutes must be found. A vegan diet is likely to be deficient in vitamin B12, and supplements may need to be taken to avoid this.

FOOD ADDITIVES

Rather than list the confusing (and daunting) chemical names of food additives, an international numbering code has been adopted so that a particular three or four digit number represents the appropriate additive. Additives may be **used** to enhance colour, flavour or shelf life, prevent foaming, and emulsify, thicken or stabilise different foods. This enables those who are allergic to, or react to a chemical, to avoid it. There are also people who wish to avoid all additives and they can identify whether a food has any by the absence (or presence) of these numbers. Hundreds of chemicals have been assigned numbers, and only some will be listed here.

NUMBER	CHEMICAL	USE
140	Chlorophyll	colouring
160b	Annatto extracts	colouring
200	Sorbic acid	preservative
202	Potassium sorbate	preservative
234	Nisin	preservative
260	Acetic acid	food acid
270	Lactic acid	food acid
304	Ascorbyl palmitate	antioxidant
306	Tocopherols	antioxidant
320	Butylated hydroxyanisole	antioxidant
330	Citric acid	food acid
339	Sodium phosphate	mineral salt
410	Locust bean gum	thickener
412	Guar gum	thickener
415	Xanthan gum	thickener
440	Pectin	gum
466	Sodium carboxymethylcellulose	thickener
471	Mono- and di-glycerides of fatty acids	emulsifier
472c	Citric and fatty acid esters of glycerol	emulsifier
477	Propylene glycol esters	emulsifier
500	Sodium (bi) carbonate	mineral salt
503	Ammonium (bi) carbonate	mineral salt
509	Calcium chloride	mineral salt
635	Disodium 5-ribonucleotides	flavour enhancer
1402	Alkaline treated starch	thickener
1422	Acetylated distarch adipate	thickener
1440	Hydroxy propyl starch	thickener

After reading the list, you will understand better the reason that numbers are used rather than full chemical names!

CURIOSITY

The only two things that humans regularly consume that were not originally part of a plant or animal are salt and water, both absolutely essential to our survival.

DIZZINESS

izziness (vertigo) can be one of the most annoying and distressing of symptoms. It is important to look after yourself when dizziness occurs as it may lead to falls, accidents or other injuries, as well as being a symptom of significant disease. The patient may feel otherwise well, but is unable to function because the world constantly revolves around them. It may also be associated with other symptoms, particularly vomiting and nausea.

ANATOMY

The **ear** is made of three main sections – the outer ear canal (where wax can accumulate) which ends at the ear drum; the middle ear between the ear drum and the start of the hearing mechanism which connects through the eustachian tube with the back of the nose and contains three small bones that magnify the vibrations caused by sound; and the inner ear which contains both the hearing mechanism and three semicircular canals which are responsible for balance. It is often diseases or disorders of these semicircular canals (the vestibular apparatus), or its connections in the brain, which cause dizziness, but other diseases which indirectly affect the balance mechanism and brain may also cause the problem.

CAUSES

A middle ear **infection** (otitis media) is a very common cause of temporary deafness, pain, fever and dizziness, particularly in children. It is often associated with a

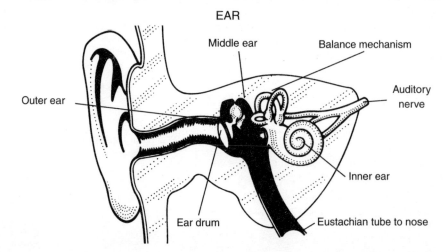

EAR

Middle ear

Balance mechanism

Auditory nerve

Outer ear

Inner ear

Ear drum

Eustachian tube to nose

common cold, and if left untreated, may progress to a permanent partial loss of hearing.

Ménière's disease may occur after a head injury or ear infection, but in most patients it has no apparent cause. It causes a constant high-pitched ringing noise (tinnitus) in the ear, dizziness, nausea and slowly progressive permanent deafness.

Motion sickness is due to an effect on the brain that is unable to reconcile the motion being seen by the eyes and that felt by the balance mechanism. Dizziness, nausea and vomiting may result.

Dizziness due to motion sickness in rear seat car passengers
can often be stopped by sitting in the centre of the rear seat
so that the road ahead can be seen.

The semicircular canals that control balance are known as the labyrinth. If this structure becomes inflamed or infected (**labyrinthitis**) the patient will become dizzy, abnormal eye movements will occur and noises may be heard in the ear.

The **Eustachian tube** connects the middle ear to the back of the nose and enables the air pressure in the ear to equalise with that outside when there is a change in altitude. If the tube becomes blocked, pressure in the ear will increase, causing pain, deafness and dizziness.

UNCOMMON EAR CAUSES OF DIZZINESS MAY INCLUDE:

- mastoiditis (infection of the mastoid bone behind the ear)

- benign paroxysmal positional vertigo (inflammation of the inner ear)

- eighth (auditory) nerve inflammation or tumour

- shingles (herpes zoster infection) involving the ear

- vestibular neuronitis (inflammation of the nerve endings in the inner ear)

- endolymphatic hydrops (increased pressure in the inner ear)

- fractured skull involving the inner ear.

OTHER CAUSES OF VERTIGO THAT OCCUR OUTSIDE THE EAR MAY INCLUDE:

- migraines (often associated with visual symptoms, nausea and vomiting)

- stroke (cerebrovascular accident)

- transient ischaemic attacks (temporary disruption to part of brain's blood supply)

- temporal epilepsy (localised form of epilepsy)

- a serious head injury

- rapid shallow breathing (hyperventilation)

- altitude sickness

- hypotension (low blood pressure)

- hardening of the arteries (arteriosclerosis)

- brain tumour, cyst, cancer or abscess

- bleeding into the brain (after a head injury)

- brain infection (e.g. meningitis, encephalitis) affecting the parts of the brain responsible for balance (particularly the cerebellum at the bottom back of the brain).

Many different heart diseases (e.g. infection, irregular rhythm) and anaemia may affect blood pressure, and cause dizziness as well as chest pain and other symptoms.

Any medication or activity that lowers blood pressure excessively may cause dizziness.

Some **medications** may have dizziness as an unwanted side effect. Examples include phenytoin (for epilepsy), benzodiazepines (e.g. Valium), barbiturates (strong sedatives), gentamicin and streptomycin (antibiotics), nonsteroidal anti-inflammatory drugs (for arthritis), and high doses of aspirin.

There are many other uncommon and rare conditions that may cause vertigo.

TREATMENT
The best way to treat the problem is to fix the cause.

If this is not possible, the most widely used medication for the management of dizziness is prochlorperazine (Stemetil) which can be given as a tablet, suppository (through the anus) or injection.

CURIOSITY
The Hall-Pike test is a diagnostic test for the cause of dizziness. It involves lying the patient down with the head hanging down off the top of a bed. The head is then rotated and abnormal eye movements (nystagmus) are noted if the test is positive. A positive tests indicates the presence of benign paroxysmal positional vertigo.

EARACHE

Look after your ears and therefore yourself by treating them kindly (don't use cotton buds, bobby pins etc. in the ears) and have any ear pain medically assessed if it persists for more than a day.

ANATOMY

The ears are the organs of hearing and of balance. The ear consists of three parts – the outer, middle and inner ear. The outer and middle parts are concerned with hearing, and parts of the inner ear are concerned with balance as well as hearing.

The **outer ear** consists of the part we can see, i.e. the ear flap (pinna) guarding the ear canal, which links the outer ear with the middle ear. The ear canal is also protected by tiny hairs, sweat glands and oil glands which produce wax to stop particles of dust and dirt from getting in. The ear canal is about 2.5 cm long.

The only thing you should ever put in your ear is your elbow.

At the end of the ear canal is a six-sided box which is the **middle ear**. Four sides of the box are made of bone but the fifth side opens into the Eustachian tube and the the sixth side, which is the one facing into the ear canal, is covered by the thin, transparent membrane that forms the eardrum. Inside the box are the three tiniest bones in the human body, commonly called after their respective shapes; the hammer, the anvil and the stirrup, but more correctly known as the malleus, incus and stapes. The stapes is the smallest bone in the body. Sound waves are collected by the outer ear, passed down the ear canal to vibrate the eardrum and then into the middle ear where the sounds are amplified by the tiny bones.

The **Eustachian tube** connects the middle ear to the back of the nose. In essence, sound consists of small fluctuations in air pressure and this tube enables the same pressure to be maintained in the middle ear as in the outside atmosphere, so that the middle ear can pick up the sound waves. If the outside pressure alters more quickly than the middle ear can adjust to, such as when we are flying or diving, the ear will hurt. The familiar pop of the ears in these circumstances is the pressure adjusting by air suddenly moving through the Eustachian tube. The connection of the tube to the throat means that phlegm and mucus sometimes travel along it and cause middle-ear infections.

The **inner ear** is filled with fluid and contains the cochlea (named because it is shaped like a cockle or snail shell), which is the part where hearing occurs. Sound passes from the middle ear through a fluid-filled chamber and into the cochlea

EAR

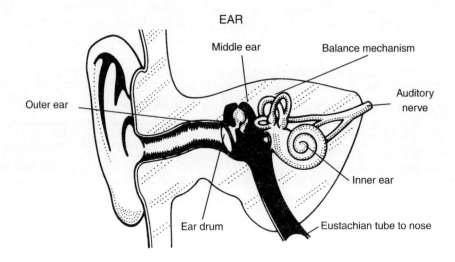

where, in a tiny hair-lined section called the organ of Corti, it is converted into nerve impulses. These nerve impulses are then transmitted to the brain by the auditory nerve which registers them as sounds.

The inner ear is also the organ of balance. Above the cochlea are three semi-circular canals set at different angles (the vestibular apparatus). These are filled with fluid which moves as the head moves. Highly sensitive hairs pick up the movement and send impulses to the brain indicating the position of the head and body.

People with a diagonal crease across the ear lobe have a
statistically increased risk of hardening of the arteries
in the heart and therefore of heart attack.

EARACHE CAUSES

Ear pain is a very common problem, particularly in children, and because the pain is often caused by a build-up of pressure inside the middle ear, normal (and even prescribed) pain killers are often not effective. Only reducing the pressure will ease the pain.

A direct **injury** to the ear from a blow, fall or sudden loud sound may cause bleeding, bruising, swelling and pain to the ear and surrounding tissues.

Otitis externa (**swimmer's ear**) is a bacterial or fungal (tropical ear) infection of the ear canal. The ear becomes very painful, and as the infection progresses, a smelly discharge usually develops.

Middle ear infections (otitis media) are a very common cause of temporary deafness in children, that if left untreated, may progress to a permanent partial loss of hearing. The ear is painful, the child is feverish, and when a doctor examines the ear, a red bulging ear drum can be seen.

If phlegm from the nose enters the middle ear cavity through the Eustachian tube, or other secretions accumulate in the cavity, it is difficult for them to escape back through the Eustachian tube to the back of the nose, particularly if the adenoids which surround the opening of the tube into the nose are swollen. This is **glue ear**, and may be responsible for recurrent infections in the ear, deafness and low grade ear discomfort.

A **Eustachian tube blocked** with phlegm will prevent pressure equalisation between the middle ear and the outside if there is an altitude change (e.g. taking off in an aircraft) or pressure change (e.g. scuba diving). Intense pain will be felt in the ear because of distortion of the sensitive ear drum with the pressure difference. In the worst cases, the ear drum will burst, the pain will ease, but the ear will be deaf until the ear drum heals.

If bacteria or viruses enter the sinuses, an infection (**sinusitis**) may result and thick pus is produced. The sinuses become very painful and tender, then waste products from the infection enter the blood stream, and cause a fever, headaches and the other unpleasant sensations of any major infection. It is quite easy for the infection to spread through the Eustachian tube from the back of the nose to the middle ear.

The **common cold** (coryza) may be caused by one or more of several hundred different viruses. It may cause a sore throat, runny nose, cough, fever, headache, earache and general tiredness.

The sensory nerves that supply the **teeth** run along the top and bottom jaws to a point just in front of the ear where they enter the skull. Any infection or disease of a tooth can inflame the nerve running from that tooth, but the pain may be felt in the ear because of the course the nerve follows to the brain. Babies who are teething often pull at their ears because of this phenomenon.

LESS COMMON CAUSES OF EARACHE MAY INCLUDE:

- foreign body in the ear canal (e.g. a small toy, nut, insect)

- mastoiditis (infection in the bone behind the ear)

- furuncle (boil in the ear)

- cholesteatoma (foul smelling growth in the ear canal)

- parotitis (infection of the parotid salivary gland below the ear)

- arthritis, diseases or other inflammations of the jaw joint

- shingles (*Herpes zoster* virus infection) involving the ear (Ramsay Hunt syndrome)

- nerve inflammation or tumour (neuroma)

- temporal arteritis (inflammation of an artery in the temple).

EAR WAX

Technically, ear wax is known as **cerumen**. It is secreted naturally in the outer ear canal by special glands, and slowly moves out to clear away dust and debris that enters the ear. It also acts to keep the skin lining the canal lubricated and to protect it from water and other irritants. The ear is designed to be self-cleaning, and attempts to clean it may pack the wax down hard on the eardrum or damage the ear canal.

Ear wax may cause problems if excess is produced, the wax is too thick, the ear canal is narrow, or the person works in a dusty and dirty environment. When wax builds up on the eardrum, it cannot transmit vibrations on to the inner ear, and so causes varying degrees of deafness, itching, and sometimes pain. Water entering the ear during bathing or swimming may cause the wax to swell.

Women who have soft ear wax have a much higher risk
of breast cancer than those with hard ear wax.

Cerumen may be **removed** by syringing, suction or fine forceps. In syringing, warm water is gently squirted into the ear to dislodge the wax, with large lumps being removed by forceps. The use of wax-softening drops may be necessary to facilitate the removal of particularly large or hard accumulations of wax. Those with recurrent problems should use wax-softening drops on a regular basis.

Ear wax normally causes no problems, and merely fulfils its cleaning role, but sometimes an infection may start in the skin of the outer ear canal under the wax causing significant pain.

CURIOSITY
It is often difficult to tell if a child has an ear infection, but this trick may help. If moving the outer ear causes pain, a middle ear infection is a possibility. If pressure on the tragus (the firm lump of cartilage immediately in front of the ear canal) causes pain, an outer ear infection is possible. If neither causes pain, an ear infection is unlikely.

EXERCISE

Taking regular exercise is one of the most important ways in which you can look after yourself, but the correct exercise for your age, weight and fitness is also important.

There is little doubt that regular exercise is beneficial to the long-term health of an individual. On the other hand, excessive exercise may be detrimental, but the degree of excess must be very high to be significantly detrimental.

EXERCISE INTENSITY

The intensity of an exercise activity can be measured by comparison to the resting metabolic rate (the rate at which the body uses energy when at rest) as shown in the table below.

ACTIVITY	METS
Sleeping	1
Walking slowly (3 kph)	2.5
Walking moderately (5 kph)	3.5
Rowing lightly (50 watts)	3.5
Golf, pulling buggy	4.5
Painting walls	4.5
Mowing lawn	4.5
Dancing rapidly	5
Aerobics – low impact	5
Cricket – bowling or batting	5
Tennis doubles	5.5
Walking briskly (6.5 kph)	5.5
Cycling, stationary (100 watts)	5.5
Chopping wood	6
Walking moderately uphill	6
Aerobics (high impact)	7
Backpacking	7
Jogging	7
Skiing	7
Tennis singles	7.5
Cycling moderately (20 kph)	8
Walking up stairs steadily	8

ACTIVITY	METS
Step aerobics	9
Running (10 kph)	10
Swimming fast freestyle	10
Cycling fast (25 kph)	10
Running fast (12 kph)	12

METS = metabolic equivalents

The general rule of 'all things in moderation' should apply to exercise as much as anything else. While regular exercise is good for general health, excessive amounts can be harmful, as can be seen by the heart failure, premature arthritis, psychiatric disturbances and other chronic wear and tear injuries suffered by elite and endurance athletes (for example, fitness guru James Fixx who died from a heart attack in his fifties).

Four hundred kilojoules (100 calories) will be used
by walking briskly for 20 minutes, swimming for
ten minutes, or running flat out for seven minutes.

Moderate exercise can make a significant difference to a person's moods. Individuals feel more energetic and able to look after themselves. There's also the added benefit of looking fit and toned, which is a confidence booster, and physical exercise can distract from worrying thoughts.

Exercise may be the last thing someone feels like doing when they are tired, depressed or anxious. They may feel they haven't got the energy to get out of the armchair, never mind swim ten lengths. However, exercise can make a person feel relaxed, stretched and energised. It has beneficial effects on the heart, helps to reduce anxiety and depression, lose weight and feel fitter.

Vigorous activity stimulates the body into releasing endorphins, the body's natural antidepressants. Aerobic exercises (which raise the pulse rate) have received most praise as a stress antidote. A minimum of ten minutes a day spent walking, swimming, playing tennis, cycling, or taking exercise classes is all that is needed. For maximum benefit to the general health, slowly increase the daily dose to 20 or 30 minutes.

Exercise doesn't have to be gruelling to be beneficial. Build up slowly and don't be overambitious to begin with. Choose something enjoyable, or it won't be continued. Taking exercise classes can bring a bonus – it's a good way of meeting people as well as keeping fit.

The **best** forms of **exercise** are cycling (mobile or fixed) and swimming, as they evenly, and with minimal stress, exercise all muscle bundles and joints in the body. Brisk walking is the best exercise for those of more mature years. Those who are completely idle are more likely to develop obesity, heart disease, high cholesterol levels, osteoporosis, diabetes and clinical depression than those who exercise regularly, but it doesn't have to be an enormous amount of exercise. Just climbing stairs or jogging for ten minutes a day is sufficient to significantly reduce the risk of all the medical conditions just listed.

The body and mind need time to relax and recuperate from the effects of everyday activity and stress. Everyone has their favourite method. Taking time to soak in a warm bath, listening to music, walking in the park, spending time with a favourite hobby or pastime can all help the wind-down process and recovery from the day.

Those who exercise and control their weight after a heart attack do much better, and survive far longer than those who remain sedentary.

MAXIMAL HEART RATE

The maximum desirable heart rate during exercise can be calculated by the formula: 220 minus age.

Therefore a 40-year-old should not exercise beyond the point when the heart rate reaches 180, and a 60-year-old should not exceed 160 beats a minute.

YOGA

Yoga is an excellent way to relax, but ordinary relaxation exercises practised every day are also very beneficial. Those described below take an average of 20 minutes and can be done at home, at work, on the bus and train, or anywhere you won't be interrupted.

- Find a comfortable position to sit or lie in.

- Close your eyes, if possible, and breathe slowly and deeply in a relaxed and even manner.

- Locate any areas of tension and try to relax those muscles, visualising the tension disappearing from that area. Feel that you are softening the muscles and letting go.

- Consciously relax each part of the body in turn, starting with your feet, slowly working up through the body, until you reach the top of your head.

- As you focus on each part of your body, think of warmth, heaviness and relaxation.

- Push distracting thoughts to the back of your mind. Thoughts may pop into your head. It can help to feel that you are letting them go, safe in the knowledge that if they are important they will come back to you later.

- After a while (20 minutes or so) take deep breaths and then open your eyes. Stay sitting or lying still for a few moments before you get up.

CURIOSITY
When people take ten minutes of moderate exercise, such as pedalling a bike, their mood improves.

The average person walks 250,000km in a lifetime.

EYES

THE MOST IMPORTANT WAYS IN WHICH YOU CAN LOOK AFTER YOUR EYES ARE:

- ALWAYS wear sunglasses when outdoors in bright sunlight

- wear protective glasses when playing sport such as squash

- wear protective glasses when using machinery such as weed slashers and grinders

- use correctly prescribed spectacles for any vision problems

- seek early medical care for any eye symptoms.

ANATOMY

Light enters the eyes and stimulates nerves which in turn transmit impulses to the brain where the information is interpreted as visual images. Light travels in straight lines, but it can be bent if it passes through a lens, be that in a camera or the human eye. The degree of bending can be precisely controlled by the shape of the lens and the shape of the lens in the human eye can be changed by tiny muscles attached to it.

The eye is the most complex organ in the anatomy of any animal.

EACH EYE IS A SLIGHTLY FLATTENED SPHERE CONSISTING OF THREE LAYERS:

- The outer layer is called the sclera and forms the white of the eye, except for the very front section, which is transparent to allow light in and is called the **cornea**.

- The second layer is the choroid and contains the blood vessels that service the eye. The front of the choroid forms the **iris**, which is the part that gives the eyes their colour depending on the inherited genes. In the centre of the iris is a small gap called the **pupil**. Muscles in the iris enlarge or reduce the size of the pupil according to the amount of light – the more light the smaller the pupil. Just behind the iris is the lens.

- The innermost layer of the eye, curving around the back of the sphere, is the **retina**. This is a light-sensitive structure containing nerve cells, commonly called rods and cones because of their shapes. The rods are sensitive to light and will function in dim light but do not produce a very sharp image. The cones are sensitive to colour. When you go into a dark-ened room such as a theatre, it is difficult to see for the first few moments. This is the time it takes the rods to adjust to the change in light.

THE EYE

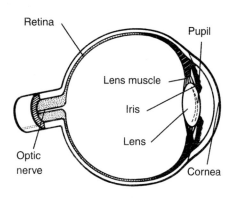

The nerves in the retina all meet together to form the optic nerve, which connects to the brain. The **fovea** is a small depression in the retina at the back of the eye where the light sensitive cells which detect vision are very highly concentrated. Light focused on this point has the greatest degree of definition. It is directly opposite the pupil.

Between the lens and the cornea is a chamber filled with a watery fluid, called the **aqueous humour**. The ball of the eye behind the lens and in front of the retina is filled with a jelly-like substance called **vitreous humour**. It is this that gives the eyeball its firmness and maintains its spherical shape.

A glass of wine a day (but not more) promotes better vision as it helps to prevent the eye disease macular degeneration.

The eye is one of the most mobile organs in the body. Each eye has a set of six external **muscles** so that it can move in all directions.

Because the eyes are so sensitive, the body provides a great deal of protection for them. They are set in two bony sockets in the skull. Externally they are guarded by the eyebrows and the eyelids. The eyebrows help to ward off blows, shield the eyes from sunlight and deflect sweat so that it does not run into the eyes.

The eyelids form a protective covering, while the fringe of eyelashes stops dust and dirt getting in. When an eyelid blinks, it wipes a film of antiseptic tears over the eye. The inner surface of both upper and lower eyelids, as well as the eyes them-selves, are covered by a transparent membrane called the conjunctiva. This helps to keep the eyes moist so that they can move freely.

VISION

Light passes through all the transparent layers starting with the cornea, then through the pupil and aqueous humour, the lens, followed by the vitreous humour to finally impinge on the retina. All these layers refract (bend) the light so that light from the large area outside is focused in the small area of the retina.

EYE FROM FRONT

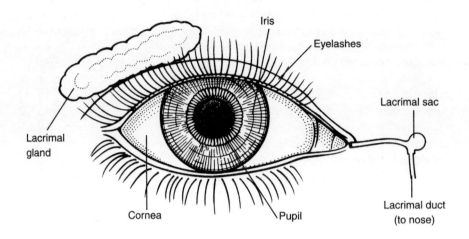

The most important refractive body is the cornea, which is responsible for about 70 per cent of the process. The lens focuses the light according to whether it is for near or distance vision. When the light reaches the retina, the nerve cells convert it into electrical impulses and send these along the optic nerve to the brain, which records visually the objects we are looking at.

Just like the lens of a camera, the lens of the eye produces an upside down image. The brain is responsible for the right-side-up, three-dimensional view that we eventually get. If the optic nerve is damaged, it can cause blindness even though the eyes themselves are still functioning. The point where the optic nerve leaves the retina has no rods and cones and so forms a blind spot.

SYMPTOMS

DISCHARGE

The eye may discharge **tears** when the person is emotionally upset or the eye is inflamed, or pus with an eye infection.

The causes of a **watery discharge** include allergic conjunctivitis (the eye reacts to a pollen, dust, chemical or other substance with itching, redness and watering), a foreign body (e.g. speck of dirt, inturned eyelash), flash burn (from watching a welding arc), ultraviolet lights, iritis (inflammation of the coloured part of the eye), scleritis (inflammation of the whites of the eyes), glaucoma (increase in the pressure of the jelly-like fluid inside the eye), and an infection of the eye with the virus *Herpes simplex.*

A creamy or green **thick discharge** may be caused by bacterial conjunctivitis, viral conjunctivitis, and trachoma (a type of conjunctivitis caused by *Chlamydia*).

CURIOSITY

Common sore eyes may be cured by washing them with breast milk (1830 medical text).

DRY EYE

Tears are produced in glands (lacrimal glands) beyond the outer corner of the eye, and are released onto the eye surface through a small tube (duct) to keep the eye surface moist. Excess tears drain through the tear duct at the inner corner of the eye into the back of the nose. If too many tears are produced, they will overflow the eye and the person will be seen to be crying. If too few tears are produced, the eye will dry out and become itchy and irritated. Technically, dry eyes are called xerophthalmia.

Dry eyes are a very common problem with old age, as the lacrimal glands wear out. The lower lid may also become slack, and separate from the eye surface with age (a condition called **ectropion**), allowing tears to escape from the eye. Lubricating drops and ointments are used to overcome the problem.

A deficiency of **vitamin A** in the diet will cause dry skin, dry eyes, shallow ulcers on the eye surface and poor night vision.

Keratoconjunctivitis sicca is an inflammation of the eye surface similar to eczema on the skin, with which it is often associated.

A viral **infection** of the eye (viral conjunctivitis) may affect tear production and cause eye drying, as well as redness and soreness.

Trachoma is a type of conjunctivitis (superficial eye infection) caused by an organism known as *Chlamydia*. It is very common in areas of low hygiene where flies can transmit the infection from one person to another. A mild trachoma infection may not be very noticeable and may cause no symptoms at all. In more severe cases, eye pain, intolerance to bright lights, and a weeping swollen eye may develop. The lacrimal gland can also be damaged so that the eye dries out.

Damage to the lacrimal gland from an injury, infection or irradiation (e.g. treatment of a skin cancer) may prevent tear production.

Some **medications** may have dry eyes as a side effect. Examples include antihistamines, blood pressure medications, pseudoephedrine (used for a runny nose) and some psychiatric drugs.

Uncommon causes of a dry eye include cirrhosis (liver failure), rheumatoid arthritis, diabetes, erythema multiforme (an acute inflammation of the skin), Sjögren syndrome (an autoimmune disease) and Riley-Day syndrome.

*Eye pain is a symptom that should never be
ignored as it may have serious consequences.*

EYE PAIN

Eye **pain** my come from the eye itself, structures around the eye, or from nerve irritation associated with other conditions.

A **foreign body** (e.g. speck of dirt, loose eyelash) in the eye will irritate it to cause pain (particularly on eye movement), redness and watering from the affected eye. After the irritant is removed, an ulcer may be left behind that will cause eye irritation for some days until it heals.

Bacterial **conjunctivitis** is very common in children but may occur at any age. The eyes (and both are usually involved) are red, sore and a yellow/green discharge forms that may stick the eyelids together overnight. Viral conjunctivitis is a viral infection of the eye surface. It is far less common than a bacterial infection, but much harder to treat. A watery, pale yellow, slightly creamy discharge occurs and the eyes are itchy, slightly sore and sometimes red.

Glaucoma is due to an increase in the pressure of the jelly-like fluid inside the eye. This may come on gradually, or may be quite sudden. Early symptoms include an eye ache or pain, blurred vision, seeing halos around objects, red eye, a gradual loss of peripheral vision and watering of the eye.

Iritis is an inflammation of the iris (the coloured part of the eye). The inflammation can be due to an infection such as toxoplasmosis, tuberculosis or syphilis, or it may be associated with inflammatory diseases in other parts of the body, including psoriasis, ankylosing spondylitis, and some bowel conditions. Almost invariably, only one eye is involved. It will suddenly become red and painful, a watery discharge will develop, and the vision will become blurred.

Other eye causes of pain include scleritis (inflammation of the whites of the eyes), looking at a welding arc (flash burn) or ultraviolet lights, trachoma (a type of conjunctivitis caused by *Chlamydia*), and an infection of the eye with the virus *Herpes simplex*.

Eye pain originating outside the eye may be due to sinusitis, migraine, cluster headache (usually associated with excess sweating of one or both sides of head), Ramsay Hunt syndrome (form of shingles affecting the face), excess thyroxine (hyperthyroidism), Reiter syndrome, Sjögren syndrome and ankylosing spondylitis (long-term inflammation of the small joints between the vertebrae that may sometimes involve the eyes).

PARALYSED EYE

The inability to move the eye in one or more directions is a rare but serious symptom.

Reasons for this problem may include a stroke affecting the part of the brain that controls eye movement, Steele-Richardson-Olszewski syndrome (a variation of Parkinson's disease), Parinaud syndrome (tumour or inflammation of the pineal gland at the front of the brain), Wernicke-Korsakoff psychosis (vitamin deficiency usually from alcoholism) and Tolosa-Hunt syndrome (painful paralysis of one eye, a drooping eyelid and enlargement of the pupil because of pressure on nerves to the eye caused by an aneurysm on the carotid artery).

Normally the eyelid just touches the top of the iris (coloured part of the eye) when the eye is relaxed. If white can be seen above the iris, the eye is probably protruding.

PROTRUDING EYE

A patient with slightly protruding eyes in comparison to the face is said to have proptosis or exophthalmos.

The thyroid gland in the front of the neck produces the hormone thyroxine, which acts as an accelerator for every cell in the body. Excess thyroxine (**hyperthyroidism**) will cause sweating, weight loss, diarrhoea, malabsorption of food, nervousness, heat intolerance, rapid heart rate, warm skin, tremor and prominent eyes.

A **tumour**, cancer or infection of the eye, the eye socket, surrounding tissues, skull or the brain behind the eye will cause one eye only to become more prominent.

Other possible causes of exophthalmos include Cushing syndrome (over production of steroids in the body, or taking large doses of cortisone), very severe high blood pressure (malignant hypertension), clots in the veins behind an eye, Hand-Schueller-Christian syndrome, Apert syndrome and Sturge-Weber syndrome.

RED EYE

Red eyes are a very common problem, and may be due to overuse, inadequate rest and too much alcohol, as well as any one of a number of diseases.

A **foreign body** (e.g. speck of dirt, loose eyelash) in the eye will irritate it to cause pain (particularly on eye movement), redness and watering from the affected eye. After the irritant is removed, an ulcer may be left behind that will cause eye irritation for some days until it heals. Chemical irritation from a substance splashed in an eye, or pool chlorine that is too strong, will cause a similar effect.

Bleeding into the white of the eye after an injury will cause a dramatic red patch.

Bacterial **conjunctivitis** and viral conjunctivitis (see eye pain entry page 143) are very common causes of a red eye in children but may occur at any age.

Allergic conjunctivitis, in which the eye is reacting to a pollen, dust, chemical or other substance that has entered the eye, will cause itching, redness and watering. Often only one eye is affected.

Iritis is an inflammation of the iris (the coloured part of the eye). The eye will suddenly become red and painful, a watery discharge will develop, and the vision is blurred. Bright lights will aggravate the eye pain and the pupil is small.

A **pingueculum** or pterygium (growth on the eye surface) may become irritated and red.

Uncommon causes of a red eye include trachoma (eye infection caused by *Chlamydia*), glaucoma, cluster headaches, episcleritis, Reiter syndrome, Behçet syndrome and Stevens-Johnson syndrome.

The use of the illegal drug cocaine is also associated with eye redness.

Bleeding into the white of the eye is much more serious
if the back edge of the red area cannot be seen.

SUNKEN EYE

The eyes may appear sunken in (enophthalmos) because of tiredness or prolonged illness of any sort, but there are some significant medical conditions that may be responsible.

Dehydration because of lack of fluid intake, or excess fluid output (e.g. diarrhoea, sweating) will result in a loss of tissue tone, and cause the eyes to sink into the head.

Malnutrition from the unavailability of food, or diseases such as anorexia nervosa, will decrease body fat, including the fat pad which normally sits behind each eye.

A significant **weight loss** due to serious disease (e.g. cancer, heart failure), or deliberate dieting, will also shrink the eye fat pad.

The thyroid gland in the front of the neck produces the hormone thyroxine, which acts as an accelerator for every cell in the body. If there is a lack of thyroxine (**hypothyroidism**), all organs will function slowly, and symptoms will include intolerance of cold, constipation, weakness, hoarse voice, heavy periods, sunken eyes, dry skin, hair loss, slow heart rate and anaemia.

A tumour of the tear producing lacrimal gland at the outside corner of the eye may put pressure on the front of the eye, and cause swelling of the tissue around the eye, to make it appear sunken into the head.

ULCER

Ulceration of the cornea, the transparent outside covering on the front of the eye, may be caused by injuries to the surface of the eye (e.g. scratch), or infections. *Herpes simplex*, the virus that causes cold sores and genital herpes, is the most common cause of all eye ulcers. Fungal infections causing ulcers are commonly seen in farm workers, but may develop in others when steroid eye drops are being used. Bacterial conjunctivitis seldom causes ulcers unless treatment is neglected.

Two rare causes are a deficiency in vitamin A (e.g. in people on fad diets, or with inability to absorb vitamin A because of diseases of the bile duct) which results in a very dry eye, and prolonged exposure of the eye in unconscious patients who do not blink.

Pain and watering occurs in the eye, there is redness of the whites of the eye, and a discharge of sticky pus occurs if an **infection** is responsible. Permanent scarring of the cornea and reduced vision may occur if the ulcer is left untreated. A swab may be taken from the eye to identify the organism responsible for an infection.

Appropriate eye drops are prescribed for bacterial and fungal eye infections. Serious *Herpes* virus infections can be treated with special antiviral eye drops and ointment, and through a microscope, minor surgery to remove the active viral areas at the edge of the ulcer may be undertaken. If necessary, a scarred cornea can be surgically replaced by a corneal transplant.

The prognosis depends on the cause and response to treatment. Ulcers caused by an injury usually heal within a few days without treatment. Most viral infections settle without treatment after a few weeks of discomfort, but in some patients, particularly those who are otherwise in poor health or on potent drugs for other serious diseases, the infection can steadily worsen to cause severe eye ulceration. Bacterial and fungal infections respond rapidly to treatment, and there is usually a good result from corneal transplantation.

Ophthalmologists are doctors who have
specialised in eye diseases.
Optometrists are scientists who measure vision
and prescribe spectacles.

DISEASES

BACTERIAL CONJUNCTIVITIS

Conjunctivitis is an inflammation of the outer surface (cornea) of the eye, due to an allergy, or a viral or bacterial **infection**.

A bacterial conjunctivitis is the most common form, and is due to bacteria infecting the thin film of tears that covers the eye. It is very easily passed from one person to another (e.g. a patient rubs their eyes with a hand, then shakes hands, and the second person then rubs their eyes). Babies suffering from a blocked tear duct may have recurrent infections. Tears are produced in the lacrimal gland beyond the outer edge of the eye, move across the eye surface and then through a tiny tube at the inner edge of the eye that leads to the nose. If the duct is too small in an infant, or is blocked by pus or phlegm, the circulation of tears is prevented and infection results.

Bacterial conjunctivitis causes the formation of **yellow or green pus** in the eyes which may stick the eyelids together. The eyes are bloodshot and sore, and almost invariably the infection involves both eyes. If allowed to persist, it may cause scarring of the eye surface and a deterioration in sight.

Rarely, resistant infections make it necessary to take a swab from the eye to determine the exact bacteria or virus responsible, but in most cases, no investigations are necessary.

Bacterial conjunctivitis is easily treated with **antibiotic** drops or ointment on a regular basis until the infection clears. A blocked tear duct may be probed and cleared if conjunctivitis persists in a baby for several months, but most grow out of the problem.

VIRAL CONJUNCTIVITIS

Any one or more of a number of viruses may infect the cornea to cause conjunctivitis. This form is not quite as easily transmitted as bacterial conjunctivitis.

Viral conjunctivitis causes slight pain or an itch, redness of the eye and often a clear sticky exudate.

Viral conjunctivitis is the more difficult form to treat, as there is no cure for most viral infections, but *Herpes* virus infections can be cured by antiviral drops. Soothing drops and ointment may be used, but time is the main treatment, and the infection may persist for several weeks until the body's own defences overcome it.

ALLERGIC CONJUNCTIVITIS

Allergic (or atopic) conjunctivitis is an allergy reaction involving the surface of the eye.

If a pollen, dust or other substance to which a person is allergic lands on the eye, an allergy reaction will occur. Allergic conjunctivitis is often associated with hay fever and often only occurs at certain times of the year.

The symptoms include redness, itching, blurred vision and watering of the eye. In severe cases the white of the eye may swell dramatically and balloon out between the eyelids. There may be a **clear, stringy discharge** from the eyes, as well as excessive tears, and if the lower eyelid is turned down it appears to be covered with a large number of tiny red bumps. Rarely, ulceration of the eye surface may occur.

Blood and skin tests can be undertaken to identify the responsible substance in some patients who are repeatedly affected.

It can be prevented by the regular use of sodium cromoglycate drops throughout the allergy time of year. Attacks can be treated by antihistamine tablets and eye drops such as olopatadine or levocabastine. Simple eye drops available over the counter from chemists and containing artery-constricting medications can be used in milder cases. Appropriate treatment usually settles the symptoms rapidly.

FLOATER

A floater is a collection of cells or protein in the thick fluid that fills the eyeball, which casts a **shadow** on the light-sensitive retina at the back of the eye. The floater forms because of bleeding into the eye, a detached retina, infection, or no cause may be found. Diabetes, leukaemia, high blood pressure, and rarer conditions may cause bleeding into the eye.

Patients notice a spot in the field of vision that may continue to move across the visual field after the moving eye comes to rest – thus the name floater. Because a serious condition may be responsible, all patients with floaters must be investigated to exclude any disease. A detached retina can be repaired by a laser in the early stages, but if left, may cause permanent blindness.

They are only treated if causing significant trouble, but if necessary, a laser can destroy the floater while a doctor uses a microscope to look into the eye. Most floaters dissipate with time.

Some people notice a black spot in their vision that moves precisely as the eyes move. This may be the blind spot, where the optic nerve passes through the retina at the back of the eye.

GLAUCOMA

Glaucoma is an increase in the pressure of the half-set jelly-like fluid inside the eyeball that damages the eye and affects the vision. The eye is filled with a thick clear fluid (vitreous humour) that is slowly secreted by special cells within the eye, while in another part of the eye the fluid is removed, allowing a slow but steady renewal. If there is a blockage to the drainage of the fluid from the eye while new fluid continues to be secreted, the pressure inside the eye increases, and damage occurs to the light-sensitive retina at the back of the eye. Other conditions may also cause glaucoma including eye tumours, infections, injury and, in rare cases, drugs (e.g. steroids) may be responsible.

THREE **TYPES** OF GLAUCOMA OCCUR – CHRONIC, ACUTE AND CONGENITAL:

- Chronic glaucoma (open-angle glaucoma) is the most common type with a slow onset over years. It usually occurs in both eyes simultaneously and runs in families. Initially it affects the peripheral vision, which is how far can be seen to the sides and up and down while looking straight ahead. One in every 75 people over 40 years have this type of glaucoma.

- Acute glaucoma (angle-closure glaucoma) is the worst type, as it develops in a few hours or days, but usually involves only one eye. There is a rapid deterioration in vision, severe pain, rainbow-coloured halos around lights, nausea and vomiting. It may start after a blow to the eye, or for no discernible reason. Immediate treatment of acute glaucoma is essential if the sight of the eye is to be saved, but even with good treatment, permanent blindness can occur.

- Congenital glaucoma occurs in babies who are born with the condition. The earliest sign is the continual overflow of tears from the eye, and the baby turns away from lights rather than towards them as a normal.

Glaucoma is **diagnosed** in most cases by measuring the pressure of the fluid within the eye. This can be done by anaesthetising the eye surface with eye drops and then resting a pressure measuring instrument (tonometer) on the surface of the eye while the patient is lying down, or by using a machine that directs a puff of air onto the eye to measure the pressure. Glaucoma may also be detected by measuring deterioration in peripheral vision using a computerised device, charts or by following a white dot on a large black screen. More complex tests, including examining the eye through a microscope to determine the nature and seriousness of the glaucoma.

The excessive pressure in the eye caused by glaucoma can be reduced by eye drops, which are usually betablockers, and/or tablets that remove some fluid from the eye.

Betablocker eye drops include betaxolol (Betoptic), latanoprost (Xalantan), levobunolol (Betagan), and timolol. Their side effects may include blurred vision, headache and a small pupil. They should be used with caution in asthma and heart disease. The other commonly used eye drop for glaucoma is carbachol pilocarpine (Pilopt). It may cause blurred vision but otherwise has minimal side effects.

The tablet used to treat glaucoma is acetazolamide (Diamox). Side effects may include pins and needles, excess urination and a poor appetite. It must be used with caution in pregnancy, and not in patients with liver disease.

In serious cases, laser microsurgery to the tiny drainage canals in the front of the eye is necessary. Congenital glaucoma always requires surgical treatment.

Without treatment, glaucoma progresses inexorably to total blindness, but if the disease is detected early, glaucoma in most patients can be successfully controlled but not cured.

CURIOSITY

In case a film should grow over the sight of the eye, you may take it off by drying human dung in the sun, and having reduced it to a very fine powder, blow it thro' a quill two times a day into the eye (1830 medical text).

CATARACT

A cataract is a **clouding of the lens** in the eye, which usually occurs slowly over a number of years and gradually reduces vision until it is the equivalent of looking through frosted glass. A lens affected by a cataract can usually be surgically replaced with an artificial lens.

By far the most common **cause** of a cataract is a slow clouding of the lens with advancing age. There is no specific cause for this, but people who live and work outdoors in very sunny climates seem to get the problem more. A small number of children have a genetic or inherited predisposition to develop a cataract early in life. Some babies are born with the problem. Patients with diabetes suffer the premature development of cataracts.

Uncommon causes of cataracts include ultraviolet, X-ray or gamma ray irradiation to the eye, exposure of a foetus to German measles (rubella) caught by the mother, damage to the eyes at birth due to lack of oxygen and a number of rare syndromes.

The condition can be diagnosed by examining the eye with an ophthalmoscope (magnifying light).

A patient who survives an electrocution may develop cataracts in the eyes (cause dimmed vision) several months later.

Cataracts are initially **treated** with powerful spectacles, but eye surgery to replace the damaged lens is the best solution. Only one eye (usually the worst one) will be operated upon initially. Once this has recovered, the second eye may be repaired. The procedure can be done under a general or local anaesthetic, and involves cutting open the top of the eye at the edge of the iris (the coloured part of the eye), removing the damaged lens by gentle suction, and inserting an artificial lens in its place. This new lens is not mobile, and cannot change shape, thus spectacles are normally still required for close work, and sometimes distant vision as well.

The most noticeable effect after the operation is the brightness of the world. Colours in particular appear far brighter than the washed-out appearance they have through a cloudy lens.

Complications may include dislocation of the new lens, or infection of the eye, but they are uncommon.

More than 95 per cent of patients achieve excellent results with surgery.

INJURY

Any injury to the eye is potentially serious and should receive expert assessment and treatment. An injured eye should not be rubbed, nor should it be opened and examined since it is very easy to do further damage. If the victim is wearing contact lenses, they may be able to remove the lenses themselves, but otherwise it is best left to a doctor. It is especially important to act quickly if any chemical has entered the eye.

*A foreign body that hits the eye but cannot be seen on
examination may have passed into the centre of the eye.*

Foreign bodies in the eye are relatively common and can usually be dealt with at home. Simply washing the face with cool water, ensuring some gets into the eyes, will often remove loose bits of grit. If a single bit is embedded in the under-surface of the upper lid and the lid is pulled back over a match, it may be possible to remove it with a moistened cotton bud. Do not touch the eye surface. If bits of grit adhere to the eye itself, unless they can be washed away easily, a doctor's attention is needed.

A bruised or **black eye** can be relieved by an ice pack (not the traditional piece of steak). Be careful not to bring the eye into direct contact with the ice. Wrap the ice in a damp cloth and alternatively leave it on and remove it from the eye for about 20 minutes at a time. If the eyeball seems to be injured or the victim is unable to see properly, get a doctor. The eye can be padded and bandaged shut while travelling to the doctor or hospital.

It is essential that **chemicals** in the eye are washed out immediately. Tilt the victim's head to the affected side, hold the eyelids gently apart and rinse the eye for at least ten and preferably 20 minutes. Make sure that the water does not splash or flow into the other eye.

Eyelids

There are two eyelids on each eye, an upper and lower. The upper one is much larger and more active than the lower. The eyelid consists of skin, a moist membrane on the inside of the lid (which folds back to form the conjunctiva over the front of the eye), a fibrous plate (tarsal plate) that gives rigidity to the eyelid, eyelashes (which shade the eye), sweat glands, Meibomian glands (oil glands that lubricate the eyelashes) and the tiny tarsal muscles.

The epicanthus is the fold of skin that covers the inner corner of the eye (the canthus). This is more prominent in Asian people.

The eyelashes are hairs growing at the leading edge of the eyelids that act to shade the eye and reduce the amount of sweat and skin oils dropping into the eye.

The medical term for the eyelid is the palpebrae.

EYELID DISEASE

Any of the structures that make up the eyelid may become affected by injury, infection, inflammation or disease.

The eyelid muscles may become fatigued by excessive hours without sleep, and start **twitching** uncontrollably.

A **sty** is a bacterial infection of one of the superficial tiny sweat or oil glands on the margin of the eyelid. There is often no apparent reason for a sty developing, but rubbing the eye, or an injury to the eye, makes it easier for a sty to develop. The infected gland becomes painful, red and swollen, and fills with pus. A sty is really a miniature abscess.

A **chalazion** is a bacterial infection of a deeper gland (Meibomian gland) within the eyelid that causes a painful red tender swelling. The upper and lower eyelids each contain about twenty Meibomian glands, which secrete an oily substance that lubricates the surface of the eye. If the tiny tube leading out of a gland becomes blocked, it will swell up into a cyst that is felt and seen as a lump in the eyelid. The problem is more common in those over 40 years of age, and may follow a period of eye irritation or conjunctivitis. A small cut into the cyst will drain out the contents.

Blepharitis is a superficial bacterial infection of the eyelid margin around the base of the eyelashes. It is often associated with dandruff.

Entropion is the in-turning of the eyelid, which results in eyelashes rubbing irritatingly on the eye surface. It may be caused by eyelid injury or infection.

Ectropion is the out-turning of the lower eyelid, which allows tears to trickle down the cheek, and is a common problem in the elderly.

Other causes of eyelid disease include allergic dermatitis, xanthelasma (yellow fatty deposits on the eyelid), skin cancer, ptosis (see below) and hyperthyroidism (excess thyroxine production).

DROOPING EYELID

Drooping of the eyelid(s) is known as **ptosis**, and may be caused by damage to the nerve controlling the eyelid muscle or a number of rarer syndromes.

Bell's palsy is a peculiar condition in which the nerve that controls the movement of muscles on one side of the face stops working. The cause is unknown. The onset is quite sudden, and a patient may find that one side of their face becomes totally paralysed in a matter of hours. They feel well, and have no other medical problems or areas that are affected.

Bell's palsy must be treated as soon as possible with steroids to speed its recovery. Every hour counts.

Myasthenia gravis causes a varying weakness of the muscles that control the eyelids, the movement of the eyes (double vision results) and swallowing. The weakness varies in severity during the day and may disappear entirely for days or weeks before recurring, but over a period of months or years the attacks become more severe. It is most common in young women and the symptoms are caused by a blocking of the nerves that supply the affected muscles.

UNCOMMON CAUSES OF PTOSIS MAY INCLUDE:

- Guillain-Barré syndrome (progressive symmetrical weakness of the limbs and face)

- Horner syndrome (nerves are compressed in the brain, neck or upper chest)

- Wernicke-Korsakoff psychosis (due to vitamin deficiencies caused by an inadequate diet while on alcoholic binges)

- Dubowitz syndrome (also causes mental retardation)

- damage to the nerve from the brain (third nerve) which controls eyelid movement by a tumour, bleed, abscess or other disease in the nerve, brain or skull.

SWOLLEN EYELID

Swelling (oedema) of an eyelid can be due to an injury, bruise or bite, but sometimes more significant conditions may be responsible.

The most common cause is angioneurotic oedema, which is a sudden, severe swelling of the eyelid and other tissues around the eye caused by an **allergy** reaction. The trigger is usually a pollen, dust, chemical or other substance that has blown into the eye, or from rubbing the eye with a contaminated finger. The affected tissue may be slightly itchy, but is not usually painful or tender.

Other causes may include hypothyroidism (an under-active thyroid gland), and obstruction of the major veins draining the head because of a tumour, clot, cancer, abscess or other disease, which will cause blood to be retained in the head, headache, and swelling of many facial tissues, including the eyelids.

EYE SURGERY

Most eye surgery is undertaken by ophthalmologists (eye doctors) who have undertaken many further years of training in this specialised area. Because of the small size of the eye, most eye surgery is carried out through an operating microscope and using extremely fine instruments, needles and threads.

Most procedures require a general **anaesthetic**, but in older people who are not good anaesthetic risks, quite major eye surgery (e.g. cataract removal) can be done using a local anaesthetic.

Because the operation is limited to a very small area of the body, the patient recovers very rapidly from eye surgery, but special drops and eye protection may be necessary for some weeks. A lot of eye surgery is now performed as day surgery, with the patient arriving at the hospital in the morning and returning home the same day.

Eye surgeons operate on the front half of the eye as far back as the lens, and on the muscles and blood vessels around the outside of the eye. They can rarely operate directly on the inside of the eyeball itself, but they can use lasers in this area. The retina is the light-sensitive area at the back of the eyeball, and if this bleeds, separates from the back of the eye, or is otherwise damaged, lasers can be shone through the pupil and onto the bleeding or damaged area to repair it.

Incisions into the eye may be repaired by tiny sutures, or by special glues that bind together the edges of the wound.

CURIOSITY

Horus was the Ancient Egyptian sky god who was depicted in the form of a falcon, and whose eyes were the sun and the moon. During a battle between Horus and the earth god Seth, the left eye of Horus (the moon eye) was blinded. The eye was then cured by the healing god, Thoth. This battle continued every month, explaining in myth the waxing and waning of the moon. Because of this recurring miracle, the eye of Horus became a powerful symbol of healing in the ancient world.

The eye of a falcon is oval in shape, with a trailing taper leading to the lacrimal gland, and the eye covets (markings) are a vertical triangular slash, and a lazy trailing marking below the eye, as shown in the diagram below.

The left eye of Horus was used throughout Ancient Egypt, and later in modified form in Ancient Greece, to signify the healing power of a potion or medication.

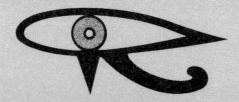

With time and abbreviation, the full symbol became modified to the Rx symbol we know today, which is often interpreted to mean 'recipe'. It is often written in a flowing Old English style script to differentiate it from the main part of the prescription, and is still used to mark the start of a prescription for twenty-first century treatments.

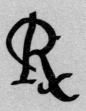

FAECES

E ven though it may sound rather disgusting to many people, you really should look after yourself by observing your own faeces from time to time. Any persistent or unexplained change in bowel habits should be investigated as it may be a sign of significant bowel disease.

There are specialist pathologists and microbiologists
who spend their entire careers studying our
fundamental excretory material.

The body disposes of solid wastes as faeces through the anus. It consists mainly of fibre (cellulose), fats, protein and small amounts of inorganic substances such as iron and phosphorus. At least two thirds of the total weight of faeces is made up of water, but more commonly it is three-quarters water, and if the person has diarrhoea, water may make up over 95 per cent of the faeces. Bacterial debris also makes up a very large part of faeces.

Faeces is usually passed once or twice a day, but some people are comfortable passing faeces only two or three times a week. The amount passed varies markedly from one person to another, and depends greatly upon the diet. The more fibre in the diet, the greater the volume of faeces.

SYMPTOMS
ABNORMAL DESIRE TO PASS FAECES
Tenesmus is the technical term for the desire to pass faeces, even though there is no faeces present in the rectum (last part of the large intestine). Diarrhoea causes the sensation, but in this case, there is good reason to go to the toilet so that the watery faeces can escape.

The most common cause is a mass in the anal canal. This may be a swollen internal pile (haemorrhoid), a tumour or cancer, polyps, or inflammation of the anal canal or rectum from infection or ulceration (e.g. ulcerative colitis).

Inflammation and infection of organs in the pelvis such as the bladder and uterus which rest on the rectum, can cause irritation in the rectum and this inflammation results in tenesmus.

A foreign body inserted into the rectum will also give this sensation.

Because the range of conditions that can be responsible for tenesmus include some very serious ones, it is essential to be checked by a doctor to determine the exact cause of the sensation.

BLOOD IN FAECES

Faecal blood may be fresh (bright red), old (dark red or black), on the outside of the stool, or mixed in with the faeces. It is a problem that must always be checked by a doctor to ensure that there is no serious cause for the bleeding.

Persistent bleeding of small amounts of blood into the gut may first be detected because the patient is anaemic, and only on special tests can the blood be detected in the faeces.

> *Bloody faeces is a sinister sign and must always be investigated*
> *by a doctor, although there are many causes that are not serious.*

Bright red blood on the outside of the faeces may be due to bleeding piles (haemorrhoids) when the bleeding tends to occur for a minute or two after passing a motion, a fissure in the anus (the anus has overstitched and torn during an episode of constipation), and disorders of coagulation (faulty blood clotting mechanism).

Bright red blood mixed in with the faeces may be due to dilated blood vessels and polyps in the rectum, a cancer in the rectum, ulcerative colitis (lining of the large intestine becomes inflamed and ulcerated), polyps in the large intestine, and diverticulitis (formation of numerous small outpocketings of the large gut due to increased pressure in the intestine from inadequate fibre in the diet).

Dark blood in the faeces (melaena) is due to blood that has been altered by the digestive process to appear very dark or black. Bleeding anywhere from the mouth down may appear in the faeces in this form. Common causes include a peptic ulcer in the stomach, oesophageal ulceration, cancer of any part of the intestine, Crohn's disease (thickening and inflammation of the small or large intestine), increased pressure of the blood in the veins draining the intestine (portal hypertension) and excessive doses of drugs such as warfarin and aspirin. The colour of the blood in the faeces depends upon the part of the gut affected.

> *Steatorrhoea is the medical term for fat in faeces, which*
> *causes the floaters that are hard to flush away.*

ABNORMAL FAECES COLOUR

More can be learnt from the colour of your faeces than you may care to know. Most changes in the colour of the faeces are due to changes in diet, but occasionally may be due to serious disease. Any persistent change in the colour of the faeces needs to be checked by a doctor. Take along a sample in a clean clear glass bottle so that it can be inspected and analysed.

Dark faeces may be due to iron and bismuth medications. Red wine and certain fruits may be responsible for dark faeces, but blood is another possibility which can herald serious disease.

Green/yellow faeces is caused by excess bile in the faeces. Bile is produced in the liver, stored in the gall bladder, and released onto food in the first part of the small intestine to aid in digestion. Excess can be caused by diarrhoea (the bile moves through the gut too quickly to be digested), bowel infections and starvation (inadequate food for the bile to work on).

Bright yellow faeces occurs in bottle-fed babies, and rarely older children and adults, who have dairy products as the main source of their diet.

Faeces takes its usual **mid-brown** colour from digested bile. If this is lacking, due to obstruction of the bile duct from the gall bladder to the intestine or because liver disease is preventing its production, the stools will be an **off-white** clay colour. Determining the cause of the lack of bile is essential.

Excess fat in the faeces (steatorrhoea) causes the faeces to be **pale yellow**.

Only blood can cause **red** faeces.

Excess iron in the diet, particularly in the form of iron tablets, may cause **black** faeces, but blood is a serious possible cause. Even if the patient is taking iron supplements, black faeces must be checked by a doctor to ensure the discolouration is not due to blood from a cancer or other disease in the intestine.

Some children and psychiatric patients indulge
in coprophilia, the eating of faeces.

INVESTIGATIONS
FAECES OCCULT BLOOD TEST
A test may be performed on faeces to detect the presence of microscopic amounts of blood. This faeces occult blood test (FOBT) can be used as a screening test for bowel cancer, but some cancers do not bleed, and some bleeding may be due to causes other than cancer.

Occult merely means hidden, so this is a test for blood that is not visible in the faeces. A chemical that detects the haem molecule (part of haemoglobin in blood) is used in one form of the test, while an immunochemical test that detects only the whole intact haemoglobin molecule is used in another, allowing differentiation between bleeding that comes from the upper and lower parts of the intestine as the haemoglobin molecule is broken down as it moves through the gut. Three tests on consecutive days are necessary.

FAECES ANALYSIS
Like urine, because faeces have passed through much of the body, an analysis of its composition can be an indication of abnormalities and disorders existing in the body. A faeces sample is collected by using a disposable plastic spoon to place a small amount of faeces into a sterile plastic container.

One of the most straightforward reasons for testing the faeces is the suspected presence of **parasites** or **worms** in the intestines. In such a case, the eggs, body parts or entire bodies can often be seen quite easily in the faeces.

Even if nothing untoward can be seen in the faeces, an analysis of the fat and salt content of the faeces provides a means of assessing if food is being properly digested and absorbed, or if there is some digestive disorder present. A culture test performed on the faeces may be carried out to determine a possible infectious cause of diarrhoea.

CURIOSITY
A morbid fear of being contaminated by faeces is called coprophobia.

FAINTING

A faint (**syncope**) is a sudden, unexpected loss of consciousness that may be preceded for a few seconds by a feeling of light headedness. Look after yourself by having any unexplained faint, or any repeated faint, assessed carefully by a doctor.

FIRST AID

If a person has fainted, they should be made to lie flat with their legs raised to increase the flow of blood to the brain. Tilt the head backwards and make sure the airways are clear. Loosen any tight clothing.

The person should regain consciousness within a minute or two. If the victim does not recover spontaneously within a short period, turn them on their side in the coma position and get medical help. Recovery usually occurs quickly, and is not associated with any convulsion or passing of urine or faeces.

CAUSES

Low blood pressure (**hypotension**) and poor blood supply to the brain are the absolute causes of a faint, and these in turn may be due to a number of conditions, including stress, anxiety, fright, over-exertion, lack of sleep, lack of food, heat, dehydration, lack of ventilation, prolonged standing and hormonal fluctuations.

A significant **infection** of any sort, from a bad dose of influenza to pneumonia or gastroenteritis, may lead to a faint, particularly if the patient is trying to push on and not rest.

Stokes-Adams attacks are caused by a sudden change in the heart rate, with the heart slowing down markedly for a few seconds or minutes, and then recovering. It is due to a problem with the conduction of electrical impulses through the heart muscle.

If someone complains of feeling faint, immediately help them to sit on the ground or floor, and encourage them to lie down if they still feel faint.

OTHER CAUSES OF A FAINT MAY INCLUDE:

- vasovagal syndrome (response to stress)

- heart attack (myocardial infarct)

- pulmonary thrombosis (blood clot in the lung)

- stroke (cerebrovascular accident)

- sudden changes in emotional state

- transient ischaemic attacks (temporary blocking of a small artery in the brain)

- low blood sugar (from starvation, or overuse of insulin or medication in a diabetic)

- micturition syncope (faint that occurs when urine passed)

- pregnancy

- hardening of the arteries (arteriosclerosis)

- severe anaemia

- dehydration

- alcohol intoxication

- effects of many drugs (e.g. those that lower blood pressure, narcotics, sleeping tablets, anxiety-relieving medications).

THERE ARE MANY LESS COMMON CAUSES OF FAINTING INCLUDING:

- narrowing (stenosis) of the main artery from the heart to the body (the aorta)

- sudden episodes of irregular heart beat

- high blood pressure (may sometimes cause a faint as the increased pressure on the brain prevents it from working properly)

- migraines

- epilepsy (may be mistaken for a faint)

- severe allergy reaction (anaphylaxis)

- Wolf-Parkinson-White syndrome (peculiar abnormality of the electrical conduction system in the heart).

Some people may fake a faint as an attention-seeking device.

TREATMENT

The patient usually recovers quickly once lying down, but should only rise slowly and when completely well.

The next step is to determine the cause of the faint. If one of the simple causes above is obvious, then no further investigation is necessary, but if there is no obvious cause or the cause is likely to be serious, and certainly if the problem is recurrent, a doctor must be consulted and appropriate investigations such as blood tests and electrocardiograms must be performed.

CURIOSITY

Upper class women in the nineteenth century who seemed to constantly faint from 'the vapours' often did so because they were so tightly corsetted that it interfered with their circulation.

FEVER

L ook after yourself by having a thermometer at home and noting the level of any fever, its changes and duration.

A fever under 39°C can be observed for a few days, from 39°C to 40°C obtain medical attention within a day, and over 40°C see a doctor as soon as possible. A fever over 42°C is a medical emergency.

EXPLANATION

The normal active human has a temperature of about 37°C. The word 'about' is used advisedly, because the temperature is not an absolute value.

A woman's temperature rises by up to half a degree after she ovulates in the middle of her cycle. Many people have temperatures up to a degree below the average with no adverse effects. The body temperature will also vary slightly depending on the time of day, food intake and the climate. All these factors must be taken into account when the notion of a normal temperature is considered.

A fever (**pyrexia**) is a sign that the body is fighting an infection, inflammation, or invasion by cancer or foreign tissue. A fever over 40°C, though, should be reduced by using paracetamol or aspirin and cool baths.

CAUSES

An **infection** by a bacteria (e.g. pneumonia, tuberculosis, tonsillitis, ear infection, urinary infection), virus (e.g. common cold, influenza, hepatitis, chickenpox, AIDS) or fungus (e.g. serious fungal infections of lungs) is by far the most common cause of a fever.

A **viral** infection usually causes a fever that comes and goes during the day, often with a sudden onset in the morning and evening, followed by a slow decline to normal over the next couple of hours.

Bacterial infections tend to cause a constant fever, usually over 38.5°C. This is because bacteria reproduce like all animals, at random times. Viruses tend to reproduce all at once, so the body is subjected to a sudden doubling of the number of viruses, which stimulates the brain to increase the body temperature.

Infections can occur in any tissue or organ of the body, and other symptoms will depend upon where the infection is sited. An untreated bacterial infection will result in pus formation, and an abscess full of pus may form at any site of infection (e.g. under the skin, in the lung, at the root of a tooth, in the bowel) and continue to cause a fever.

A fever may be beneficial to the patient, because many germs (viruses particularly) are temperature sensitive, and are destroyed by the fever.

OTHER CAUSES OF A FEVER MAY INCLUDE:

- appendicitis

- malaria (caused by a mosquito-borne parasite)

- many different cancers (usually when well advanced)

- leukaemia

- inflammation of tissue

- severe allergy reaction

- rejection of a transplanted organ

- autoimmune diseases (e.g. rheumatoid arthritis, systemic lupus erythematosus)

- rheumatic fever (rare inflammation affecting the heart)

- haemolytic anaemia (the body destroys its own blood cells)

- blood clot in the lung (pulmonary embolus)

- liver failure from cirrhosis (hardening of the liver).

RARE CAUSES OF A FEVER MAY INCLUDE:

- toxic shock syndrome

- brain tumour

- stroke

- head injury

- Felty syndrome (a complication of rheumatoid arthritis that causes intermittent arthritis in numerous joints and enlargement of liver, lymph nodes and spleen)

- Stevens-Johnson syndrome (ulceration of the eyes, mouth inflammation, and ulcers in the vagina, urethra and anus)

- very high blood pressure

- neuroleptic malignant syndrome (a side effect of the over- or excessive use of tranquillising medication in psychiatric conditions)

- Riley-Day syndrome (occurs predominantly in Jewish people and is associated with a lack of tears, fever, sweating and high pain tolerance).

Medications can sometimes cause a fever as a side effect (e.g. methyldopa used for blood pressure).

Illegal drugs such as amphetamines, cocaine and LSD are well known to cause a fever, as well as tremors and sometimes convulsions.

A patient with a persistent fever over 40°C needs to be checked by a doctor within a few hours. A patient with a fever of 42°C needs to be seen by a doctor immediately!

THERMOMETERS
A thermometer is an instrument used to measure temperature.

IN MEDICINE, IT MAY BE:
- -

- a graduated glass tube filled with alcohol or (less commonly these days due to its toxicity) mercury that is placed in the mouth, anus or (less accurately) armpit.

- an infrared sensitive electronic probe placed in the ear.

- a temperature-sensitive electronic probe placed anywhere in or on the body that is accessible.

- a heat-sensitive strip placed on the skin (not very accurate).

CURIOSITY
The abuse of illegal drugs such as heroin, other narcotics and LSD can cause a fever.

FITS AND CONVULSIONS

A fit or a convulsion is a result of a disturbance in the functioning of the brain. In looking after yourself and your family, ensure that anyone who has a fit or convulsion is thoroughly assessed by a doctor to determine the cause.

FIRST AID

The main task of anyone present at a seizure is to protect the sufferer from harm. Do not restrict their movements, since the spasms and jerking are automatic and trying to stop them may cause injury. Simply move any objects that may be a danger and, if necessary, remove false teeth (but do not prise the mouth open or force objects into it). Protect the head from banging against the floor by putting something flat and soft (such as folded jacket) under it. If necessary, loosen the person's collar so they can breathe more easily. Artificial respiration will probably be impossible, and the sufferer will breathe normally again at the end of the seizure, generally after a minute or so.

The sufferer may fall asleep once the seizure has ended, in which case place them in the coma position (on side with legs bent) and allow them to wake naturally. There may be a card or tag on the person saying what to do in case of a seizure – look for this and follow the instructions.

CAUSES

Although relatively uncommon, and very distressing when they do occur, there are scores of causes for a convulsion that vary from the obvious to the extremely obscure.

Everyone thinks of epilepsy and other serious diseases when fitting occurs, but a simple **faint**, severe bacterial and viral **infections**, high fever and a sudden shock or intense **fear** can trigger a convulsion. **Overdoses** of numerous prescribed and illegal drugs, as well as alcohol, strychnine and cyanide poisoning may also be responsible.

Children sometimes have convulsions because of a sudden rise in temperature. These **febrile convulsions** consist of body rigidity, twitching, arched head and back, rolling eyes, a congested face and neck, and bluish face and lips. Generally the seizure will end quite quickly, but the carer should ensure that the airway is clear, turn the child on to the side if necessary, remove clothing, bathe or sponge the child with lukewarm water, and when the convulsion has eased obtain medical attention.

*Febrile convulsions do NOT lead to the development of
epilepsy or other forms of convulsions in later life.*

Epilepsy is a condition that causes recurrent seizures (fits). Some people are born with epilepsy, while others acquire the disease later in life after a brain infection, tumour or injury. Brain degeneration in the elderly, removing alcohol from an alcoholic or heroin from an addict, or an excess or lack of certain chemicals in the body can also cause epilepsy. Fits can vary from very mild absences in which people just seem to lose concentration for a few seconds, to uncontrolled bizarre movements of an arm or leg, to the grand mal convulsion in which an epileptic can thrash around quite violently and lose control of bladder and bowel.

A **head injury** may cause immediate or delayed fitting because of injury to the brain, or bleeding into or around the brain. Bleeding may also be caused by the spontaneous rupture of a weakened artery or vein in the skull, and the resultant pressure on the brain can have many varied effects.

The brain is supported and completely surrounded by a three-layered membrane (the meninges), which contain the cerebrospinal fluid. If these meninges are infected by a virus or bacteria (**meningitis**), the patient may experience headache, fever, fits, neck stiffness and in severe cases may become comatose.

Encephalitis is an infection of the brain itself, which may be confused with meningitis. The symptoms include headache, intolerance of bright lights, fever, stiff neck, lethargy, nausea, vomiting, sore throat, tremors, confusion, convulsions, stiffness and paralysis.

Severe **dehydration** caused by excess sweating and/or lack of fluid in a hot environment, particularly if exercising, may cause collapse and fitting. This may be combined with excessive body temperature (hyperthermia), which aggravates the problem. Marathon runners who collapse and start twitching are often suffering from these problems.

Low blood sugar levels (**hypoglycaemia**) caused by excessive doses of insulin or other sugar-lowering medications in diabetics may starve the brain of essential nutrients and affect its function.

Children who have behaviour problems may have severe temper **tantrums** which can appear to be similar to a convulsion. If the child is a very determined breath-holder, the end stage may be collapse and fitting due to lack of oxygen reaching the brain, which usually settles quite quickly.

A lack of oxygen from near drowning, **suffocation** or smoke inhalation may also have adverse effects on the brain that trigger fitting.

Hysteria may occur because of fear, stress, anxiety or some other type of stress, and the hysterical reaction may result in collapse, convulsions and coma.

UNCOMMON CAUSES OF CONVULSIONS MAY INCLUDE:

- stroke (cerebrovascular accident)

- tumour or cancer affecting the brain or surrounding structures within the skull

- significant liver or kidney disease

- abnormal migraines

- hydrocephalus (increased fluid within the skull)

- malignant hypertension (extremely high blood pressure)

- eclampsia (a rare complication of pregnancy)

- lack of thyroxine (hypothyroidism) from an under-active thyroid gland in the neck.

Rapid shallow breathing may alter the balance of carbon dioxide and oxygen in the lungs, and thus the blood. The blood becomes more alkaline, and irritates small muscles, particularly in the hands, which go into spasm and may appear to be a convulsion. This is known as **tetany** (totally different to tetanus infection) and patients have fingers and sometimes wrist, forearms and feet pointed in a firm spasm. Hormonal and calcium imbalances in the blood may also cause tetany.

EPILEPSY

Epilepsy is a brain condition causing recurrent seizures (fits). It may be congenital or acquired later in life after a brain infection, tumour, injury or with brain degeneration in the elderly. Fits are caused by a short-circuit in the brain after very minor and localised damage. This then stimulates another part of the brain, and then another, causing a seizure. Triggers such as flickering lights, shimmering televisions, certain foods, emotional upsets, infections or stress can start fits in some patients.

> *Epileptics are not mentally retarded, but some forms of*
> *mental retardation have epilepsy as a complication.*

The symptoms vary depending on the type of epilepsy.

THERE ARE SEVERAL DIFFERENT TYPES OF EPILEPSY THAT ARE SPECIFICALLY DESCRIBED:

- **Petit mal absences**. The mildest form of epilepsy. These may vary from stopping in mid-sentence for a second or two and loss of concentration, to fluttering of the eyelids or other milder unusual muscle movements. There is no loss of consciousness or collapse. They are more common in children.

- **Abnormal absences**. These are similar to petit mal, but may be associated with partial seizures or a fugue state.

- **Simple partial seizures** (also known as focal seizures). Start with abnormal activity within one nerve cell in the brain, and the symptoms depend on the area of brain affected. There may be spasm of an arm or leg, strange smells, hallucinations or other phenomena. There is no loss of consciousness.

- **Complex partial seizures** (also known as temporal lobe or psychomotor seizures). These are the same as simple partial seizures, but there is some change in consciousness or loss of awareness.

- **Jacksonian epilepsy**. This is a simple partial seizure in which there is a progression in the muscle spasm or seizure from one area to another (e.g. a muscle spasm may spread up the arm from the fingers to the shoulder). Occasionally there may be loss of power in the affected muscles (Todd paralysis) for hours or days afterwards.

- **Myoclonic seizures**. Sudden, short-lasting muscle contractions involving just a single muscle, a limb, or sometimes the whole body. The patient may fall, but there is no loss of consciousness, and recovery is immediate, but the problem may recur.

- **Atonic seizures** (also known as drop attacks). A brief loss of all muscle strength, and loss of consciousness. Usually occur in children.

- **Secondary seizures**. These occur when a partial seizure progresses to become a generalised seizure.

- **Tonic-clonic seizures** (also known as grand mal seizures). Sudden onset of generalised muscle spasm, rigidity, loss of consciousness and collapse which last for a minute or two. The patient may go blue due to the cessation of breathing for the duration of the attack. The patient usually urinates and may pass faeces during the attack. After recovering from a grand mal fit, the patient has no memory of the event, is confused, drowsy, disoriented and may have a severe headache, nausea and muscle aches.

- **Status epilepticus**. A condition where one grand mal attack follows another without the patient regaining consciousness between attacks.

- **Tonic seizures**. These are a milder and briefer form of tonic-clonic seizures that last only a few seconds.

Many patients with epilepsy develop warning **auras** before an attack, which can be a particular type of headache, change in mood, tingling, light-headedness or twitching.

Epilepsy can be **investigated** by an EEG (electroencephalogram) to measure the brain waves, blood tests to exclude other diseases and a CT scan of the brain to find any structural abnormality.

Many different anti-epileptic drug combinations in tablet or mixture form are used to **control** epilepsy, and regular blood tests ensure that the dosage is adequate. Medication must be continued long-term, but after several years without fits, a trial without medication may be undertaken. Epileptics must not put themselves in a position where they can injure themselves or others.

CURIOSITY

Extract from an 1821 medical text book.

'A person subject to epilepsy is often able to prevent a fit from coming on by tying a cord between the part where the preceding aura is first felt and the rest of the body'.

FOOD POISONING

Food poisoning is an illness involving the intestine, caused by eating food contaminated by a bacteria, or a toxin produced by bacteria. Many different types of bacteria may be responsible. Look after yourself by thinking twice about the food and drink you are consuming, particularly in developing countries and in fast food outlets that may not appear as clean as you would wish. In these situations, avoid the foods most likely to be contaminated.

FOODS THAT ARE PARTICULARLY LIKELY TO BE RESPONSIBLE ARE:

- dairy products

- seafood

- cold, cooked chicken that has been poorly stored

- other meat that has been inadequately refrigerated

- fried foods

- meat dishes that have been reheated

- stale bread.

Patients develop the **symptoms** of nausea, vomiting, diarrhoea, a fever and stomach cramps, and small amounts of blood may be vomited or passed in the motions. Most attacks develop suddenly within 30 minutes to eight hours of eating the contaminated food, but may take up to 24 hours.

No specific **investigation** can diagnose the cause in an individual, but a suspect food can be tested to see if it is contaminated. Food poisoning is strongly suspected when a number of people are affected simultaneously, but it may be confused with gastroenteritis. Faeces tests may be performed if another cause is suspected and blood tests are sometimes necessary for dehydration.

Usually no **treatment** is necessary other than a clear fluid diet to replace the fluids and vital salts that are rinsed out of the body by the vomiting and diarrhoea, and then careful reintroduction of foods. In the very young and elderly, dehydration may be a problem, and intravenous drips in hospital may be required. Antibiotics are rarely necessary, and most attacks settle within six to twelve hours.

There are three unusual and severe forms of food poisoning that must be considered – botulism, ciguatera and scombroid.

BOTULISM

Botulism is an extremely severe form of food poisoning. **Home-preserved fruits** and vegetables and, very rarely, commercially canned foods may be responsible for harbouring the bacterium *Clostridium botulinum*, which is capable of producing an extremely potent poison (toxin) that attacks the nervous system.

> *Whole families have tragically died from botulism*
> *after eating grandma's special home preserve.*

Twelve to 36 hours after eating inadequately preserved food, the patient develops double vision, difficulty in swallowing and talking, a dry mouth, nausea and vomiting. The muscles become weak, and breathing becomes steadily more difficult. The patient must be hospitalised immediately and put upon an artificial breathing machine (ventilator) to maintain lung function once the paralysis occurs. An antitoxin is also available for injection.

Death occurs in about 70 per cent of patients unless adequate medical treatment in a major hospital is readily available. In the best circumstances, up to 25 per cent of patients will still die.

CIGUATERA

Ciguatera is a form of seafood poisoning caused by eating **reef fish** that contain the ciguatera toxin. The fish itself is not affected, and there are no tests for differentiating safe from toxic fish. The poison is produced at certain seasons by a microscopic animal (Dinoflagellida) that proliferates on tropical reefs. This is eaten by very small fish, who are then eaten by bigger fish, who are then eaten by still bigger fish. There may be a dozen steps along this chain, with the poison being steadily concentrated in the fish tissue at every step. Ciguatera is present in a low concentration in most reef fish, but only when it exceeds a certain concentration does it cause problems in humans.

There are far higher concentrations of toxin in the gut, liver, head and roe of reef fish, which should never be eaten or used to make fish soup, and they cannot be destroyed by cooking.

> *The larger the fish, the more likely it is to be affected by ciguatera.*

Symptoms vary dramatically from one patient to another, depending on the amount of toxin eaten, the size of the victim, and the individual reaction. They may include unusual skin sensations and tingling, diarrhoea, nausea, abnormal sensation, headaches and irregular heartbeats. Unusual tingling sensations may persist for years, and subsequent serious attacks may be triggered by eating tiny amounts of ciguatera that may be present in fish that others can eat without adverse effects.

There are no diagnostic tests, and no specific treatment or antidote, but medication may be used to control symptoms.

Patients with a mild reaction usually recover in a few days as the toxin is naturally eliminated from the body, but severe attacks may cause symptoms for a couple of months. Death is rare but possible, usually occurs within 36 hours of the onset of the attack, and is caused by the effects of the toxin on the heart and blood vessels.

SCOMBROID

Scombroid (or histamine fish poisoning), is a reaction to eating **contaminated fish**. It is very common around Hawaii and the western United States, but also occurs in the South Pacific. Tuna, mackerel and dolphin fish are more commonly responsible.

Symptoms, which start suddenly and usually settle quickly, include flushing of the face and neck, itchy skin, low blood pressure, headache, intestinal cramps, vomiting, diarrhoea, palpitations and skin pain. Rarely, a serious anaphylactic reaction may occur. The onset of symptoms occurs between five and 60 minutes after eating fish.

It is caused by eating fish that have been infected by specific bacteria that were introduced either in the marine environment or during handling and poor storage. The bacteria produce high levels of histamine in the fish flesh. No method of preparation destroys the histamine, and it may affect fresh, frozen, cooked and canned fish.

Antihistamine tablets or injections are used in treatment, and although the condition settles in a few hours without treatment, it will resolve within half an hour with appropriate treatment.

CURIOSITY

Queensland, home to the Great Barrier Reef, has more cases of ciguatera than the rest of the world combined, and most research into the disease has been performed at Brisbane's University of Queensland.

FRACTURES

L ook after yourself and your family by knowing how to deal with a fracture when one occurs – and almost invariably, at least one child in a family will suffer a fracture before reaching maturity.

A fractured bone is usually caused by abnormal violence, pressure, force or twisting being applied to a bone.

With a fracture, patients experience pain that is worse with use of the bone, swelling and tenderness at the site of the fracture, bruising over or below the fracture and loss of function of the limb or area. Pathological fractures (see fracture types below) may be relatively pain free in some cases.

FIRST AID

FIRST AID FOR A FRACTURE INVOLVES:

- keep the victim as warm and comfortable as possible

- gently remove clothing from any open wound and cover it with a clean (preferably sterile) dressing

- do not try to manipulate the bone or joint, as further (potentially very serious) damage may be caused

- move the affected area as little as possible and immobilise the fracture

- if the injury is in the arm, use a sling or strap the arm to the body. If the leg is injured, strap the injured leg to the uninjured leg. Alternatively, make a splint from a broom handle, branch or a rolled-up newspaper (remembering to protect any open wound)

- do not give the victim anything to eat or drink, as the setting of the fracture may require an anaesthetic.

A break and a fracture are different terms for the same thing.

FRACTURE TYPES

THERE ARE SEVERAL DIFFERENT TYPES OF FRACTURE:

- -

- **hair line** fracture – tiny crack part-way through a bone

- **greenstick** fracture – abnormal bend in a child's soft bone wrinkling one surface only

- **simple** fracture – a single break across the whole width of a bone

- **avulsion** fracture – a small fragment of bone is pulled off at the point where a muscle, tendon or ligament attaches

- **impacted** fracture – the forcible shortening of a bone as one fragment of bone is pushed into another

- **comminuted** fracture – two, three or more breaks in the one bone

- **depressed** fracture – a piece of bone (often in the skull) is pushed in below the level of the surrounding bone

- **compound** fracture – the skin over the fracture is broken by a bone end

- **pathological** fracture – a break in a bone bone weakened by osteoporosis, cancer or other disease

TYPES OF BONE FRACTURE

Skin

Bone

Simple

Stress

Compound

Impacted

Greenstick

Comminuted

TREATMENT

For healing, the bone fragments must be aligned as perfectly as possible after manipulation (under an anaesthetic if necessary), and fixed in position with plaster, pins, plates, or screws. It is normally necessary to prevent movement in the joints at either end of the broken bone. The exact treatment will vary considerably from one bone to another, with some fractures requiring minimal fixation (e.g. fracture of humerus – upper arm bone), while others require major surgery (e.g. fracture of hip). Movement at the fracture site may cause failure to heal, and chronic pain may occur at fracture site. Fractures requiring surgery and compound fractures are susceptible to infection. Death of bone tissue can occur if small fragments of bone are present.

Any movement between the fracture ends slows healing.

Fracture healing times vary significantly but the following can be used as a rough guide for the time required to heal a simple fracture sufficiently to allow it to be used:

FRACTURE LOCATION	TIME REQUIRED
distal phalange (end bone of finger or toe)	one week
middle phalange (middle bone of finger or toe)	two weeks
proximal phalange (nearest bone in finger or toe)	three weeks
metacarpal (hand bone)	four weeks
wrist bone	five weeks
foot bone, forearm bones (ulna, radius), clavicle (collar bone), skull, rib	six weeks
elbow, fibula (smaller lower leg bone), patella (knee cap)	seven weeks
humerus (upper arm bone), shoulder blade (scapula), sternum (breast bone)	eight weeks
tibia (larger lower leg bone)	nine weeks
knee	ten weeks
femur (thigh bone), pelvis	twelve weeks

Double these times over 70 years, and halve them under five years of age. Proportional times apply for the middle aged and teenagers. Complete pain-free healing may take three times as long.

The majority of fractures can be successfully treated with an eventual return to full function of the bone.

PLASTER

The traditional plaster cast is made from plaster of paris, although lighter, stronger, more durable and expensive fibreglass casts are available.

If a plaster cast is applied, it is important to look after it properly while it does its job.

UNDER NO CIRCUMSTANCES SHOULD THE PATIENT:

• get the plaster wet (it will get soft)

• walk on or put pressure on the plaster (it will crack or weaken)

• poke sticks under the plaster to ease any skin irritation (this will roll up the padding and cause pressure sores).

It is important to return to see the doctor the day after the plaster is applied to ensure that it is correctly fitted, and not too tight or loose.

If fingers or toes become swollen, bright red, blue, stiff or cannot be moved, contact a doctor immediately, as the plaster may have become too tight as the injured tissue swells. Do not wait until morning if this happens at night.

Elevate the affected limb. If the plaster is on a leg, keep it up on a pillow in bed, and on a footstool whenever sitting. If on an arm, keep the arm in a sling so that the hand is as high as possible. Elevation prevents swelling, stiffness and pain.

A soft or loose plaster may be more comfortable,
but is less effective and must be changed.

Some plasters are made of **fibreglass**. These have to be treated in the same way as normal plaster, although they are much lighter and are not badly affected by water.

Wiggle the fingers and toes regularly while the plaster is applied to maintain circulation and mobility.

If the plaster becomes soft, loose or cracked, return to the doctor as soon as possible to have the plaster reinforced or replaced.

A walking heel is sometimes attached to a plaster. These are designed to be used over short distances around the house only, and not on long expeditions to the shopping centre or into the garden. Crutches must still be used in these situations.

SLINGS

Slings are used to rest, support or immobilise injuries to an upper limb or shoulder. They are triangular in shape and can be adapted from any suitably shaped piece of material.

An **arm sling** is used to support an injured forearm in a position roughly parallel to the ground. The victim should support the injured arm, with the wrist and hand raised higher than the elbow. Place the open sling between the chest and forearm, with the apex of the triangle stretching well beyond the elbow, the top point hanging over the shoulder on the uninjured side. The bottom point is towards the ground so that the long side of the triangle hangs down, parallel to the body. Bring the apex round the elbow so that it lies flat along the arm. Bring the base point up over the forearm and the top point around the neck so that the two points meet in the hollow just above the collar bone on the injured side. Tie the two ends in a reef knot.

A picnic table cloth, folded diagonally, makes a perfect emergency sling.

An **elevation sling** is used if the hand or forearm is injured, or to provide support for an injured shoulder without causing pressure on the shoulder or upper chest. The victim should rest the hand of the injured side on the opposite shoulder, with the elbow and upper arm held close against the chest. Cover the forearm and hand with a sling, with the apex of the triangle pointing towards the bent elbow, and the top point over the victim's shoulder on the uninjured side. The base point should be hanging down, so that the long side of the triangle extends down the length of the body. Gently push the base of the sling under the hand, forearm and elbow of the injured limb. Then bring the lower end of the base up and around the victim's back on the injured side. Bring the two ends of the sling together around the back of the victim and secure with a reef knot on the uninjured side. Fold the top of the sling at the elbow, and fasten it with a pin or tape, or tuck it in.

Check the victim's fingernails after applying a sling to make sure they have not turned blue. If they have, loosen the sling or bandage.

CRUTCHES

Crutches are used to assist walking in patients with foot and leg disabilities from pain and fractures to a missing limb.

CRUTCHES MAY BE MADE FROM WOOD OR METAL, AND COME IN TWO MAIN TYPES:

- axillary crutches have a padded curved bar that sits in the armpit and two shafts that join below a hand piece. Both the length of the crutch and the position of the hand piece can be adjusted.

- Canadian crutches are usually metal, have a hoop shaped piece that surrounds the upper arm, and a hand piece that protrudes from the metal shaft. The length of the crutch is the only adjustment.

It is important that crutches are adjusted to prevent complications. When using axillary crutches, there should be a gap of at least two centimetres between the top of the crutch and the armpit. NEVER put weight onto the armpit when walking or resting as damage to the nerves in the armpit may occur.

The crutch length should allow the person to use the crutches with minimal stooping. The arms should be straight, and the weight of the body should be taken easily on the hands and arms.

When using crutches, always go up steps and slopes foot first and bring the crutches up to the level of the grounded foot before taking the next step. When descending steps and slopes, always put the crutch down first and bring the good foot down to the level of the crutches (but no further) before taking the next step. On level ground, swing through the crutches so that in each step, the crutches finish the same distance behind the body that they started in front.

SPECIFIC FRACTURE TYPES

COLLES' FRACTURE

A Colles' fracture is a common fracture of the **forearm** bones (ulna and radius) which are bent back and broken just above the wrist. It is usually caused by landing on the outstretched hand during a fall. The fracture is diagnosed by an X-ray.

Symptoms include pain, swelling, tenderness and a backwards deformity of the forearm bones just above the wrist.

The bones must be put back into place under an anaesthetic if the deformity is significant, and held in position by plaster. Persistent deformity will occur if the bones are incorrectly aligned.

The fracture normally heals well after six weeks in plaster in an adult, or three to four weeks in a child.

COLLES' FRACTURE OF FOREARM BONES

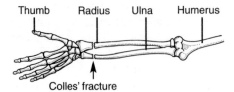

Thumb   Radius   Ulna   Humerus

Colles' fracture

MARCH FRACTURE

March fracture is a stress fracture of a **forefoot** (metatarsal) bone caused by prolonged running, jumping or walking, usually on hard surfaces (e.g. soldiers on a route march). More significant metatarsal fractures may occur with direct injury.

Severe pain is felt in the ball of the foot and excruciating pain on attempting to walk. There may be minimal changes on X-ray and a bone scan may be necessary to detect the fracture. Six weeks rest in plaster and on crutches heals these fractures.

The hash symbol (#) may be used as a notation in medical records for either a fracture or to indicate a number.

PATHOLOGICAL FRACTURE

Any bone can obviously fracture if excessive force is applied to it, but sometimes a bone may break with **minimal force**. This is considered to be an abnormal (or pathological) fracture.

The most common reason for such a fracture is osteoporosis, which is a thinning of the bone structure caused by a lack of calcium in the bone. This usually occurs in elderly women, and can be corrected by adequate calcium in the diet at younger ages, or special medications that place calcium in bones.

All other causes are rare, and include osteomalacia (softened bone due to lack of vitamin D), osteogenesis imperfecta (a genetic condition resulting in fragile bones) and Riley-Day syndrome (occurs only in Jewish people, and is associated with a lack of tears, fever and sweating).

POTT'S FRACTURE

A Pott's fracture is a fracture above the **ankle**, when the bottom ends of the two bones in the lower leg (the tibia and fibula) are broken off by a twisting force to the lower leg, often after catching the foot in a hole while running.

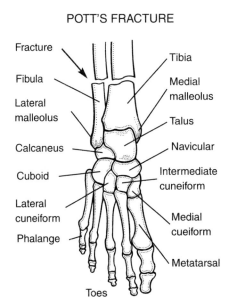

POTT'S FRACTURE

Fracture
Fibula
Lateral malleolus
Calcaneus
Cuboid
Lateral cuneiform
Phalange
Toes

Tibia
Medial malleolus
Talus
Navicular
Intermediate cuneiform
Medial cueiform
Metatarsal

There is pain, swelling, tenderness and loss of function of the lower leg and ankle. The fracture is diagnosed by an X-ray.

Manipulation of bone ends under anaesthetic is undertaken to achieve good alignment, then the ankle is encased in plaster. Sometimes open operation and fixation of the bones by plates and screws is required. The complications that may occur include failure to heal, poorly aligned bone ends and infection after open operation.

These fractures require up to three months rest to heal adequately.

SCAPHOID FRACTURE

A fracture of the scaphoid bone, one of the eight small **wrist** bones, which lies on the thumb side of the wrist. It is usually caused by falling on the outstretched hand.

BONES OF THE HAND

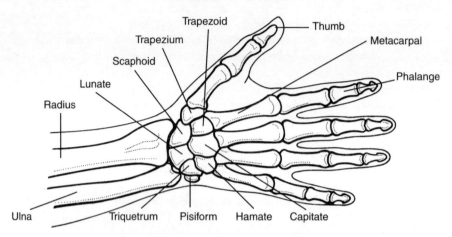

Although there may be pain and tenderness on the thumb side of the wrist, these fractures are often hard to detect, and X-rays ten to 14 days apart may be necessary.

Even if an initial X-ray is normal, a wrist that is
persistently painful after an injury must be
X-rayed again after ten to 14 days.

Immobilisation of the wrist in plaster for four to six weeks is the usual treatment, but in a small number of cases, part of this small bone may die after a fracture and result in a constantly painful wrist joint. An artificial scaphoid bone can be inserted if complications occur.

SMITH'S FRACTURE

A Smith's fracture occurs if the wrist is bent forward excessively to cause a fracture of the **forearm bones** (ulna and radius) just above the wrist. Falling onto the back of the outstretched hand is a common cause.

There is pain, tenderness, swelling, deformity and loss of function of the forearm and wrist.

The fracture is diagnosed by an X-ray, and then the bones must be put back into place under an anaesthetic and held in position by plaster. A persistent deformity may occur if incorrectly aligned.

This fracture normally heals well after six weeks in plaster in an adult, and three to four weeks in a child.

STRESS FRACTURE

A stress or fatigue fracture is an abnormal break of a bone, often in the foot (march fracture) or lower leg (fibula or tibia), due to repeated excessive stress on a bone. Pain and tenderness develops in the affected bone that is worsened by use.

The fracture is diagnosed by X-ray, CT or radionucleotide scan, and treated by rest in a plaster cast.

CURIOSITY
Plaster was used to set fractures by the physicians in ancient Egypt, 4000 years ago.

GASTROENTERITIS

It is important to look after yourself during epidemics of gastroenteritis by being extremely careful with your personal hygiene. Even so, it can be impossible to avoid.

CAUSE

Gastroenteritis is a **viral infection** of the gut. The Rotavirus and Norovirus (previously known as the Norwalk virus) are the most common viruses responsible, particularly in children. They often appear in epidemics, and usually in spring or early summer. The infection passes easily from one person to another through contamination of the hands and food, on the breath, in vomitus and faeces, and on surfaces contaminated by the patient.

Contaminated surfaces should be cleaned with 0.1 per cent household bleach or a strong detergent and then not touched for at least an hour.

Institutions such as aged care facilities and boarding houses are notorious for the spread of this virus.

A Rotavirus vaccine is currently being developed and may be available by the time this book is published.

SYMPTOMS

Patients develop an uncomfortable feeling in the stomach, gurgling, cramping pains and then vomiting. A few hours later the **vomiting** starts to ease, and **diarrhoea** develops. Young children may become rapidly dehydrated and require urgent hospitalisation.

The illness usually lasts only one to three days in healthy adults, but the patient may remain infectious for up to two days after their apparent recovery, and so should not return to work or school until at least a day after recovery, and should be scrupulous with their personal hygiene.

Food handlers should be excluded from work until two days after recovery.

INVESTIGATION

Usually no investigations are necessary, but faeces tests may be performed if another cause is suspected and blood tests are sometimes necessary for dehydration.

TREATMENT

The treatment involves a specific diet to replace the fluid and vital salts that are rinsed out of the body by the vomiting and diarrhoea, and then careful reintroduction of foods. In adults, medications can be used to slow diarrhoea, and paracetamol can be used for belly pain at all ages. Some children develop an intolerance to milk sugar (lactose) after the infection, and this may prevent them from returning to a normal diet for weeks or months.

GASTROENTERITIS DIET
Take small amounts of food and fluids very frequently (every hour), rather than large amounts three times a day.

DAY 1 CLEAR FLUIDS ONLY
Electrolyte solutions (e.g. Repalyte, Hydralyte and Gastrolyte) available from chemists (taste better if cold) are best, but white grape juice, clear soups, Bonox, very dilute flat lemonade, very dilute cordial, and frozen cordial may be used for a short time in milder cases. Average 50mLs an hour for a child, 100mLs an hour for an adult.
Do NOT drink plain water.
Soy drinks (e.g. Isomil, Prosobee, Infasoy) can be used as a milk substitute in infants.
Lactose free milk ('Lactaid') may be used.
Breast milk is perfect for infants even with gastroenteritis.

DAY 2 LIGHT DIET
Continue clear fluids and add bread, toast, boiled rice, dry biscuits (e.g. quarter slice of bread, half a dry biscuit every half hour).

DAY 3 ADD NUTRITION
Boiled vegetables, fruits, white meats (chicken breast, fish), cereals.

DAY 4 GRADUALLY INCREASE FOOD INTAKE
Until return to normal.

AVOID
All dairy products (e.g. milk, cream, cheese, butter, ice cream, custard, yoghurt)
Eggs
Red meat
Fatty and fried foods
(until completely better).

DEHYDRATION
Dehydration is a lack of water in the body. As the human body is almost 70 per cent (seven tenths) water, even a small drop in the total amount of water in the body can have significant effects.

Patients who lose less than five per cent (one twentieth) of their body water will feel thirsty, have a dry mouth, but few other symptoms.

More severe dehydration resulting in a loss of five per cent to ten per cent (one tenth) of the body water will cause sunken eyes, loose skin, rapid heart rate, minimal passing of urine, and, in babies, depression of the soft spot at the front of the skull.

In a child, to test for severe dehydration pinch up a small bit of loose skin on the belly. It should snap back flat immediately when released. If it does not, seek urgent medical care.

Dehydration in excess of ten per cent may be life-threatening, particularly in children. **Symptoms** include altered mood, poor concentration, drowsiness, irritability, weak pulse, cold white hands and feet, loose folds of skin and eventually loss of consciousness.

Dehydration may be caused by loss of fluid in diarrhoea, copious vomiting, excessive sweating (e.g. exercise, heat), which also causes a loss of sodium in salt, passing excess urine (e.g. taking too many fluid tablets, diabetes insipidus and other diseases); or by lack of fluid intake, usually when fluids are not readily available.

Blood tests can accurately determine the degree of dehydration.

Treatment involves giving a solution of water and electrolytes (vital elements) by mouth if possible, or intravenously. In an emergency, a mixture containing a level teaspoon of salt and eight level teaspoons of sugar or glucose into a litre of boiled water may be given by mouth. Plain water should not be given as it will pass straight through the body. Because of their lower body weight, children will dehydrate far more rapidly than adults.

CURIOSITY

Viral gastroenteritis is very contagious, and once established in an institution, may be very difficult to eliminate. This was well demonstrated by the epidemic of gastroenteritis that attacked Caribbean cruise ships in 2002–3, devastating the industry.

HAIR LOSS

The best way in which people (particularly men) with hair loss can look after themselves is to protect the exposed scalp from injury, particularly from the sun, by regularly wearing a hat.

A healthy adult loses at least 100 hairs a day from their head, so only excessive hair loss above this level is abnormal. Hair may be lost in small patches (alopecia areata), large areas (alopecia totalis, baldness), or there may be diffuse loss of hair from all over the head (telogen effluvium).

CAUSES

BALDNESS

By far the most common form of scalp hair loss is that caused by **hereditary** tendencies in men. If your father or grandfather was bald, you have a good chance of developing the same problem. Baldness is a gender-linked genetic condition that is very rare in women, but passes through the female line to men in later generations. There are no cures available, and none are likely for some time to come.

Almost always, male pattern baldness commences with gradual hair loss, starting at the front of the scalp on either side, or in a circular area on top. It is usually accompanied by excess hair on the body due to higher levels of testosterone. The connection between baldness and sexual potency is unproven.

Minoxidil or finasteride tablets or minoxidil scalp lotion may slow or stop hair loss, but the only real treatments are hair transplants, scalp flap rotation or a wig.

*Hypotrichosis is the medical term for a reduced
amount of hair on the scalp and body.*

TELOGEN EFFLUVIUM

Telogen effluvium is a form of **diffuse** hair loss. Both men and women have fewer hairs as they grow older, but excessive generalised hair loss from the scalp, and sometimes other hairy areas of the body (e.g. eyebrows, pubic area, chest), may be a symptom of disease such as sex hormone disturbances (e.g. pregnancy, menopause), an over- or under-active thyroid gland, pituitary gland diseases, many other serious illness, drugs used to treat cancer, radiation therapy, too much vitamin A, and sudden and excessive loss of weight (e.g. anorexia nervosa). Extreme mental or physical stress may also be responsible. Blood and other tests may be done to exclude specific causes but are often normal.

If a cause can be found, this should be treated. When the cause is medication, the hair usually grows back when it is ceased.

ALOPECIA AREATA

Alopecia areata is a common cause of **patchy** hair loss. There is a family history in about 20 per cent of patients, or fungal infections and drugs used to treat cancer may be responsible, but in most cases no specific cause can be found. Stress and anxiety are not usually a cause. Alopecia areata is different to baldness in that it can occur at any age, in either sex, in any race, and is more common under 25 years of age.

Victims have a sudden loss of hair in a well-defined patch on the scalp or other areas of body hair (e.g. pubic area, beard, eyebrows), and a bare patch 2cm or more across may be present before it is noticed. The hairless area may slowly extend for several weeks before stabilising. Several spots may occur simultaneously, and may merge together as they enlarge. If the entire body is affected, the disease is called alopecia totalis, which is not a different disease, just a severe case of alopecia areata. Patients need to be careful to avoid sunburn to exposed scalp skin.

Treatment involves strong steroid creams, injections of steroids into the affected area, and irritant lotions.

In 90 per cent of patients, regrowth of hair eventually recurs, although the new hair may be totally white and it may take many months or years. The further the bare patch is from the top of the scalp, the slower and less likely the regrowth of hair. It is rare to recover from total hair loss.

OTHER CAUSES

The hair density tends to decrease with **age**, and older people will have fewer hair growing follicles on their scalp than when they were young. This occurs far more after the **menopause**, which in women occurs about 20 years earlier than in men. Unfortunately there is nothing that can be done to reverse this process, but there are products available which will thicken the remaining hair to make it appear that more is present.

A sudden **loss of weight**, either by diet or disease, is often associated with diffuse hair loss.

After **pregnancy**, the combination of a sudden change in hormone levels with the delivery of the baby and breast development for milk production, and the physical and mental stress of looking after and breast feeding an infant may result in diffuse hair loss.

LESS COMMON CAUSES OF HAIR LOSS MAY INCLUDE:

- fad diets lacking in essential nutrients (e.g. proteins, iron, zinc)

- diseases of the hormone-secreting glands of the body (e.g. pituitary gland in the brain, thyroid gland in the neck, testes and ovaries)

- autoimmune diseases in which the body inappropriately rejects some of its own tissue (e.g. systemic lupus erythematosus)

- excessive intake of vitamin A either as vitamin supplements or eating large quantities of orange-coloured foods (e.g. carrots, paw paw)

- diabetes mellitus.

Drugs used to combat cancer are well known to cause serious hair loss, often involving the entire scalp, but other drugs may also cause the problem, although usually not as significantly. Examples include anticoagulants that prevent blood clots (e.g. warfarin), lithium (for psychiatric conditions), betablockers (for heart disease and high blood pressure) and the oral contraceptive pill.

There are many rarer causes of scalp hair loss, some of which include liver failure, uraemia (kidney failure), tumours or cancers anywhere in the body (particularly those involving the testes or ovaries), trichotillomania (psychiatric condition in which the patient pulls out handfuls of their own hair) and Fröhlich syndrome (late onset of puberty, thin wrinkled skin, obesity around the genitals and buttocks).

*Don't forget wigs as a form of treatment. They are now
almost indistinguishable from real hair.*

BALDNESS TREATMENT
HAIR TRANSPLANT
Through the centuries, thousands of treatments have been tried to cure baldness. None has been particularly successful, until the development of hair transplants in the 1980s.

Many bald men are not happy with the state of their scalp, and wish to reverse the inevitable progress of the condition. The first stop in treatment should be a general practitioner, who will discuss the pros and cons of hair transplants. If you decide to proceed further, you will be referred to a plastic surgeon. The surgeon will examine the scalp, and the remaining hair, and explain what can be done to help you. If you decide to proceed, it will take several operations over several months to give you a reasonable head of hair, and in the meantime, your scalp will look rather moth-eaten.

The procedure involves taking small plugs of hair, skin and underlying tissue from the hairy part of the scalp, and transplanting them into the bald area. The plugs are only two or three millimetres in diameter, and two or three hundred may eventually be taken and transplanted.

The transplanted hair will grow like normal hair, and, although far thinner than normal growth, will give a very respectable appearance in due course.

The complications will include the failure of some of the transplanted hair plugs to survive, and the possibility of infection. Fortunately, the scalp has a very poor nerve supply, and so there is only minimal discomfort and virtually no pain involved.

FINASTERIDE
Finasteride is a medication in tablet form that can be used for two extraordinarily different purposes – reducing benign enlargement of the prostate gland and increasing hair growth in male pattern baldness.

It must never be used in pregnant women, as severe damage may be caused to the foetus. Pregnant women whose male partner is using finasteride must avoid sex during pregnancy, as even contact with semen may cause deformities in the foetus.

Side effects may include impotence, decreased libido, breast enlargement in men and a rash.

It is quite expensive, extremely dangerous in pregnancy, but otherwise safe and effective. It may take some months for an improvement in symptoms.

MINOXIDIL

Minoxidil is a medication used as a tablet to treat severe high blood pressure and as a lotion for baldness. Although the tablets may have some problems with their use, the lotion is very safe but reacts with steroid creams and acne preparations. The ability to reverse male baldness was found by accident in patients taking the drug for blood pressure. Success in baldness varies greatly between patients, and long-term use is required.

CURIOSITY

From a 1915 diary:

- The local doctor treats diphtheria with doses of salts, senna and calomel. The hair is cut off and cold compresses are applied to the head.
- Today, our sweet child's hair was cut off as a a last resort treatment for head lice.

HEADACHE

A headache is probably the most common symptom to be experienced by mankind. Look after yourself by not putting up with a headache which may affect your mood, ability to concentrate, work or enjoy yourself, but treat it effectively and appropriately. This may include seeking medical advice if the headache is persistent, recurrent or fails to respond to simple remedies.

CAUSES

GENERAL

A headache may be associated with problems of any of the multiple complex structures in the head, or disorders of many of the body's other organs.

Fatigue, stress and anxiety may in themselves cause a headache, or may trigger muscle spasms in the temples and scalp that are responsible for the pain.

Any **infection**, by a bacteria (e.g. tonsillitis, sinusitis, ear infection, bronchitis, urinary infection), virus (e.g. influenza, common cold, glandular fever, hepatitis), fungus or parasite (e.g. malaria), may cause a headache, as may a fever of any cause.

Injury to any part of the head may cause a headache, but sometimes, and very seriously, the headache may occur some days after the injury due to slow bleeding from a leaking vein within the skull.

A headache is more significant when not associated with any other symptoms elsewhere in the body

The most common headaches are tension headaches, migraine and cluster headaches.

TENSION HEADACHE

A tension (muscle spasm) headache causes a dull, persistent pain with varying intensity that is often described as a **pressure** or tightening around the scalp. It occurs as a localised band around and across the head, and is not aggravated by exercise or alcohol.

The muscles at the top of the neck, in the forehead and over both temples go into prolonged contraction, which tightens the scalp, causing pressure on the skull, and further increases the strain on the muscles. Tension headaches are episodic, often in association with stress. Depression and anxiety are common accompanying symptoms. The pain may last for 30 minutes or a week.

Muscle spasm headaches usually have a **cause** (e.g. stress, infection, psychiatric disturbance, eye strain), and if possible this should be rectified. Simple medications such as aspirin or paracetamol, sometimes in combination with muscle relaxants, are readily available to ease both the muscle spasm and pain. Commercially available combinations (e.g. Fiorinal, Mersyndol, Panalgesic) are useful in the short-term, but often cause drowsiness. Mild heat and massaging the tense muscles will give temporary relief. Relief of chronic anxiety by talking through the problems with a doctor or counsellor, accepting help to deal with a stressful situation, and using an anti-anxiety medication may also be useful.

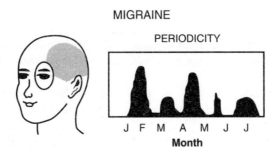

TENSION HEADACHE

MIGRAINE

Migraines are often associated with **visual** symptoms including flashing lights, shimmering, seeing zigzag lines and loss of part of the area of vision. They usually occur on only one side of the head, are described as throbbing, and cause intolerance of exercise, light and noise. **Nausea** and vomiting are common. Migraines occur periodically, and may last for a few hours to several days. The patient often looks pale and drawn.

MIGRAINE

PERIODICITY

J F M A M J J
Month

CLUSTER HEADACHES

Cluster headaches are not common, but cause a very characteristic pattern of headache, usually associated with excess **sweating** of one or both sides of the head. They occur in episodes once or twice a year, causing severe pain around or behind one eye that spreads to a temple, the jaw, teeth or chin. They often begin during sleep, and other effects may include a red, watery eye, drooping eyelid, altered pupil in the eye, stuffy nose and flushed face.

Cluster headaches may be triggered by alcohol, temperature changes, wind

CLUSTER HEADACHE

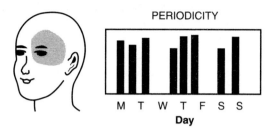

blowing on the face or excitement. They usually last for 15 minutes to three hours, and are named because of their tendency to occur in clusters for several weeks. They can be cured in a doctor's surgery by breathing pure oxygen for 15 minutes.

OTHER CAUSES

Many people fear that their headache may be due to a **brain tumour**, but this is actually very rare, with most brain tumours causing other symptoms that lead to their diagnosis well before a headache develops. Cancerous and benign tumours may develop not only in the brain tissue itself, but in the other structures within the skull such as the pituitary gland, membranes around the brain (meninges), sinuses and eyes. Most brain tumours are benign and can be cured by surgery.

Snoring and sleep apnoea (brief stops in breathing during sleep)
may be the cause of an early morning headache.

Anything that puts abnormal pressure on the brain may cause headaches. An **abscess** caused by an untreated infection in the brain or an injury that penetrates the skull is one possibility.

Bleeding inside the skull caused by an injury or rupture to a blood vessel is another. An aneurysm is the ballooning out of one side of an artery. The aneurysm may put pressure on the brain to cause a headache, or rupture to cause very severe effects on the brain function.

Viral or bacterial infections of the brain (**encephalitis**) or surrounding membranes (meningitis) will almost invariably cause a headache.

Inflammation of nerves in the scalp and face may appear to be a headache, when really it is the tissue outside the skull that is affected. Trigeminal neuralgia is one relatively common example, as is the pain of neuralgias associated with pinched nerves in the neck that spread from the base of the skull up the back of the head and as far forward as the hairline.

Psychiatric disorders as varied as phobias (abnormal fears), depression, post-traumatic stress disorder and excessive anxiety may cause headaches.

The brain cannot feel pain as it has no sensory nerves.
Headaches come from the skull and its surrounding
muscles, ligaments, membranes and nerves.

OTHER COMMON CAUSES OF HEADACHE MAY INCLUDE:

- increased pressure within the eye (glaucoma)

- poor vision (resulting in eye muscle strain)

- inflammation of the eye (iritis)

- menopause

- menstrual periods (premenstrual tension)

- contraceptive pills

- pregnancy

- other fluctuations in the level of the sex hormone oestrogen

- sexual intercourse, either during arousal or with orgasm/ejaculation

- inflammation or infection of the teeth (e.g. abscess or dental decay)

- jaw joint disorders (e.g. arthritis)

- neck disorders (e.g. arthritis or ligamentous strain)

- nose problems (e.g. large polyp)

- sinus problems (e.g. polyp or infection – sinusitis)

- cancer of any tissue in the body may cause headaches due to the release of toxins into the blood (e.g. leukaemia)

- under-active and over-active thyroid gland (hypothyroidism and hyperthyroidism)

- diseases of other glands (e.g. adrenal glands, testes, parathyroids)

- extreme high blood pressure

- anaemia (a lack of haemoglobin and/or red blood cells).

A wide range of medications (e.g. for control of high blood pressure, epilepsy and cancer) may cause headache as a side effect.

The SUNCT syndrome's name is an acronym of its major symptoms – Short lasting headache, Unilateral, Neuralgiform (nerve pain), Conjunctival injection (red eyes), Tears.

UNCOMMON CAUSES OF HEADACHE MAY INCLUDE:

- SUNCT syndrome (variant of cluster headache)

- poorly controlled diabetes (either high sugar levels from lack of treatment, or low blood sugar from excess medication)

- severe allergy reactions (anaphylaxis)

- acromegaly (thickening and enlargement of the bones in the skull and legs)

- Cushing syndrome (over-production or over-dosage of steroids)

- low blood pressure (e.g. from excessive medication, sudden change in position, shock or fright)

- failure or inflammation of any of the body's major organs (e.g. kidneys, spleen or liver)

- pre-eclampsia (complication of pregnancy associated with a rise in blood pressure)

- autoimmune diseases (e.g. systemic lupus erythematosus, rheumatoid arthritis, scleroderma)

- inflammation of arteries in the neck (carotodynia) or temples (temporal arteritis)

- Paget's disease (softening of bone throughout the body)

- toxic shock syndrome

Bruxism is the term used to describe grinding the teeth.
This can cause head pains as well as dental problems.

There are many other causes that have not been included, because almost any abnormality in the body may result in some kind of headache as our brain, or its surrounding structures, perceives the disorder in body function.

CURIOSITY

Extract from 1789 medical text:

'Trephining of the skull (boring a hole) and replacement of the bone that is missing with a silver plate is sometimes useful in the cure of repeated headache'.

Ouch!

HEAD INJURY

L ook after yourself with any head injury, as neglect can have very serious consequences. Any patient who sustains a head injury, even if it appears to be mild, should be checked by a doctor. If after being checked he or she shows no serious signs of damage, they can go home and expect that recovery will follow within 24 hours. However, rarely, complications may follow at any time over the next few days.

The brain is housed, very compactly, in the rigid skull, and cannot tolerate any increase in pressure. If pressure increases due to bleeding or swelling from fluid, then pressure is exerted on the base of the brain which contains the vital centres controlling such functions as breathing and heart action.

FIRST AID

The first-aider should lie the patient down, keep them warm and comfortable, apply cold compresses applied to the brow or the site of injury, and not give anything to eat or drink for the first few hours after the injury. Medical attention should be sought. Paracetamol may be used for pain, but aspirin should be avoided. Keep the victim under observation for at least 24 hours for signs of more serious injury.

A deteriorating level of consciousness and increasing confusion are serious signs.

OBSERVATION

Someone should keep the patient under close observation over the next 24 hours at least, and take them to a doctor immediately if any of the features below are noticed. The problems may occur gradually and certain warning signs will develop that indicate the pressure will have to be relieved by surgery.

WATCH FOR:

• Unconsciousness or undue drowsiness

• Confused irrational or delirious behaviour

• Headache which continues

• Bleeding from an ear

- Repeated vomiting

- Fits or spasms

- Blurred or double vision.

OTHER POINTS TO CONSIDER:

- Diet – Food and drink should be consumed in moderation for 24 hours

- Alcohol – Nil for 24 hours

- Drugs – No medication unless instructed by doctor. Paracetamol is allowed.

- Rest – No physical exercise for 24 hours. Use a flat pillow. Do not drive a vehicle.

*No one who has suffered a significant head injury
should be left alone for the first 24 hours.*

CONCUSSION

Concussion is due to **bruising** of part of the brain, from a moderate to severe blow on the head (generally at the back) or a severe shake of the body. Symptoms can vary in severity from mere giddiness and a headache for an hour or two to a complete loss of consciousness, sometimes lasting for weeks. The range of symptoms includes temporary, partial or complete loss of consciousness, 'seeing stars', shallow breathing, nausea and vomiting, paleness, coldness and clamminess of the skin, blurred or double vision, and possibly loss of memory.

A skull X-ray and CT scan may be performed to exclude fracture or other complications, but do not specifically diagnose concussion.

In most cases, complete recovery within a few hours or days is normal.

SUBDURAL HAEMATOMA

A subdural haematoma is a collection of **blood** between the brain and the skull that puts pressure on the brain and affects its function. The dura mater is the outermost of the three meninges (membranes) that surround and support the brain, so by definition this is a bleed between the dura mater and the arachnoid mater, which is the middle membrane. The innermost membrane is the pia mater.

*A patient who suffers mental deterioration within a week of
a significant head injury requires urgent hospital care.*

The bleeding is usually due to a significant head injury, but sometimes may be due to the rupture of a blood vessel affected by arteriosclerosis (hardening of the artery), high blood pressure or for no obvious reason. The onset may be sudden, or may be delayed for some weeks after a head injury if the bleed and build-up of pressure is very gradual.

The symptoms may include confusion, vomiting, dizziness, headache and abnormal brain function (e.g. partial paralysis, strange sensations) depending on the position of the blood collection and the pressure it applies to the brain.

A CT or MRI scan is used to find blood collection, and this is followed by urgent surgical removal of the blood collection.

It may be fatal or cause permanent disability if left untreated, but there are good results from surgical treatment.

CURIOSITY

A fall of over five metres onto the head is fatal in more than 90 per cent of cases.

HEARING

ook after yourself by protecting your ears from loud noises, be it jet engines, music or grinders, from a young age. This is the best way to preserve good hearing into old age.

It is hard for most of us to imagine a totally silent world, and there are actually very few people classified as deaf who can hear absolutely nothing. Most deaf people hear a blur of noise that is not quite comprehensible, and this can be more annoying than total silence. The worst affected are those who cannot hear any intelligible sound, and are sufferers from tinnitus (a constant buzzing in the ears).

HEARING TESTS

The most basic test for hearing simply involves the doctor talking to the patient and making sounds to see if they can be heard. An experienced doctor can assess hearing loss quite accurately using this method. A similar test uses a ticking watch. The patient covers first one ear and then the other, and the doctor determines at what distance the sound of the watch can be heard.

A **tuning fork** may be used to test the ability to hear tones conducted by air and by the bones of the head.

A more scientific way of evaluating hearing is using an **audiometer**. This is a device that produces pure tones of a certain pitch and loudness. The first part of the test measures the ability to hear air-conducted sounds and involves listening through ear-

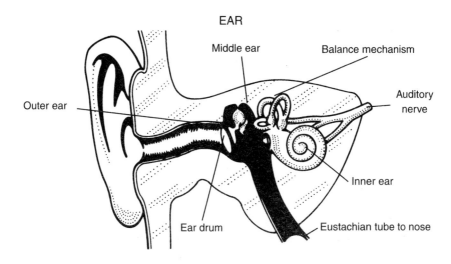

EAR

Middle ear

Balance mechanism

Outer ear

Auditory nerve

Inner ear

Ear drum

Eustachian tube to nose

phones to tones of different pitch and volume, or to spoken words. The patient signals when they can hear something, or to repeat the words. The second part of the test measures the ability to hear bone-conducted sounds. For this, a vibrating device is placed on the bone behind each ear, and the patients signals when a tone is heard.

A young child's hearing can be tested by measuring brain waves with an electroencephalogram (EEG) as sounds are played through earphones.

If a parent feels their child may be deaf, careful
investigation is always essential.

CAUSES OF DEAFNESS

If excessive quantities of **wax** or a foreign body (e.g. tiny toy or foam packing ball in children) block the outer ear canal, hearing will be reduced in that ear.

The gradual decrease in hearing associated with advancing **age** is the most common form of deafness. This is basically due to thickening of the ear drum, wear and tear on the tiny bones that conduct the vibrations of the ear drum to the hearing apparatus in the inner ear, and a loss of sensitivity in the spiral tube that senses the vibrations and turns them into nerve impulses in the brain. The higher frequencies of sound disappear first, and this cuts out a lot of hearing discrimination, so that conversation in a noisy room melts into a constant blur of sound.

Middle ear **infections** (otitis media) are a very common cause of temporary deafness in children, that if left untreated, may progress to glue ear and a permanent partial loss of hearing.

Any infection of the nose, sinuses or throat may cause partial deafness due to pressure on the **Eustachian tube**, which connects the middle ear to the back of the nose, and normally opens to allow equalisation of air pressure with changes in altitude.

The ear drum may be damaged and rupture with changes in air pressure (**barotrauma**) that cannot be equalised because of a blocked Eustachian tube. Diving and flying are the common causes for this problem, particularly if there is a rapid change in pressure.

Direct **injury** to the ear drum may occur from trying to clean the ear with a bobby pin or cotton bud, or a sharp object accidentally entering the ear. Rarely, the delicate bony mechanism inside the ear may also be injured, leading to permanent deafness.

Ménière's disease may occur after a head injury or ear infection, but in most patients it has no apparent cause. It is more common in men, and with advancing age. The cause is a build-up in the pressure of the fluid inside the hearing and balance mechanisms of the inner ear. The increase in pressure causes a constant high-pitched ringing noise (tinnitus) in the ear. Other symptoms include dizziness, nausea and slowly progressive permanent deafness.

Ménière's disease is one of the most difficult conditions to treat,
and may be so annoying that it leads to suicide.

Uncommon causes of deafness include otosclerosis (arthritis like degeneration of the tiny bones in the ear), a cholesteatoma (foul smelling growth in the ear), bony growths in the outer ear canal (exostoses), a fracture of the skull around the ear and a lack of thyroxine (hypothyroidism).

A number of **medications** may have temporary (or very rarely, permanent) deafness as a side effect. These include aspirin, betablockers (used for high blood pressure and heart disease), quinine, aminoglycosides (an antibiotic) and cancer treating drugs (cytotoxics).

Numerous generalised **infections**, such as measles, mumps and meningitis, may cause temporary or permanent deafness.

Infection of a woman in the early months of pregnancy with german measles (**rubella**), cytomegalovirus or toxoplasmosis may affect her unborn child to cause permanent and total deafness.

Total deafness in an ear is usually associated with congenital (developmental) defects, surgery to the ear, severe head injuries or tumours in or around the ear.

EUSTACHIAN TUBE
The Eustachian tube is a thin tube that passes through the centre of the head from the back of the nose to the bottom of the middle ear. Its opening into the nose is surrounded by lymph tissue called the adenoids. Its purpose it to **equalise pressure** between the middle ear cavity and the outside air when a person changes altitude. The pop you feel when changing rapidly (e.g. taking off in an aircraft) is caused by air passing through this tube.

It may become blocked with phlegm and mucus, or allow these to pass into the middle ear to cause a glue ear or middle ear infection (otitis media), both of which reduce hearing.

The Eustachian tube is named after the Italian anatomist and student of Versalius, Bartolommeo Eustachio (1524–74).

TINNITUS
A persistent, high pitched **ringing** noise in an ear, when there is no sound actually present, is called tinnitus. It is a very annoying symptom, as the noise may continue day and night without relief, and drown out quieter noises that the person is trying to hear.

Ménière's disease (see above) is one quite common cause of tinnitus. Avoiding prolonged episodes of loud noise (e.g. jet engines, loud bands) helps to reduce the incidence of the condition.

Damage to the **blood supply** of the inner ear from a head injury, aneurysm (swelling of an artery) or hardening of the arteries (arteriosclerosis) will affect the sensitive hair cells in the inner ear that detect sound, and cause them to trigger off inappropriate nerve signals that are interpreted by the brain as a high pitched noise.

The tiny semicircular canals of the inner ear that control balance are known as the labyrinth. If this structure becomes inflamed or infected (**labyrinthitis**) the patient will become dizzy, abnormal eye movements will occur and noises may be heard in the ear.

OTHER CAUSES INCLUDE:

- degeneration of the hearing mechanism (cochlear in the inner ear) with age

- middle ear infections (otitis media)

- direct injury to the ear

- sudden change in pressure on the ear (with decompression of an aircraft or sur-facing too quickly from a scuba dive)

- acoustic neuroma (tumour of hearing nerve)

- endolymphatic hydrops (increased pressure in the inner ear)

- otosclerosis (a form of arthritis in the bones of the middle ear).

Rare causes may include persistent high blood pressure, some neuroses (e.g. schizophrenia), altitude sickness (ascending rapidly to heights over 3000m) and Costen syndrome (abnormal stresses are placed on the jaw joint and muscles of chewing).

Medications such as stimulants, excess aspirin and quinine (used for malaria) may cause tinnitus as a side effect.

Excess caffeine from coffee and cola drinks can cause tinnitus.

EAR DRUM RUPTURE

The rupture of the ear drum (tympanic membrane) leaves it with a slit or round hole. The **cause** may be increased pressure in the middle ear (e.g. Eustachian tube blockage), infection (e.g. otitis media), glue ear or direct injury to the ear (e.g. extremely loud sudden noise, poking stick into ear).

Pain and deafness occur, and if infection is present there may be a discharge. Infection in the ear may lead to permanent deafness.

It is diagnosed by examining the ear with an otoscope (magnifying light). Anti-biotics are then prescribed to prevent or treat infection, and in persistent cases, surgery is performed to place a tiny skin graft is put over the defect.

Most ruptured ear drums heal in a few days to weeks, depending on size of hole and cause.

CURIOSITY
Extract from a 1797 medical text:
'When deafness proceeds from dry wax in the ears it may be cured by syringing with warm milk'.
A treatment that would work just as well today.

HEPATITIS

L ook after yourself and your family by preventing hepatitis A and B (and sub-sequently D) by having vaccinations against these diseases, particularly if travelling to developing countries or working in close contact with people (e.g. nurses, hairdressers).

Hepatitis is a term that indicates any inflammation or infection of the liver. There are many different types and causes of hepatitis.

ANATOMY

The liver is the largest **gland** and internal organ in the body. Wedge-shaped, smooth and rubbery, it lies behind the lower few ribs on the right side, weighs about 1.5kg and has the same reddish brown colour as the animal livers we are familiar with in the butcher shop. The liver plays an integral part in the processing of food (metabolism).

The liver is the body's **chemical processing plant**. It regulates the amount of blood sugar, assists in producing the blood clotting mechanisms, helps to nourish new blood cells, destroys old blood cells, breaks down excess acids to be eliminated as urine, stores and modifies fats so they can be more efficiently utilised by cells all over the body, stores certain vitamins and minerals, and removes poisons from harmful substances such as alcohol and drugs. The liver is also an important source of heat, which is essential to maintain the body's temperature.

The liver has an amazing ability to repair itself if damaged.

The liver aids the **digestive process** by manufacturing bile, which mixes with the digestive juices in the duodenum. Bile is a thick yellowy green liquid containing salts that break down fat into small droplets so that it can be more easily digested. It is manufactured constantly, but because it may be required only a few times a day, it is carried from the liver through ducts to the gall bladder, a small pear-shaped bag lying just under the liver, where it is stored until it is needed.

Once **bile** salts are manufactured, the body makes the most of them. Having fulfilled their digestive purpose in the small intestine, they are not simply discarded but are recycled through the blood and back to the liver to be used again. It is estimated that this recycling process takes place about 18 times with only about five per cent of salts being eliminated in the faeces each time.

One of the functions of the liver is to remove a yellow pigment called **bilirubin**, produced by the destruction of old red blood cells, from the blood. If the liver

THE LIVER AND GALL BLADDER

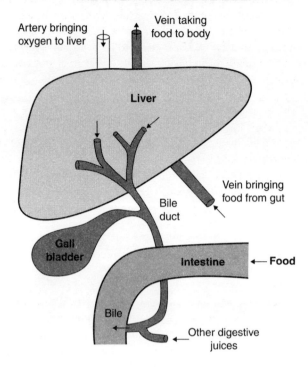

Artery bringing
oxygen to liver

Vein taking
food to body

Liver

Vein bringing
food from gut

Bile
duct

Gall
bladder

Intestine   ←— Food

Bile

Other digestive
juices

becomes diseased and cannot function properly, this yellow pigment stays in the bloodstream and gives a yellowish tinge to the skin and whites of the eyes – the jaundice that is a striking symptom of liver diseases such as hepatitis.

It is possible to survive quite normally on one quarter of a liver.

The chemical processing capabilities of the liver are amazingly complex and wide-ranging. Substances which enter as one thing frequently leave as something else, depending on the body's needs. For example, most amino acids are converted into **proteins**, but if the body is short of glucose, the liver will combine some of the amino acids with fat to make extra sugar. Similarly if the level of blood sugar is too high, glucose is converted into a substance that can be stored.

The liver's **storage** capacity is equally attuned to the body's specific needs at any given time. If more vitamins are consumed than the body immediately needs, certain types of them will be stored to be released if the supply falls off. A person could survive as long as 12 months without taking in any vitamin A, and for up to four months without new supplies of vitamins B12 and D.

HEPATITIS A

Hepatitis A (infective hepatitis) is a viral infection of the liver caught by **eating food that has been contaminated** by someone who has the disease. The virus lives in the liver, but large numbers pass down the bile duct and into the gut, and into the faeces. If sufferers are not careful with their personal hygiene, the virus may be passed on to someone else. When hepatitis A virus particles are swallowed, they are absorbed with the food into the bloodstream and migrate to the liver, where after an **incubation** period lasting two to six weeks they start multiplying and cause damage to liver cells. Patients may pass on the virus for a week or two before they develop any symptoms. The vital preventative factor is the standard of hygiene in the community.

The liver is used by the body to process food and eliminate waste products through bile which passes into the gut. If the liver is damaged, it cannot work efficiently, and the main constituent of bile (bilirubin) builds up in the blood stream. Because of the yellow colour of bilirubin, the skin slowly turns a dark yellow (jaundice). The whites of the eyes are affected first, and this may be the only sign of the disease in a dark-skinned person. Other symptoms are nausea, vomiting, marked tiredness, loss of appetite, generalised aches and pains, fever and a large tender liver.

Hepatitis A may be a significant risk to travellers
in developing countries and vaccination is advised.

Blood tests are available to detect antibodies against the various hepatitis viruses and diagnose the type of hepatitis and monitor its progress.

Hepatitis A can be **prevented** by a vaccine that may be combined with the vaccine against hepatitis B. Two injections at intervals of six to twelve months give at least five years, and possibly far longer, protection against hepatitis A. It is not designed to be used in pregnancy, but unlikely to cause serious adverse effects if given inadvertently. It may be given with caution in breast feeding and children over five years. The first injection takes effect after 14 days, and lasts for at least six months, while boosters give long-term protection. The most common side effect is a local reaction at injection site, while unusual reactions may include a headache, fever, tiredness, nausea, loss of appetite and general unwellness.

The main **treatment** is bed rest, and a diet that is low in protein and high in carbohydrate, and alcohol is forbidden. Sometimes it is necessary to give medication for nausea and vomiting and to feed severely affected patients by a drip into a vein for a short time. If it continues to worsen, drugs may be used to reduce the liver damage. In rare cases (two in 1000), the disease may progress despite all efforts of doctors and result in death, but this is more common in the elderly.

There is usually an initial worsening of the symptoms, followed by a slow recovery period that may take from one to four months. In children, it may be present, and recovery may occur with no symptoms ever being present. Permanent liver damage is uncommon.

HEPATITIS B

Hepatitis B (serum hepatitis) is a viral infection of the liver that can only be caught by **intimate contact** with the blood or semen of a person who has the disease or is a carrier of the disease. Examples include receiving blood from a carrier, using a contaminated needle, rubbing a graze or cut on an infected person's graze or cut, being bitten by an infected person, or most commonly, by having sex (homosexual or heterosexual) with them. Ninety per cent of babies born to mothers who are carriers catch the disease. The highest incidences are amongst homosexual men, drug addicts who share needles, Australian Aborigines, and the disease is widespread in South-East Asia. Blood banks screen all donations for hepatitis B. Splashes of blood into an eye or onto a cut or graze can spread the disease, and doctors, dentists, nurses and other health workers are therefore at risk.

There is a long **incubation** period of six weeks to six months, and the infection cannot be detected during this period. Once active, it causes the patient to be very ill with a liver infection, fever, jaundice (yellow skin), nausea and loss of appetite. Some patients develop only a very mild form of the disease but they are still contagious and may suffer the long-term effects.

Blood tests are available to detect antibodies against the various hepatitis viruses and diagnose the type of hepatitis and monitor its progress.

It has been possible to **vaccinate** against hepatitis B since the first vaccine was introduced in 1986. Three injections at intervals of one month and six months give at least five years protection. It should not be used during pregnancy unless essential, but accidental vaccination during pregnancy is unlikely to cause any significant problem. It may be used in children from birth onwards. Local soreness, swelling, redness and tissue hardness are the most common side effects. Unusually, a headache, dizziness, fever, muscle aches, tiredness, nausea, diarrhoea, joint pain and a rash may occur.

The hepatitis B vaccine is now given routinely to all infants.

Treatment involves bed rest and a diet that is low in protein and high in carbohydrates, and alcohol is forbidden. Sometimes it is necessary to give medication for nausea and vomiting and to feed severely affected patients by a drip into a vein for a short time. If it continues to worsen, drugs may be used to reduce the liver damage.

Patients must ensure that they are no longer infectious before having sex with anyone and have regular blood tests throughout their life to detect any liver damage. Nine out of ten patients recover completely after a few weeks, but one in ten become chronic carriers. Ten per cent of patients develop cirrhosis, failure of the liver or liver cancer, and about one per cent of patients develop a rapidly progressive liver disease that causes death.

HEPATITIS C

Hepatitis C is a viral infection of the liver transmitted from one person to another through **blood contamination** such as the sharing of needles by drug users. All blood donations are screened for this virus. Sexual transmission is possible but uncommon, and the incubation period is six to seven weeks.

The symptoms are usually mild, and the patient may only be vaguely unwell for a few days, but a minority progress to develop jaundice, liver enlargement and nausea. About a quarter of patients develop permanent liver damage, often after many years.

Hepatitis C is less easily caught by sex than the other forms of hepatitis.

Blood tests are available to detect antibodies against the various hepatitis viruses and diagnose the type of hepatitis and monitor its progress.

Treatment involves bed rest and a diet that is low in protein and high in carbohydrates, and alcohol is forbidden. Sometimes it is necessary to give medication for nausea and vomiting and to feed severely affected patients by a drip into a vein for a short time. If it continues to worsen, drugs may be used to reduce the liver damage. Unfortunately, it is not yet possible to vaccinate against hepatitis C.

No cure is available, but many patients lead normal long lives, although about half eventually develop cirrhosis and liver failure.

HEPATITIS D

Hepatitis D is a viral infection of the liver that can only be caught by patients who already **have hepatitis B**. The two diseases may be caught at the same time or separately. Hepatitis D is much more common in intravenous drug users with hepatitis B than in patients who have caught hepatitis B in other ways, and it is also more prevalent in countries around the Mediterranean.

If hepatitis D is caught at a later time than hepatitis B, there are usually no symptoms, but infection increases the risk of developing serious liver disease in those who already have hepatitis B. Blood tests are available to detect antibodies against the various hepatitis viruses and diagnose the type of hepatitis and monitor its progress.

You can only catch hepatitis D if you already have hepatitis B.

Usually no **treatment** is necessary, but in severe cases, drugs may be used to reduce the liver damage. There is no specific vaccine against hepatitis D, but vaccination against hepatitis B will effectively prevent both diseases.

No cure is available, and most patients lead normal lives, but many eventually develop cirrhosis, liver failure or liver cancer.

HEPATITIS E

Hepatitis E is a viral infection of the liver caught from **contaminated food** and water in the same way as hepatitis A. It is rare in Western countries with the highest incidence being in central Asia, Algeria and Mexico. Patients becomes jaundiced, are nauseated and tired, vomit, have no appetite, and develop aches, pains, a fever and a large tender liver. Blood tests are available to diagnose the type of hepatitis and monitor its progress.

Hepatitis E is particularly serious in pregnant women,
whom it can kill within hours of symptoms appearing.

The immediate death rate from hepatitis E is far higher than in other types of hepatitis, and may occur within a day or two of symptoms appearing. The death rate is far higher in pregnant women. Even so, most patients recover completely, and there are no long-term liver problems. There is no vaccine available, but a gammaglobulin injection will give short-term protection. Scrupulous personal hygiene is vital.

HEPATITIS F
There is no form of hepatitis known as hepatitis F.

HEPATITIS G
The GB virus was at one time thought to be a cause of **hepatitis G**, but recent research has found that although present in some patients with hepatitis, it was not actually responsible for the symptoms. The GB virus is transmitted from one person to another through blood contamination such as the sharing of needles by drug users, and probably by sex. The GB virus is found in about two per cent of all people, and interestingly, it seems to confer some resistance to the progression of the AIDS virus from the early stages of the disease to the more serious later stages. Hepatitis G is a disease that was once thought to exist, but has now been removed from the list of liver infections.

JAUNDICE
Jaundice is a yellow colour in the skin caused by high levels of bilirubin in the blood. Bilirubin is a waste product of the body, caused by the breakdown of the oxygen-carrying haemoglobin in red blood cells. It is removed from the blood by the liver, before passing into the gall bladder, and then onto the food in the small intestine to assist in digestion. Bilirubin also gives faeces its dark yellow/brown appearance.

The original term for jaundice was icterus.

Jaundice may be confused with **carotenaemia**, which is a yellowing of the soles and palms caused by excessive levels of vitamin A (carotene) in the blood, and is due to eating excessive quantities of yellow food (e.g. carrots, pumpkins, paw paw) or supplements with large amounts of vitamin A.

There are numerous medical conditions that may cause jaundice.

An **obstruction** to the bile duct drainage from the liver to the small intestine will prevent bilirubin from escaping into the gut. It continues to build up in the liver, and overflows back into the blood from where it is deposited in the skin. The obstruction may be caused by a gall stone in the bile duct, cancer in the liver (hepatoma), secondary cancer in the liver that has spread from elsewhere (e.g. breast, bowel), or a tumour in the pancreas which presses on and constricts the bile duct.

Cholecystitis is an inflammation or infection of the gall bladder, usually caused by gall stones that have formed within it. In most cases it causes pain and indigestion, but if the gall bladder becomes very swollen it may obstruct the bile duct to prevent bilirubin from leaving the liver.

Many newborn **infants** are jaundiced for a short time after birth. This is caused by immaturity of the liver, and the change from a primitive form of haemoglobin (foetal haemoglobin – HbF) which breaks down to form bilirubin, while a more mature form of haemoglobin is made in the spleen and bone marrow to replace it. In severe untreated cases, the high levels of bilirubin may damage the brain, so careful monitoring and treatment if bilirubin levels rise too high is essential. The jaundice can be eased by ultraviolet light, which penetrates the child's delicate skin to destroy bilirubin. Sun will destroy bilirubin, as can be demonstrated by dog faeces, which turns white after being out in the sun for a week or so.

In dark skinned people, jaundice may only be seen
as a yellowing of the whites of the eyes.

Cirrhosis is damage to the liver that results in its normal tissue being replaced by scar tissue. As the disease progresses the liver is unable to function successfully, and it cannot clear bilirubin out of the blood, resulting in jaundice. Cirrhosis may be caused by serious long-lasting infections (e.g. hepatitis B), poisons or excessive alcohol intake over a long period.

Hepatitis is an infection of the liver by a virus. There are many different types of hepatitis, but the most common are hepatitis A (caught from contaminated food) and hepatitis B (caught by intimate contact with an infected person's blood or semen). In their acute stages, all types of hepatitis will cause jaundice, but the long-term consequences will depend upon the type of hepatitis and the individual's response to it.

Other causes of jaundice include **malaria** (transmitted by mosquitoes in tropical areas), severe viral infections (e.g. cytomegalovirus of babies, glandular fever), severe bacterial infections (e.g. syphilis, leptospirosis, *Clostridia*), Gilbert syndrome (an inherited condition in which the liver fails to adequately clear bilirubin from the blood), yellow fever (severe infection of the liver transmitted by mosquitoes in central Africa and tropical America), pancreatitis (excruciatingly painful inflammation of the pancreas), and severe anaemia caused by the rapid breakdown of red blood cells (e.g. sickle cell anaemia, haemolytic anaemia).

Some **medications** may have jaundice as a side effect. Examples include medications that include chlorine, sulpha antibiotics and the general anaesthetic halothane.

There are many rarer causes of jaundice including Hodgkin's disease (cancer of the lymph tissue), a thrombus (clot) in the vein leading from the liver, sclerosing cholangitis (progressive blockage of the drainage tubes of the liver with inflamed scar tissue), parasites that invade the liver (e.g. Hydatid cysts, Echinococcus), thalassaemia major (an inherited condition that causes the red blood cells to be fragile and break down very rapidly) and the Dubin-Johnson syndrome (children who are born without a gall bladder).

CURIOSITY

Antarctic explorers who were starving and ate their sled dogs, also ate the dog's liver, which gave them a near fatal overdose of vitamin A and yellow skin.

HERPES

The term 'herpes' refers to any inflamed spreading skin eruption caused by the herpes virus. Most appear initially as small blisters, but these may break down rapidly into a sore. Looking after yourself depends on which form of herpes is being considered. Genital herpes and shingles require urgent medical attention (within 12 hours) and correct, rapid treatment in order to prevent complications.

HERPES SIMPLEX VIRUS

Herpes simplex is a virus that causes infections of moist membranes and skin. The most common areas affected are around the nose, lips, vulva, vagina and penis, but the skin anywhere on the body may be involved. The herpes virus is widely distributed in the community, and infections are very common.

The herpes simplex virus (HSV) comes in two main types, labelled simply 1 and 2. Herpes simplex 1 tends to cause infections around the nose and mouth (cold sores) and herpes simplex 2 tends to cause genital infections, but they are interchangeable and not mutually exclusive. A distantly related virus, Herpes zoster, is responsible for shingles and chickenpox.

Specific antibody blood tests are available to detect the form of virus present, and its degree of activity.

The term is Herpes is derived from the Greek word for
creep (herpes), as the rash appears to creep across the skin.

COLD SORE

Cold sores are a common skin infection, usually around the nose or mouth, caused by the virus **Herpes simplex type 1**.

Initially, the infection is caught as a child, when it is a simple mouth infection. The virus then migrates to the nerve endings around the lips and nose, and remains inactive there for many years. It may later reactivate at times of stress or illness to cause cold sores. It is passed from one person to another by direct contact (e.g. kissing). Sixty per cent of the population are infected and remain carriers throughout their lives. Sores are uncommon before five years of age, and the incidence decreases in old age. Recurrences tend to develop at the same spot.

Active infection is characterised by redness and soreness of the affected area, followed a day or two later by an eruption of small blisters, which rapidly burst to leave a shallow, weeping, painful ulcer. In severe cases, there may be a mild fever, and the lymph nodes in the neck may become tender and enlarged. An additional bacterial infection is the only common complication. If necessary, the diagnosis can be confirmed by taking special swabs from the sore.

If treated by appropriate antiviral creams and lotions (e.g. aciclovir, idoxuridine) as soon as the redness and discomfort is felt and before the blisters form, it may be possible to stop further progress. Once the cold sore is established, a cure is not normally possible, but drying, antiseptic and anaesthetic creams or lotions may be used. Patients who are severely affected on a regular basis may use expensive aciclovir or famciclovir tablets continuously to prevent infections.

Cold sores affect only one quarter of the population. Some people may be carriers, but have a natural resistance to the infection.

The sore heals and the pain eases in about a week. Some patients have only one attack of cold sores in their lives, while others develop one every month. Over many years, most patients find that their attacks become less frequent.

WHITLOW

A whitlow is a skin infection beside a finger nail, caused by the virus **Herpes simplex type 1**. Initially, the infection is caught as a child, when it is a simple mouth infection. The virus then migrates to the nerve endings around the finger or toe nail, and remains inactive there for many years. It may later reactivate at times of stress or illness. Recurrences tend to develop at the same spot.

Redness and soreness of the skin occurs, usually besides a nail, followed a day or two later by an eruption of small blisters, which rapidly burst to leave a shallow, weeping, painful ulcer. In rare cases, the infection can spread into the throat and lungs, and these patients become extremely ill.

If treated by appropriate creams and lotions as soon as the redness and discomfort is felt and before the blisters form, it may be possible to stop further progress. Once established, a cure is not normally possible, but drying, antiseptic and anaesthetic creams or lotions may be used. The sore heals and the pain eases in about ten days.

GENITAL HERPES

Genital herpes is a contagious viral infection of the genitals caused by the **Herpes simplex type 2** virus, which is caught by sexual contact with someone who already has the disease. It is possible, but unlikely, for the virus to be caught in hot spa baths and from a shared wet towel. If sores are present, there is a good chance of passing the disease on, but a patient is also infectious for several days before a new crop of sores develop. Condoms can give some protection against spreading the disease.

Once a person is infected with the virus, it settles in the nerve endings around the vulva or penis, and remains there for the rest of that person's life. With stress, illness or reduced resistance, the virus starts reproducing and causes painful blisters and ulcers on the penis or scrotum (sac) in the male; and on the vulva (vaginal lips), and in the vagina and cervix (opening into the womb) of the female. The first attack may occur only a week, or up to some years, after the initial infection. An attack will last for two to four weeks and then subside, but after weeks, months or years, a further attack may occur. Women are affected more severely and frequently than men. The incidence of gynaecological cancer is increased in women with the infection and in rare cases it can cause encephalitis (brain infection).

Oral sex may transfer Herpes simplex type 1 to the · genitals, and Herpes simplex type 2 to the lips.

If a baby catches the infection from the mother during delivery, it can cause severe brain damage in the child. For this reason, if a woman has a history of repeated herpes infections, she may be delivered by caesarean section.

The infection is diagnosed by taking a swab from the ulcer or a blood test.

Antiviral tablets and ointments will control an attack, but must be started within 72 hours of its onset, or they can be taken for months or years to prevent further attacks. Good control is possible with modern medications.

HERPES ZOSTER VIRUS

Herpes zoster (HZV) is the virus responsible for the chickenpox infection, and subsequently may cause shingles.

CHICKENPOX

Chickenpox (varicella) is a generalised infection caused by the virus Herpes zoster. Infection occurs when the virus passes to another person from the fluid-filled blisters that cover the body of patients, or in their breath and saliva. Patients are **infectious** for a day or two before the spots appear, and remain infectious for about eight days. The incubation period is ten to 21 days.

Early **symptoms** are similar to those of a cold, with a vague feeling of being unwell, headache, fever and sore throat. The rash usually starts on the head or chest as red pimples, then spreads onto the legs and arms, and develops into blisters before drying up and scabbing over. New spots may develop for three to five days, and it may be two weeks or more before the last spot disappears. The diagnosis can be confirmed by blood tests, but none are usually necessary.

Chickenpox gained its name because the skin of sufferers resembled that of a freshly plucked chicken.

Treatment involves bed and home rest until the patient feels well, and medications to relieve the itch (e.g. calamine lotion, antihistamines), fever and headache. There is a vaccine available to prevent the disease.

Complications are more common in adults, and include chest infections and a type of meningitis. It is unusual for the pock marks to scar unless a secondary bacterial infection occurs.

Complete recovery within ten days is normal. Once a person has had chickenpox, it is unlikely (but not impossible) that they will ever catch it again.

Once a patient has had chickenpox, the virus never leaves their body but migrates to the nerves along the spinal cord where it remains forever. The virus may be reactivated years later at times of stress to give the patient the painful rash of shingles.

SHINGLES

Shingles (varicella) is an infection of nerves and skin by the **Herpes zoster** virus, which is the same virus that causes chickenpox, and is usually caught as a child. The virus never leaves the body, but migrates to the roots of nerves along the spinal cord, where it remains inactive lifelong.

At times of stress, the virus may reactivate and move along the nerve to cause the skin and other tissues to become very painful. Shingles is far more common in older people, and uncommon in children. You cannot catch shingles from another person, but a child who has not had chickenpox may catch this from a person who has active shingles.

A painful blistering rash is a medical emergency as it may be shingles and treatment must be started immediately to ensure a cure.

An acutely tender, blistering **rash** develops, often in a belt-like line on one side of the body, and even the slightest touch causes severe shooting pain. Any nerve may be affected, and it can occur on the abdomen or chest (most common sites), or on the face or legs. Occasionally the rash leaves permanent scars, particularly on the face. A small number of elderly people can develop chronic inflammation in the nerve, and pain that persists for years (post-herpetic neuralgia). The worst complication occurs if nerves around the eye and ear are involved, when dizziness, ear noises and, rarely, blindness may occur (Ramsay-Hunt syndrome).

No investigations are normally necessary, but if required the diagnosis can be confirmed by taking special swabs from a sore.

Shingles can be **cured** by specific antiviral tablets, but only if treatment is started within 72 hours of the rash first appearing. If treatment is neglected until after three days from the onset of the rash, the only treatment is painkillers, drying antiseptic lotions and mild sedatives. Steroids may be used in severe cases.

The term shingles is derived from the Greek word cingulum, which means belt, as the shingles forms a belt-like rash around one half of the body.

The rash dries out slowly and disappears over several weeks, usually healing completely. The pain is slower to disappear, and may last a month longer than the rash, but the vast majority of patients make an excellent recovery.

RAMSAY-HUNT SYNDROME

The Ramsay-Hunt syndrome is the infection of a **facial** nerve with the Herpes zoster virus.

Shingles may affect any nerve leading out from the brain or spinal cord, but if the nerve affected (the geniculate ganglion) is the one supplying the ear and face, the patient will develop this syndrome.

It causes severe earache, dizziness, and a painful blistering rash across the upper face and ear. No investigations are normally necessary, but if required the diagnosis can be confirmed by taking special swabs from a sore.

Damage to the eye surface can result in blindness if
treatment for the Ramsay-Hunt syndrome is delayed.

Antiviral medication (e.g. aciclovir, valaciclovir) must be taken as soon as the shingles starts to prevent its spread. Steroids may also be used to reduce complications, but permanent deafness and dizziness can result if treatment starts too late.

ANTIVIRALS

Until very recently, drugs that killed viruses and cured viral infections (**antivirals**) were limited to the idoxuridine eye drops and ointments used for cold sores and herpes simplex infections. Idoxuridine is far more effective if used early in the disease when the virus is multiplying.

Aciclovir (Zovirax) was the first antiviral tablet/injection that could attack viral infections from within the body, but it (and the newer **famciclovir** and **valaciclovir**) only acts against herpes zoster and herpes simplex viruses that cause cold sores, genital herpes and shingles.

These antivirals are available as tablets, injections and creams. They are remarkably safe and effective, but should only be used in pregnancy and breast feeding if medically essential. They may be used in children. Lower doses are necessary in the elderly. Use tablets with caution in serious kidney disease, dehydration and brain disorders.

Side effects are minimal, but rarely may cause nausea, vomiting and headache. They interact with probenecid, diuretics (fluid tablets), interferon and methotrexate.

Aciclovir, famciclovir and valaciclovir have a very high success rate in treating Herpes infections, but it is vital that any patient who suspects they have shingles must see their doctor immediately, as they only work if started within 72 hours of onset of rash. Chickenpox and cold sores are normally only treated under special circumstances, as the medication is quite expensive. Eye infections with Herpes may cause blindness if not treated rapidly and effectively. The cream is only effective against cold sores if started as soon as symptoms appear.

CURIOSITY

Children who catch chickenpox before one year of age may develop the infection again later in life, as their immune system was not developed enough at the time of infection to give lifelong immunity. For this reason, the chickenpox vaccine is not given until 18 months of age.

HICCUPS

L ook after yourself by not over-indulging, eating rapidly, smoking, becoming intoxicated or becoming too stressed – the most common causes of hiccups.

Hiccups are caused by repeated spasms of the diaphragm, which is a sheet of muscle across the body between the chest and the abdomen. When the diaphragm muscle contracts we breathe in, and the muscles relax as we breathe out. When the diaphragm contracts spasmodically, a small amount of air is suddenly forced into the lungs, causing the characteristic sound.

CAUSES

Simple causes of hiccups include emotional stress, smoking, drinking excess alcohol, over-eating, rapid eating, sudden changes in temperature, swallowing air when nervous and indigestion.

More seriously, hiccups may be due to inflammation of organs that touch the diaphragm. In the abdomen, the stomach may be inflamed by a peptic ulcer or hiatus hernia (part of the stomach slips up into the chest), or a diseased liver may irritate the diaphragm. In the chest, pleurisy (inflammation of the membrane around the lungs), pneumonia or heart disease may be the cause.

Hiccoughs is the correct English spelling but it has been almost completely replaced everywhere by the American spelling – hiccups.

Irritation of the phrenic nerve, which runs from the brain to the diaphragm and controls its action, may cause hiccups. Tumours of the nerve or brain, or pinching of the nerve on its long route through the neck and chest, may be responsible.

Rarely, psychiatric disturbances may have intermittent hiccups as an attention-seeking feature.

CURES

The hiccups may be cured by a counter-irritation or relieving the stomach pressure. Drinking water, holding a deep breath, swallowing a teaspoon full of table sugar, a fright, and burping are well-known remedies.

Medications can be given to relax the diaphragm muscle in persistent cases. Rarely they may persist for days, weeks, months or years, and the causes need to be investigated and treated in these cases.

DIAPHRAGM

The diaphragm is a sheet of muscle that runs across the body to separate the chest from the abdomen (belly). It is shaped like a dome, curved upwards towards the chest. It is attached to the ribs and vertebrae.

It contracts down to aid breathing in, and relaxes back when breathing out.

There are holes in the diaphragm to allow the oesophagus (gullet), aorta and inferior vena cava (main vein from the lower body) to pass from the chest into the abdomen. If the hole for the oesophagus becomes stretched, part of the stomach may slip up into the chest to form a hiatus hernia.

CURIOSITY

Extract from an 1821 medical text:

'A draught of generous wine, or a dram of any spirituous liquor, will generally remove a hiccup'.

And why not try it?

HOME MEDICAL CHEST

Look after yourself and your family by ensuring that you have an appropriately equipped home medical chest readily available. There is no point knowing what to do if you do not have the necessary medication or equipment.

A COMPREHENSIVE HOME MEDICAL CHEST SHOULD CONTAIN THE FOLLOWING ITEMS:

- first aid book

- sterile dressing

- adhesive dressings (various sizes)

- surgical tape (to fix dressings)

- antiseptic cream

- antiseptic ear drops

- antiseptic eye drops

- antiseptic liquid

- charcoal solution (for overdose)

- cotton gauze (NOT cotton wool)

- elastic bandages (wide)

- eye pads

- lotion for bites and stings

- menthol inhalant

- paracetamol liquid and tablets

- scissors

- skin closure strips

- splinter forceps

- sunscreen

- thermometer

- triangular bandage (sling).

The home medicine chest should be located where everyone in the family knows about it, but in a position where it is not accessible to young children.

This kit should be checked annually, and any expired medications replaced. If travelling by car, take the kit with you, and if flying, take small quantities of those items you feel may suit your needs most.

CURIOSITY

As a general practitioner, I am constantly amazed how often, when giving phone advice to patients after hours, they do not have even the simplest home remedies available, resulting in discomfort, expense and inconvenience as they are obtained.

HORMONE REPLACEMENT THERAPY

W omen should look after themselves as they mature by ensuring that they understand the mechanism of the menopause (see separate entry in this book), the ways in which it can be managed, and in particular, the pros and cons of hormone replacement therapy (HRT).

Sex hormones are produced by the ovary in the woman and the testes in the man to give to each sex its characteristic appearance.

In women, the sex hormone **oestrogen** that is produced for the first time at puberty causes breast enlargement, hair growth in the armpit and groin, ovulation, the start of menstrual periods and later acts to maintain a pregnancy.

If the sex hormones are reduced or lacking, these characteristics disappear. This happens naturally during the female menopause. After the menopause, the breasts sag, pubic and armpit hair becomes scanty, and the periods cease due to the lack of sex hormones.

HORMONE REPLACEMENT METHODS

Hormone tablets are the main method of menopause control. While passing through the menopause, it is usual to take one hormone (**oestrogen**, e.g. Premarin) for three weeks, and a different hormone (**progestogen**, e.g. Provera) is added in for the last seven to ten days, and then no hormones are taken for a week. After the menopause has been completed and all periods have stopped, it is usual to take both the oestrogen and progestogen constantly. Other dosage regimes may be recommended.

If oestrogen is taken without progestogen, there is over-stimulation of the endometrial tissue in the uterus (womb) which can increase the risk of cancer of the uterus. When the two are taken together, either cyclically (progestogen for only part of the month) or constantly (both hormones all the time) there is no increased risk of uterine cancer. In a hysterectomy the uterus is removed, and so women who have had a hysterectomy cannot have an increased risk of cancer of the uterus, and these women only need to take the oestrogen, and progestogens are unnecessary.

These hormones maintain the body in a near-normal balance, while underneath the artificial hormones, the natural menopause is occurring, so that when the tablets are stopped after a year or two, the menopausal symptoms will have gone.

The emotional storm of puberty is really very similar to menopause,
although acne replaces hot flushes in the former.

215

Hormone replacement therapy can be given as tablets, skin patches, skin cream, vaginal cream, implants, nasal spray or injection.

Every woman must assess her own needs in consultation with her doctor regarding her lifestyle expectations and the risks of using HRT. Many women are now continuing hormone replacement therapy (HRT) for many years after the menopause to prevent osteoporosis (and the resultant fractured bones), and to slow ageing. Generally speaking, HRT has been a major advance in the health of women, who now outlive men by an average of more than seven years.

HRT SAFETY

Concerns about the safety of hormone replacement therapy (HRT) relate to **long-term** (greater than five years) use of **combined** (oestrogen and progestogen) HRT. Short-term use for up to five years is still apparently safe and is used to control the symptoms of menopause (e.g. hot flushes, dry vagina, aching).

Long-term use needs to be weighed for each individual woman according to her risk factors for heart disease, osteoporosis, breast cancer, stroke and blood clot.

The points for and against hormone replacement therapy are outlined as simply as possible in the following points.

BENEFITS:

- Improved sense of well being.

- Increases libido (sexual desire).

- Lubricates the vagina and enhances sexual pleasure.

- Breast shape retained for longer without drooping.

- Reduced risk of bowel cancer (risk decreases from 1.6 women in every 1000 developing bowel cancer in any one year to 1.0).

- Significantly reduced risk of osteoporosis (risk decreases from 1.5 women in every 1000 having a hip fracture from osteoporosis in any one year to 0.9).

- Slows the development of wrinkles and keeps the skin moist and more elastic.

- Improves mood and reduces irritability.

- Relieves the hot flushes, depression, bloating and other symptoms of menopause.

DISADVANTAGES:

- Increased risk of breast cancer if taken for more than four years (risk rises from 3.1 women in every 1000 developing breast cancer in any one year to 3.9).

- Increased risk of heart attacks if taken for more than four years (risk rises from 2.4 women in every 1000 having a heart attack in any one year to 3.1).

- Increased risk of blood clots in veins (leg blood clots) (risk rises from 1.1 women in every 1000 developing a blood clot in any one year to 2.9).

- Increased risk of stroke (risk rises from 1.9 women in every 1000 developing a stroke in any one year to 2.7).

- Breast tenderness and breakthrough bleeding in early stages of use.

- Nausea and belly cramps may occur and migraines may be aggravated.

Statistics are for postmenopausal women on combined oestrogen and progestogen HRT.

The risks of HRT must be measured against the better quality
of life achieved by many women who use HRT.

Except under special circumstances, women who have had **cancer** of the breast, uterus or cervix; hormonal mastitis (breast pain), endometriosis, blood clots (thromboses) or strokes, should not use HRT.

Overall, the **risk** of using HRT is very small, and the latest research shows that women who use HRT to control hot flushes, mood swings, pelvic fullness and breast discomfort are far less likely to develop serious side effects than women who use HRT with no significant symptoms. The short-term benefits of HRT on menopausal symptoms may in fact give a better long-term quality of life.

SEX HORMONES
OESTROGEN
Oestrogens include dienoestrol, ethinyloestradiol (Estigyn), oestradiol, oestriol (Ovestin), etonogestrel (Implanon), conjugated oestrogen (Premarin) and piperazine oestrone (Ogen). They are used in contraceptive pills, for hormone replacement therapy during and after the menopause, and are usually combined with a progestogen unless the woman has had a hysterectomy.

Side effects may include abnormal menstrual bleeding, vaginal thrush, nausea, fluid retention, breast tenderness, bloating and skin pigmentation. These side effects can usually be overcome by adjusting the dosage.

They should not be used in pregnancy, breast feeding, children, and patients with liver diseases or a bad history of blood clots. Care must be used in patients with breast cancer, epilepsy and hypertension.

All humans react the same way to all sex hormones.
If you give a man oestrogen he will develop breasts.

PROGESTOGEN
Progestogens include dydrogesterone (Duphaston), medroxyprogesterone (Provera), gestrinone and norethisterone (Primolut-N, Micronor, Noriday). They

are used to control abnormal menstrual bleeds, endometriosis, for preventive contraception, 'morning-after' contraception, hormone replacement therapy and premenstrual tension. Medroxyprogesterone is an injectable progesterone that may be used for contraception, to treat certain types of cancer and endometriosis. As a contraceptive it is given every three months.

Side effects include the cessation of menstrual periods, breakthrough vaginal bleeding, headaches, and possibly a prolonged contraceptive action (up to 15 months). The other progestogens usually have minimal side effects, but they may include headache, abnormal vaginal bleeding, insomnia, breast tenderness, nausea and sweats.

They should not be used in pregnancy, liver disease, and patients with blood clots or breast lumps. Care must be used in patients with with hypertension and diabetes.

DANAZOL

Danazol (Danocrine) is a special type of sex hormone that acts against oestrogen and is used to treat endometriosis, severe menstrual period pain and severe breast pain. Side effects are common and may include acne, weight gain, excess body hair, retained fluid, dry vagina, sweats and the development of a deep voice. It must never be used in pregnancy, or in patients with pelvic infection, liver disease, blood clots or heart failure.

TIBOLONE

Tibolone (Livial) is another way of treating the symptoms of menopause, and preventing osteoporosis after the menopause. It must be used with caution in high cholesterol or triglycerides, liver disease or risk of blood clots (thromboses). Do not take it if suffering from undiagnosed vaginal bleeding, hormone-dependent tumours (e.g. breast cancer), significant heart disease, recent stroke, blood clots or severe liver disorders.

Tibolone is the HRT to have when you don't want to have HRT.

It is commenced in menopause, a year after the last menstrual bleed, and not during the transition stage of menopause.

Common side effects include weight gain, dizziness, headache and belly pain, while unusual ones may include migraine, dermatitis, disturbed vision, skin irritation, nausea, constipation, breast pain and vaginal irritation. It interacts with other hormone replacement therapies used in menopause, anticoagulants (e.g. warfarin), barbiturates, carbamazepine and rifampicin.

Released in 2000 as a completely new method of managing symptoms of the menopause, it seems to suit many women very well, while others cannot tolerate it.

CURIOSITY
Recent research shows that the worse the symptoms of the menopause (e.g. hot flushes), the less likely a woman is to develop serious side effects from the use of hormone replacement therapy.

HYPERTENSION

E veryone should look after themselves by ensuring that their blood pressure is checked regularly from 30 years of age onwards.

EXPLANATION

High blood pressure (hypertension) is an excessive pressure of blood within the arteries, which occurs in 20 per cent of adults over 40 years of age.

The heart contracts regularly to pump blood through the arteries under high (systolic) pressure. When the heart relaxes between beats, the blood continues to flow due to the lower (diastolic) pressure exerted by the elasticity of the artery walls. Hypertension occurs when one, or both, of these pressures exceeds a safe level.

Blood pressure is not an absolute value, but can vary significantly with position, time of day, exercise, anxiety, eating, menstruation, pregnancy etc.

MEASUREMENT

Blood pressure readings are written as systolic pressure/diastolic pressure (e.g. 125/70) and are measured with a **sphygmomanometer**. The numbers are a measure of pressure in millimetres of mercury.

Blood pressure varies with exercise, anxiety, age, fitness, smoking and drinking habits, weight and medications. In a very elderly person, 160/90 may be acceptable, but in a young woman, 110/60 would be more appropriate. In a middle-aged person, a blood pressure of 140–160/90–100 would be watched carefully for a couple of months, then treatment started once a persistently high level was confirmed. Levels above 160/90 are usually treated sooner, and over 200/120 immediate treatment is necessary.

When treating a patient, doctors will try to keep blood pressure below 140/85, but even lower figures may be desirable in diabetics and those with a bad family or personal history of heart disease. Life insurance companies generally require the blood pressure to be under 136/86 for the person to be acceptable at normal rates.

The correct blood pressure must be individualised for each patient depending on age, history, family, occupation, weight, cholesterol, smoking and other risk factors.

CAUSES

The majority of patients have 'essential' hypertension, for which there is no single identifiable cause.

THE IDENTIFIABLE CAUSES INCLUDE:

- inherited tendency

- smoking

- obesity

- kidney disease

- oestrogen-containing medications (e.g. the contraceptive pill)

- hyperparathyroidism (over-active parathyroid glands in the neck alter calcium levels)

- phaeochromocytoma (rare tumour of the adrenal glands – see below)

- a number of other rare diseases.

High blood pressure may also be a complication of pregnancy (pre-eclampsia), when it can lead to quite serious consequences.

SYMPTOMS

The arteries of a person with high blood pressure will become hardened, brittle and may eventually rupture, causing a stroke, heart attack or other serious injury to vital organs.

The majority of patients have no symptoms for many years, but those who do have symptoms complain of **headaches** and **tiredness**, although only when the blood pressure is very high do the further symptoms of nausea, confusion, and disturbances in vision occur.

COMPLICATIONS

Untreated high blood pressure causes **strokes** and **heart attacks** at an earlier age than would be expected with normal blood pressure. Other complications may include kidney damage and bleeding into an eye. A rapidly progressive condition known as malignant hypertension can sometimes develop and cause remarkably high levels of blood pressure.

TREATMENT

Once diagnosed, blood and urine tests are performed to see if there is any specific cause, and X-rays of the kidneys and an electrocardiogram (ECG) may also be performed.

Hypertension is **Prevented** by:

• keeping weight within reasonable limits

• not eating excessive amounts of salt

• not smoking

• exercising regularly.

There is no cure, but hypertension can be successfully **controlled** by taking tablets regularly lifelong. A wide range of medications are available (e.g. diuretics, alphablockers, betablockers, calcium channel blockers, ACE inhibitors etc.), but it takes days or weeks for the tablets to work. Regular checks are essential until the correct dosage is determined, then blood pressure checks every three to six months are necessary.

The first symptom of high blood pressure may be sudden unexpected death.

Once controlled, there is no reason why the patient should not lead a full and active working, sporting and sexual life. Untreated, most patients with only moderate hypertension die within 20 years.

PHAEOCHROMOCYTOMA

A phaeochromocytoma is a rare **black-celled tumour** in the adrenal glands (which sit on top of each kidney), which releases a substance into the blood stream that causes very high blood pressure (hypertension). It is sometimes an hereditary tendency, but most arise for no apparent reason.

Patients have extremely high blood pressure, severe headaches, palpitations of the heart, abnormal sweating, nausea and vomiting, abdominal pains, blurred vision, and brain damage that may result in loss of speech, blindness or unconsciousness. Other symptoms may include increased appetite, nervousness and irritability, shortness of breath, weight loss, light-headedness and chest pain (angina). Some patients have multiple tumours in other parts of the body, and an unexplained sudden death may be due to a heart attack caused by an undiagnosed tumour.

Some forms of phaeochromocytoma are associated with cancer,
but a phaeochromocytoma is not a cancer itself.

The diagnosis is confirmed by special blood tests that measure excessive levels of catecholamines (the chemical released by the tumour). A CT scan or a magnetic resonance imaging scan (MRI) is performed to locate the tumour.

Controlling the high blood pressure with medication is the initial aim of treatment, and then surgically removing the tumour. Long-term management with medication, but without surgery, is not practical.

The prognosis depends on the damage caused by the high blood pressure before diagnosis, and how many tumours are present. If the tumour is removed early, a complete recovery is expected. Without treatment, the disease is invariably fatal, and even in the best medical centres, a small percentage of patients will die from complications of the disease or the surgery.

ANTIHYPERTENSIVES

Medications that control and reduce high blood pressure (hypertension) are called antihypertensives.

ACE INHIBITORS

Angiotensin converting enzyme (ACE) inhibitors are a class of drugs that prevent the contraction of the tiny muscles that circle around small arteries by blocking the action of the chemical that is essential for the contraction of these tiny artery muscles. They are used for the treatment of high blood pressure, heart failure, and improve survival after heart attack.

Examples include captopril (Capoten), fosinopril (Monopril), quinapril (Accupril, Asig), perindopril (Coversyl), trandolapril (Odrik), lisinopril (Prinivil) and ramipril (Tritace).

Side effects may include a dry cough, swelling of ankles, rash, headache and dizziness. They should not be used in pregnancy, or with severe kidney or brain disease.

ALPHABLOCKERS

Alpha receptor blockers are drugs that block the reception of certain nerve signals to the arteries, and if these signals are not received, the artery relaxes, allowing more blood to flow through at a lower pressure. These drugs have undergone considerable refinement over the years, and most of the earlier ones that had significant side effects are no longer used. They are used to treat high blood pressure, heart failure, enlarged prostate gland and Raynaud's disease. They are available only as tablets and must be started in a very low dose, which is slowly increased over several weeks.

Examples of medications in this class (with brand names in brackets), include prazosin (Minipress), doxazosin (Carduran) and indoramin. Side effects may include headache, drowsiness, nausea, palpitations and blurred vision. They must be used with care in pregnancy and liver disease.

Antihypertensives do NOT cure high blood pressure, they merely control it, and medication must be taken long-term.

ANGIOTENSIN II RECEPTOR ANTAGONISTS

A new class of medications introduced in 1998 for the treatment of high blood pressure and other heart diseases was the angiotensin II receptor antagonists (A2 agonists). Like ACE Inhibitors, they prevent the contraction of the tiny muscles that circle around small arteries by blocking the action of the chemical that is essential for the contraction of these tiny artery muscles, but with fewer side effects. They are available only as tablets but may be combined in the one tablet with a thiazide diuretic (hydrochlorothiazide).

Examples of medications in this class (with trade names in brackets) include candesartan (Atacand), irbesartan (Avapro, Karvea), and telmisartan (Micardis, Pritor).

Side effects may include sleep disturbances and depression. They should not be used in pregnancy, but low blood pressure is the only likely effect in overdose.

BETABLOCKERS

High blood pressure, migraine, irregular heartbeat, stage fright, prevention of heart attack, exam nerves, angina, overactive thyroid gland, tremors and glaucoma – all these diseases can be controlled, or treated, by the amazingly versatile group of drugs called betablockers. Some betablockers are very specific for particular diseases (e.g. timolol is used only in eye drop form for glaucoma while atenolol acts mainly on the heart), but others (e.g. propranolol) can act in virtually all areas. They are available on prescription in tablet and injection forms.

Beta receptors are present on certain nerves in the body, and blocking the action of these nerves with betablockers produces the desired effects. Because they can control a fine tremor and anxiety about performance, these drugs are banned in the Olympic and Commonwealth games, as they would give athletes such as archers and shooters an unfair advantage. Betablockers are generally very safe medications.

Examples include atenolol (Noten, Tenormin), metoprolol (Betaloc), oxprenolol (Corbeton), pindolol (Visken) and propranolol (Inderal).

Side effects may include low blood pressure, slow heart rate, cold hands and feet, nightmares, stuffy nose and impotence. They must not be used in asthmatics as they can trigger an asthma attack, and care must be used when giving them to diabetics.

CALCIUM CHANNEL BLOCKERS

Calcium is essential for the contraction of the tiny muscles around the arteries. When these muscles contract, the artery becomes smaller and narrower. Calcium channel blockers prevent the calcium from entering the muscle cells through tiny channels in the membrane surrounding the cell. These muscle cells cannot then contract easily, remain relaxed, and do not narrow the artery. The wider an artery, the less resistance is placed on the blood flowing through it, and the lower the blood pressure. Because they prevent the contraction of all arteries, they reduce the strain on the heart, and some of these drugs can therefore be used to treat angina (a lack of blood to the heart muscle) as well as high blood pressure and a rapid heart rate.

Calcium channel blockers are quite safe and are normally used in tablet form, although some can be given as injections. They can interact with a number of drugs, so doctors must be aware of all the patient's medications.

Examples of drugs in this class include amlodipine (Norvasc), diltiazem (Cardizem), felodipine (Agon, Plendil), isradipine, nifedipine (Adalat) and verapamil (Cordilox, Isoptin).

Side effects may include constipation, tiredness, headache, swelling of feet, dizziness, indigestion and hot flushes. They should be used only if essential in pregnancy, and not in heart failure or low blood pressure. Care should be taken when used in patients with diabetes.

If blood pressure medication is ceased, the high levels
may return within hours of the missed dose.

HYDRALAZINE

Hydralazine (with the common trade name of Apresoline) is a medication in tablet form used to treat high blood pressure, often in combination with other medications. It is particularly useful in the high blood pressure associated with pre-eclampsia of pregnancy. It should not be used in the first seven months of pregnancy, and only if medically necessary later in pregnancy. It is safe in breast feeding, but should not be used in children.

Take care in using hydralazine if suffering from angina, recent heart attack, other heart diseases, recent stroke, kidney or liver disease. Do not take it if suffering from SLE (systemic lupus erythematosus), very rapid pulse, aortic aneurysm, heart failure or cor pulmonale.

Common side effects may include slowed reactions, rapid heart rate, palpitations, dizziness, flushing, low blood pressure and angina, while uncommon effects may include headaches, joint pains and swelling, muscle aches, nasal congestion and stomach upsets. Stop the medication and consult a doctor if there is any unusual bleeding or irregular heart beat.

Hydralazine may interact with vasodilators, calcium channel blockers, ACE inhibitors, diuretics, other medications for high blood pressure, diazoxide, tricyclic antidepressants, tranquillisers, betablockers, adrenaline, MAOI (monoamine oxidase inhibitors) and alcohol.

An overdose may result in a rapid heart rate, low blood pressure, dizziness, nausea, sweating, irregular heart rate, angina, heart attack and death. If taken recently, induce vomiting then seek urgent medical assistance.

It is only used in the most severe and difficult forms of high blood pressure as it interacts with a wide range of other medications.

INDAPAMIDE

Indapamide (Natrilix) is a diuretic medication that increases urine production and is used for the treatment of high blood pressure, often in combination with other medications. It should only be used in pregnancy and breast feeding if medically essential, and is not for use in children. Use it with caution in systemic lupus erythematosus (SLE), kidney and liver disease, and do not take it if suffering from severe kidney or liver disease. Regular blood tests are necessary to check for irregularities in blood chemistry (electrolytes).

Common side effects may include tiredness, dizziness, headache, muscle cramps and diarrhoea, while unusual ones may include a rash, impotence, sleeplessness, nausea and gout. Indapamide interacts with barbiturates, narcotics, lithium, other diuretics and herbs such as celery, dandelion and uva ursi.

METHYLDOPA

Methyldopa (Aldomet) is an old fashioned medication used in the treatment of high blood pressure (hypertension). It may still be used today in patients in whom more sophisticated medications are inappropriate. It is inconvenient as it must be taken three or four times a day. It is safe in pregnancy and children, but side effects may include fever, sedation and headache.

THIAZIDE DIURETICS

Thiazide diuretics are a type of fluid tablet that has been widely used for fluid problems since the 1950s. They increase the rate at which the kidney produces urine, and therefore the frequency with which a person has to visit the toilet to pass urine. They include medications such as hydrochlorothiazide, bendrofluazide, bendrothiazide, chlorthalidone, hydroflumethiazide, benzthiazide, chlorthiazide, metolazone and clopamide, and are used to treat conditions such as high blood pressure, tissue swelling and excess fluid in the body.

They should not be used in pregnancy unless medically essential, and may reduce the volume of milk in breast feeding. They are sometimes used for this purpose in women who wish to stop breast feeding. Use thiazides with caution in gout, kidney disease, liver disease, diabetes, SLE and asthma, and not at all if suffering from complete kidney failure.

It may be necessary to take potassium supplements, or eat bananas and dried apricots, to prevent potassium depletion while taking thiazide diuretics.

Common side effects include increased urinary frequency, while unusual ones may include nausea, vomiting, gut cramps, diarrhoea, dizziness, headache and a rash. They may interact with lithium, barbiturates, digoxin, insulin, steroids, lithium, NSAIDs and tablets for controlling maturity onset diabetes. There is a beneficial interaction with most medications that lower blood pressure. The herbs guarana, liquorice, celery, dandelion and uva ursi may also interact with thiazides.

They are not permitted in high-level competitive sports as they act as masking agents for other illegal drugs.

An overdose may cause confusion, dizziness and gut spasms due to chemical (electrolyte) imbalances. Administer activated charcoal or induce vomiting if the tablets were taken recently, give extra fluids and seek medical assistance.

CURIOSITY

Syndrome X (yes, that is the correct name) is a newly recognised autoimmune condition that may be a cause of high blood pressure. The body inappropriately rejects its own tissue, in this case the cells that respond to insulin. The symptoms may include high blood pressure, a tendency to develop diabetes, obesity and cholesterol imbalances. There is a significantly increased risk of stroke and heart attack. It is diagnosed by sophisticated blood tests, then medication is prescribed to control blood pressure, diabetes and cholesterol levels. No cure is possible, but good control is normally achieved.

ILLEGAL DRUGS

Look after yourself, your health and your sanity by never using illegal drugs. They have been made illegal for good reasons, not to stop you from having fun. All of them have severe adverse effects that can significantly affect your life.

There are dozens of chemical compounds that have the potential to be addictive and are used illegally to give artificial stimulation.

Possibly one in every 100 people is dependent upon illicit drugs in Western society, and a far higher percentage have experimented with them at one time or another.

The most commonly used illegal drugs are:

COCAINE

Cocaine (**crack**, **coke**) is a naturally derived addictive stimulant substance that is manufactured from the leaves of the coca plant which is native to South America. It is available as a white crystalline powder, and can be administered by sniffing it into the nostrils (most common), injection into a vein, or smoking. It is usually diluted with sugars such as lactose and glucose to less than 50 per cent purity.

Cocaine has no recognised medical uses (although local anaesthetics and blood vessel constrictors are derived from it), but is used illegally as a psychoactive drug to cause euphoria (artificial happiness).

Users of cocaine tend to be depressed and have a poor self-image and ego.

The more refined version of cocaine, known as '**crack**', is the only form that can be smoked, and is ten times more potent than cocaine base, and is therefore more dangerous. All forms are highly addictive, and whether they are smoked, sniffed or injected, cocaine works within seconds to **cause** euphoria (artificial happiness), mood enhancement, increased energy and stimulates the brain to increase all sensations. After use many people feel worse than before, hence they want to repeat the artificial high. With continued use, the duration of the pleasant effects becomes shorter and shorter, requiring further doses every 15 to 30 minutes to maintain the desired effect.

Side effects include severe damage to nostrils (if inhaled), fever, headache, irregular heart rate, dilation of pupils, loss of libido, infertility, impotence, breast enlargement and tenderness in both sexes, menstrual period irregularities, abnormal breast milk production, and may lead to a desire for more frequent use or stronger drugs of addiction. It will also aggravate psychiatric disturbances. Cocaine should never be used in pregnancy as it increases the risk of malformation and heart disease in the baby.

Less commonly, it may cause high blood pressure, perforation of the nasal septum, difficulty in breathing, convulsions, stroke, dementia and a heart attack.

Cocaine **interacts** with may legal medications and illegal drugs, including stimulants, antidepressants, sedatives, alcohol, heroin, marijuana and other medications acting on the brain.

Blood and urine tests can detect the presence of cocaine.

An overdose can cause convulsions, difficulty in breathing, irregular heart rate and coma, and death may occur.

The long-term outcomes for addicts is reasonably good, as cocaine is not as addictive as heroin, but more addictive than marijuana.

ECSTASY

Ecstasy is a synthetic stimulant (3,4-methylenedioxymethamphetamine) that comes as a tablet and has found favour in dance clubs since the mid 1990s. There is no easy or definite way in which to determine if someone is using Ecstasy unless a specific blood test is performed. From a parent's point of view, it is almost impossible, as the symptoms of its use could also be explained by the variable moodiness of the average teenager.

The **symptoms** of Ecstasy are rapid in onset and brief in duration. The rapid onset explains its popularity, as the user gets a high quickly after taking the tablet. The effects are increased if used with alcohol, as this increases its rate of absorption, and this also explains the fatalities that can occur.

Alcohol and ecstasy can be a suddenly fatal mixture.

Serious **adverse effects** result in an irregular heart beat that may become so serious that a heart attack and death occurs. Most users experience a period of increased perception of sounds, sights and smells that makes the world seem a more exciting place. It can also result in sexual disinhibition, hallucinations and general euphoria.

After the high has worn off, the user may be moody, drowsy, have red and sore eyes, be nauseated and vomit, be poorly coordinated and have poor coordination.

GAMMA-HYDROXYBUTYRATE

Gamma-hydroxybutyrate (**GHB**) is an illegal drug that is used to give effects similar to those of alcohol. GHB is found naturally in the body and assists in the transmission of nerve signals. As with many such substances, it has many alternative names including GBH, fantasy, grievous bodily harm, Georgia home boy, liquid ecstasy and goop.

It was developed in the 1960s as an anaesthetic, but abandoned because of adverse **side effects** such as nausea, dizziness, vomiting, low blood pressure, poor coordination, collapse, disorientation, fits and loss of consciousness. It is now illegal to manufacture, posses or sell the substance in many countries.

It is available as a powder, which is often mixed with water, and is colourless and tasteless. As a result it can be used to spike drinks, and make the user comatose. It acts when taken in small doses to help in weight reduction, treat alcohol withdrawal and to induce sleep, and was sold by health shops for these purposes for many years.

GHB is colourless and tasteless and has been used as a rape drug.

If used regularly, it will increase the desire of the user for the effects that are considered beneficial such as an increase in mood, relaxation, disinhibition, and enhanced perception (particularly of music). As a result it is often used at rave dance parties.

The drug takes effect in about 20 minutes, and lasts one or two hours.

Overdoses may be fatal, particularly when combined with alcohol or other illegal drugs that affect the brain.

HEROIN

Narcotics, including codeine, pethidine, morphine and oxycodone, are all derived from heroin and can be abused if taken regularly or excessively. Heroin is normally used by addicts as an injection directly into a vein, but it may also be inhaled or eaten, when it has a much slower effect.

Heroin is refined from the milky juice of the opium poppy. Most abusers have personality disorders, antisocial behaviour, or are placed in situations of extreme stress.

It **causes** exaggerated happiness, relief of pain, a feeling of unreality, a sensation of bodily detachment, and contracted pupils that do not respond to light are a sign of use. Tolerance develops quickly, and with time, higher and higher doses must be used to cause the same effect.

Heroin is often combined with abuse of alcohol, smoking and synthetic drugs. Physiological problems include vomiting, constipation, brain damage (personality changes, paranoia), nerve damage (persistent pins and needles or numbness), infertility, impotence, stunting of growth in children, difficulty in breathing (to the point of stopping breathing if given in high doses) and low blood pressure.

Withdrawal causes vomiting, diarrhoea, coughing, twitching, fever, crying, excessive sweating, generalised muscle pain, rapid breathing and an intense desire for the drug. These symptoms can commence within eight to 12 hours of the last dose, and withdrawal peaks at 48 to 72 hours after withdrawal. Mild symptoms may persist for up to six months.

Heroin is the most addictive of all illegal drugs, and desperate addicts are responsible for a large proportion of crime as they try to raise enough money for their next fix.

As sterile techniques are often not followed when self-injecting, the veins and skin at the injection site become infected and scarred. Blood and urine tests can detect the presence of narcotics.

One quarter of heroin addicts will die within ten years of commencing the habit as a direct result of the heroin use, and a rising proportion will die from complications of the intravenous injections such as AIDS, septicaemia and hepatitis B, C and D.

KETAMINE

Ketamine was initially used as an anaesthetic, but is now rarely used on humans except in areas where an anaesthetist is not available. It is still widely used as a veterinary anaesthetic, and used illegally as a mood enhancer. It may be referred to as 'Special K'.

Ketamine is a favourite drug at rave parties where users never seem to tire.

Ketamine is colourless and odourless and may be used illegally as a tablet, liquid or injected. In low doses it acts as a stimulant, causes loss of coordination (users may dance for hours in an uncoordinated manner), and induces artificial happiness and a floating sensation.

Side effects may include nausea, vomiting, slurred speech, headache, muscle spasms and numbness. Some users may feel they are about to die, and they may be very stressed when the drug wears off. In other cases, the anaesthetic effect may cause users to unknowingly injure themselves (e.g. not be aware that a cigarette has burnt down to their fingers). Psychological dependence may occur.

In overdose, breathing slows and heart rate increases, vision is impaired and convulsions may occur.

LSD

Lysergic acid diethylamide (LSD) is a synthetic **psychedelic** drug that was first developed in 1947. Its use peaked in the late 1960s, but it is no longer widely used.

*Although LSD is still around, the hippy drug of
the sixties is no longer a cool drug to use.*

LSD is taken by mouth in pill form. It **causes** a rapid heart rate, high blood pressure, dilation of pupils, tremor, terror, panic and high fever within a few minutes of being swallowed. Addicts seek the hallucinations, illusions and happy mood that also occur. The actions last for 12 to 18 hours after swallowing the tablet.

Long-term effects include psychoses, personality changes, schizophrenia, deterioration in intelligence, poor memory and inability to think in abstract terms. Tolerance to LSD develops rapidly, and higher and higher doses must be taken to obtain the same effect. Death as a direct effect of LSD is rare, and there are no significant effects after withdrawal of the drug.

MARIJUANA

Marijuana (**cannabis, hashish, 'grass'** or **'pot'**) is an addictive drug that is taken into the body by smoking or eating. The concentrated resin from the plant (hashish) is stronger and more dangerous than marijuana, and produces a more noticeable effect. Marijuana is made from the hemp plant, *Cannabis sativa* which has as its active ingredient the chemical tetrahydrocannabinol (THC). THC occurs in all parts of the cannabis plant and is a depressant drug, not a stimulant.

Users tend to have a poor self-image and ego.

Initially the drug **causes** excessive happiness, followed by a long period of depression and drowsiness. If used daily for a few weeks it eventually ceases to have its original effect, and the user must increase the dose to reach the same level of intoxication, which is how addiction develops. Blood and urine tests can detect the presence of THC.

Most drugs dissolve in water, but THC dissolves in the body's fat, and so stores of the drug can be established in the system. This leads to a prolonged withdrawal stage, and the frightening **flashbacks** that regular users experience when a sudden release of the drug from the body's fat stores occurs. These flashbacks can occur without warning for weeks after the last use of marijuana, and may cause hallucinations while working or driving and can therefore place others at risk.

Long-term use may cause an increased risk of bronchitis, lung cancer and other respiratory diseases associated with smoking; decreased concentration, memory and learning abilities; interference with sex hormone production; and cannabis psychosis, which is similar to schizophrenia. Cannabis is often also used with other drugs to intensify its effects, often in unpredictable ways. Using cannabis and alcohol together can be much more dangerous than using either drug by itself.

Marijuana is more addictive and damaging than alcohol, but there is a better long-term prognosis than with other illicit drugs, unless the user moves to using stronger and more addictive substances.

MESCALINE

Mescaline is a naturally-occurring psychedelic drug found in several types of cactus species, but most commonly the **Peyote** and San Pedro cacti, which also contain a large variety of related psychoactive compounds. Mescaline belongs to a family of compounds known as phenethylamines, making it quite distinct from the other major psychedelics such as LSD, but the synthetic psychedelic ecstasy is also a phenethylamine.

In prehistoric times peyote was used throughout Central and South America in various rituals.

After alcohol, mescaline is probably the oldest mood-modifying drug.

Mescaline was first extracted from cacti in 1896. From 1919 it was used by psychiatrists, but in 1953 the popular novelist Aldous Huxley brought it to the attention of the public. Today, natives throughout America still perform sacred Peyote rituals that purportedly put one in touch with supernatural and divinatory powers.

In most countries Peyote and mescaline are illegal, but in the US members of the Native American Church are permitted to use it. It causes relaxation, an intensity of senses and hallucinations lasting six to 18 hours, but stomach discomfort is a common side effect of mescaline use, and the cacti are difficult to eat without processing.

STIMULANTS

The most common stimulants are amphetamines, and tablets are used in medicine to treat mild depression, disorders of excessive sleep, some types of senility and (rather strangely) over-activity in children. They have been known to be abused by long-distance truck drivers and others who wish to stay awake for long periods of time. Dependence upon these drugs can develop rapidly.

Examples include dexamphetamine and methylphenidate (Ritalin). **Side effects** may include insomnia, restlessness, nausea, dry mouth, difficult urination and tremor. They must not be used in pregnancy, depression, hypertension and thyroid disease.

Other stimulants (e.g. ephedrine, pseudoephedrine) are used in very low doses to dry up excessive nose secretions during a common cold, and have been extracted and concentrated from these medications to give an exaggerated high.

TREATMENTS

THE TREATMENT OPTIONS AVAILABLE FOR ALL TYPES OF ADDICTIVE DRUGS ARE:

- Gradual withdrawal while receiving counselling and medical support.

- Immediate drug withdrawal ('cold turkey') under medical supervision.

- Halfway houses that remove the patient from the environment in which drug taking is encouraged.

- Individual or group psychotherapy.

Addicts must want to be treated before they can be successfully treated.
A supportive environment and family dramatically increase the success rate.

The treatment options available for users of **heroin** and other addictive narcotics vary somewhat from other illegal drugs as heroin is far more addictive. The options are:

- Gradual withdrawal while receiving counselling and medical support.

- Immediate drug withdrawal ('cold turkey') while hospitalised in a specialised unit, sometimes combined with other drugs that are used temporarily to reduce the symptoms associated with the drug withdrawal.

- Substitution of heroin with a prescribed medication (e.g. methadone) on a medium- to long-term basis before it is slowly withdrawn.

- Naltrexone may be used to flush heroin from the body, and relieve the addiction within a few days, a process that must be undertaken under strict supervision in a specialised clinic. Naltrexone may also be used long-term to reduce the desire for heroin.

- Halfway houses that remove the patient from the environment in which drug taking is encouraged.

- Individual or group psychotherapy.

- Education of intravenous drug users of the dangers associated with their habit (e.g. the development of AIDS or hepatitis B).

CURIOSITY

Coca Cola derives its name from the fact that the original nineteenth century formula contained cocaine. This was removed long ago, but it still contains a significant amount of the stimulant caffeine. No wonder it was so popular!

IMPOTENCE

Impotence may become a psychological impediment for a man, significantly affecting his ability to interact with the opposite sex, and making him antisocial and depressed. This should never be allowed to happen, as men can look after themselves by obtaining appropriate advice and treatment from their general practitioner.

Impotence is the inability of a man to obtain a firm erection of the penis when sexually stimulated. It is a very common problem, and something that every man experiences at some time, particularly in middle age and older.

PENIS ANATOMY

The penis has the twin tasks of passing urine out of the body in a controlled manner, and being the organ used in male sexual intercourse. During sex, its length is designed to allow sperm to be deposited as close to the cervix as possible.

At rest, the penis is a soft sausage-like structure hanging limply down from the base of the abdomen where it is attached to the bones of the pelvis. However, it is

MALE GENITAL ANATOMY

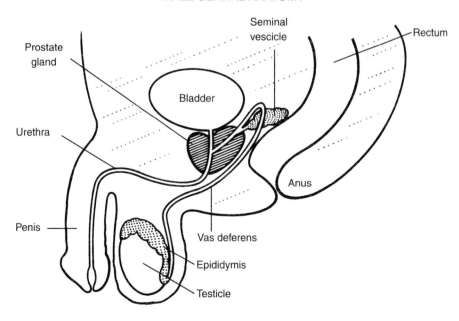

233

made up of two sausage-like tubes of spongy tissue (the corpora cavernosa) and these fill with blood under high pressure when the man is sexually aroused so that the penis becomes firm, erect and distended and is thus able to penetrate the vagina.

Sperm are manufactured in the testicles and travel through the male reproductive system, combining with a white sticky fluid to form semen. At the height of sexual excitation, or orgasm, the semen is ejaculated.

The penis discharges both urine and semen, transported along its length by the urethra. This is different from women in whom the organs for sex and the organs for urinating are separate. It is not possible, however, for a man to release both urine and semen at the same time.

Smegma acts as a lubricant between the head of the penis and the foreskin.

The head of the penis, or **glans**, is a highly sensitive zone which is easily sexually stimulated. Where the glans meets the shaft of the penis, the sensitive skin covering the penis folds back on itself to form the prepuce or foreskin. It is this part of the skin that is removed by circumcision.

Circumcision in English society started after the Crimean war, during which many men had to have circumcisions due to infections from poor hygiene.

CIRCUMCISION

Circumcision has been commonly performed in much of the English-speaking world for several generations, but in more recent times it has been seen as unnecessary surgery performed for no medical reason. Because the foreskin is the most sexually sensitive part of the penis, it is now considered possible that a man's later sexual pleasure may be diminished by the operation.

Sometimes the foreskin is so tight that the child cannot urinate properly (a condition called **phimosis**) and in this case circumcision may be essential. The condition will not usually become apparent until the age of about five.

ERECTION

The process of erection is one over which the man has no direct control as it is a local reflex in the pelvis triggered by sexual excitement.

CAUSES OF IMPOTENCE

A wide range of diseases may cause impotence, and these must be excluded by appropriate investigations before a psychological cause is diagnosed, or impotence treatment is given. If a cause is found, it should be specifically treated to resolve the problem. Only if no particular cause can be diagnosed should the various impotence treatments available be used.

A lot of impotence is caused by a **psychological** feedback mechanism. For one of the reasons listed below, a man may fail to develop an erection when attempting sex. He will feel embarrassed and ashamed about this, particularly if it is with a new partner. The next time he tries to have sex, he will be anxious as to whether he will be able to perform. This anxiety will make him concentrate on trying to get an erection, which is an almost certain way in which to prevent an erection. After two failures, the anxiety increases, which further decreases the chance of success at subsequent attempts. It requires the patient understanding of the man's partner and the continuing advice of a doctor, to overcome this erection failure cycle.

The harder a man tries to have an erection, the less likely he is to succeed.

Common causes of impotence include the overuse of **alcohol** (which increases the desire, while reducing the ability), **stress** and anxiety in any aspect of life, difficult circumstances (e.g. lack of privacy), heavy **smoking**, illegal **drugs** (e.g. marijuana, heroin) and **medications** (e.g. those used to lower blood pressure and improve depression, sedatives, cimetidine, clofibrate, digoxin).

OTHER POSSIBLE CAUSES OF IMPOTENCE INCLUDE:

• depression

• pituitary gland disease (gland in the brain which controls all other glands including the testes)

• testicular diseases or injury

• poorly controlled diabetes mellitus (sugar diabetes)

• high levels of cholesterol may cause hardening of the arteries (atherosclerosis) and make it difficult for the blood to get into the penis

• cancer of the prostate gland may interfere with the normal nerve and blood vessel reflexes that allow an erection.

Rare causes of impotence include Peyronie disease (a replacement of the blood-filled sacs by fibrous scar tissue), multiple sclerosis, paraplegia and quadriplegia, lead poisoning and Klinefelter syndrome (a chromosomal abnormality).

TREATMENT

Psychological factors may be overcome by not planning sex, but relaxing and waiting until the right circumstances occur spontaneously. Mutual heavy petting and erotic stimulation without the expectation of sex, sexual toys, pornography and vacuum pumps to create an erection may be used. Once spontaneous erections develop, sex may start again.

NUMEROUS MEDICATIONS ARE ALSO AVAILABLE INCLUDING:

• alprostadil (Caverject) injections into the penis

• alprostadil (Muse) pellets may be inserted into the urethra (urine tube in the penis)

- sildenafil (Viagra), tadalafil (Cialis) and vardenafil (Levitra) tablets.

Several other medications are under development (e.g. apomorphine).

ALPROSTADIL

Alprostadil is combined with prostaglandin e1 as an injection with the trade name **Caverject**. It is used for the treatment of impotence. An injection is given into the penis, about one-third of the way from the base, at the two o'clock or ten o'clock position. An erection usually occurs within ten minutes. Side effects may include pain and bruising at the injection site, and a prolonged erection. It should not be used in patients taking anticoagulants or with any infection in the blood or groin.

SILDENAFIL

Better known by its brand name of **Viagra**, sildenafil is a medication used for the treatment of impotence (inability to obtain erection of the penis). After the medication is taken, it may take one to four hours to be effective, and its effect may last up to 12 hours. An erection does not occur just because the tablet is taken – sexual stimulation is also necessary.

It must never be taken by patients with heart disease or angina, while taking nitrate drugs (e.g. glyceryl trinitrate) used for angina, or in patients with liver disease, high or low blood pressure or with a history of a recent stroke. Side effects may include headache, flushing, blue haze in vision and indigestion.

It has been argued that Viagra has liberated men as much as the contraceptive pill liberated women.

TADALAFIL

Tadalafil (**Cialis**) works in the same way as sildenafil and has much the same precautions and interactions. Its advantage is that it can be taken with food and alcohol, and it works faster, lasts longer, and has fewer side effects than its famous competitor.

VARDENAFIL

Vardenafil (**Levitra**) is another medication that works in much the same way as sildenafil and tadalafil. Do not take it if suffering from significant heart disease, angina, severe kidney or liver disease, low blood pressure, recent stroke or heart attack or inherited retinal diseases of the eye. It should be used with caution in liver and kidney disease, a deformed penis, sickle cell anaemia, history of priapism (prolonged erections of penis), multiple myeloma, leukaemia, bleeding disorders and active peptic ulcer. Lower doses are used in the elderly. Common side effects may include nausea, heartburn and dizziness, while unusual ones may be flushing, watery nose, headache, light-sensitive eyes and blurred vision. Rarely, muscle spasms, fainting and low blood pressure occur. There is a severe interaction with nitrates used for angina, and milder interactions are possible with erythromycin, amyl nitrate, ritonavir, ketoconazole, indinavir, itraconazole, alphablockers and even grapefruit juice.

EJACULATION
EXPLANATION

The ejaculation of semen from the penis is the culmination of sexual intercourse in men, and makes it possible for his female partner to fall pregnant. Ejaculation may also be stimulated by masturbation.

The man feels a build-up of pressure in the base of the penis and testicles, and then with a release of pressure and pleasure, the semen is forced down the urethra by contraction of the seminal vesicles in the groin and the muscles at the base of the penis. Ejaculation may last in an intense phase for ten to 30 seconds, but semen may leak from the penis for some minutes afterwards. The penis usually becomes flaccid and soft shortly after ejaculation.

EJACULATION FAILURE

An inability to ejaculate (ejaculatory failure or retarded ejaculation) during sexual intercourse is the male equivalent of a failed orgasm in the female. Some men can ejaculate when masturbating, or with oral sex, but not with vaginal sex. This problem may be a drug side effect, or due to psychological problems, an inhibited personality, subconscious or conscious anxiety, or fear of losing self-control. Any significant underlying disease should be excluded.

Treatment involves progressive desensitisation with the assistance of a co-operative sex partner, who initially masturbates their partner to ejaculation, and over a series of weeks, learns to bring him almost to the point of ejaculation by hand stimulation before allowing vaginal sex. Another technique involves additional stimulation of the penis during intercourse by the woman massaging the penis with her fingers while the man thrusts in and out of the vagina. Distracting the man from consciously holding back the ejaculation by passionate kissing or other stimulation of the face or back during intercourse may also help. Reasonable results can be achieved with commitment to the treatment program.

LACK OF EJACULATION

The male ejaculation or discharge of semen at the time of sexual intercourse sometimes goes awry, and instead of travelling from the sperm storage sac (seminal vesicle) in the groin, into the penis and out through the urethra, the ejaculate goes backwards into the urinary bladder.

Causes include prostate surgery or disease, injury to the pelvis or the spinal cord, diabetes, or a tumour of the spinal cord. It may also be due to psychological stress, a stroke, tumour or cancer in the brain, compression to or damage of the nerves in the pelvis, Parkinson's disease, or to an abnormality the individual was born with (when it will usually become evident soon after puberty).

Sometimes it may be a side effect of medications such as those used to treat high blood pressure, psychiatric conditions, and diuretics (which remove excess fluid from the body). Often no cause can be found.

Men who have difficulty in ejaculating may be helped by a change in sexual position so that the woman is on top.

PREMATURE EJACULATION

Premature ejaculation can be very embarrassing for a man. He is just about to have sex, or has just started, when he finds he is no longer able to control himself and he ejaculates his sperm. The penis then becomes soft and flaccid. This leaves his partner sexually frustrated and may damage a relationship.

The most common **cause** is psychological stress, emotional upsets and perform-ance anxiety. The more the man tries to please his partner, the more trouble he may have with the problem. The man may also be over-stimulated, excited and foreplay may have been too intense.

There are virtually no diseases or physical conditions which cause this problem.

Therapists can teach appropriate techniques, which involve the co-operation of the partner, to overcome premature ejaculation.

One simple **treatment** is the penis squeeze. If a man feels that ejaculation is imminent, he indicates this to his partner, and all sexual activity ceases. The man, or his partner, uses the thumb and forefinger to squeeze the penis firmly from above and below, about one third of the way down the shaft from the head of the penis. This will cause the sensation of imminent ejaculation to cease, and the penis may start to become less rigid. Sexual activity can then recommence.

RETROGRADE EJACULATION

Retrograde ejaculation occurs if semen is ejaculated from the sac at the base of the penis (seminal vesicle), but instead of passing along the urethra in the penis to the outside, it travels in the other direction and enters the bladder. It is usually a complication of surgery in the area (e.g. to the prostate), due to advanced diabetes or a side effect of some uncommon drugs. The man has the sensation of orgasm during sex, but no ejaculation occurs.

Unfortunately, no treatment is available, but the resultant infertility may be overcome by microsurgical techniques to remove sperm from the man and artificially inseminate a woman.

LIBIDO

Libido is the emotional desire for sexual intercourse and the natural instinct for sexual satisfaction.

LACK OF LIBIDO

Libido is controlled by the brain and not the testes or ovaries, although diseases of these glands can certainly have an adverse effect on libido as they do not respond to stimuli from the brain.

To enjoy and be successful in achieving sexual intercourse, both partners mustbe relaxed, secure and comfortable. Psychological **stress** of any sort will reduce sexual desire. Examples can be as wide-ranging as worries about work, money, pregnancy, discovery (will the children come in?), the relationship itself or disease.

Many **psychiatric** conditions, but particularly depression, will remove desire for sex. Difficulty in sleeping, loss of interest in other activities and poor self esteem are other signs of depression.

Failure of any major organ of the body (e.g. heart, liver, kidney) or any other serious disease will affect the normal hormonal and chemical balances, as well as causing stress and anxiety, and sex becomes something to be remembered rather than sought.

Lack of privacy = lack of libido.

Disease, infection, tumour (e.g. Fröhlich syndrome), injury or cancer of the pituitary gland under the centre of the brain will affect libido. This tiny gland is the conductor of the gland orchestra in the body, and is itself directly controlled by the brain. If for one of these reasons it does not produce the necessary hormones to stimulate the testes or ovaries, they will not release the appropriate sex hormones (testosterone and oestrogen) to allow appropriate sexual responses. Rarely, the pituitary gland may become over-active, and over-stimulate the sex glands to drain them of their hormones.

The part of the brain controlling the pituitary gland can itself be affected by a stroke, bleeding, injury, tumour, cancer or abscess. Parkinson's disease and other degenerative conditions of the brain will both reduce desire and ability.

In men, any disease that reduces the production of testosterone (male hormone) in the testes will reduce libido. Examples include infections (orchitis), tumours (e.g. cancer), cysts and torsion (twisting to cut off the blood supply). Other causes of low libido in men include enlargement of the prostate gland and poorly controlled diabetes mellitus.

Women find that their libido varies during the month, usually being highest at the time of ovulation (when they are most likely to get pregnant) half-way between the start of one period and the next, and lowest during a menstrual period. Pregnancy also lowers libido for its duration, and breast feeding has a similar effect on the hormones. Other causes of low libido in women include tumours or cysts of the ovary, and during the menopause, when there is a lack of oestrogen, sex may be uncomfortable as well as undesirable.

Numerous **drugs**, legal, illegal and prescribed, can reduce libido. Examples include alcohol, heroin, marijuana, steroids, antihistamines (e.g. cold preparations), benzodiazepines (e.g. diazepam, oxazepam), fluid pills and some of those used to treat depression (tricyclics) and decrease high blood pressure (betablockers).

CURIOSITY

Although it contains no bone, an erect penis can still be fractured by over-enthusiastic sex or other injury. The injury is actually a rupture of the corpora cavernosa which contain blood under pressure during an erection.

INCONTINENCE

Incontinence is an inability to control the release of bodily fluids. It usually refers to incontinence of urine, but may also refer to faeces.

The best way for women to look after themselves and avoid urinary incontinence is to perform pelvic floor exercises regularly for a couple of months after childbirth.

INCONTINENCE OF URINE

This is the inability to control the outflow of urine so that wetting of clothing or bedding occurs. It is a problem that affects women far more than men. Repeated urinary infections may be a complication.

CAUSES

In women, there is normally an acute angle between the bladder and the opening into the urethra (tube leading to the outside). If this angle is reduced for any reason, the woman will become more prone to urinary incontinence.

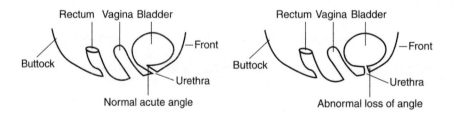

Diagrammatic cross-section through a woman's pelvis showing normal angle of urethra and bladder that prevents incontinence, and the abnormal situation after childbirth when the angle may be lost.

Alcohol and **caffeine** are both known to increase the production of urine, and if too much of the former is consumed, the person may lose their inhibitions and urinate inappropriately.

A sudden severe fright or shock, and extreme fear, may cause loss of bladder control.

An **infection** of the bladder or kidney will result in the frequent, painful passage of small amounts of urine. Women may find their control of urination to be compromised with these infections.

Although embarrassing and uncomfortable, the only health risk from urinary incontinence is an increased incidence of bladder infections.

Childbirth can cause damage to the muscles that control the release of urine, and may result in long-term problems with **stress incontinence**, so that every time the woman laughs, coughs or exercises, she passes a small amount of urine. The loss of muscle tone in the floor of the pelvis can result in the same problem. The muscle tone in this area is maintained by the female hormone, oestrogen, so the lack of oestrogen at menopause is usually responsible. Obesity will further aggravate the problem. Pelvic floor exercises supervised by a physiotherapist, hormone replacement therapy, weight loss and surgery can all help control these causes of incontinence.

A number of **medications** may aggravate incontinence. Examples include blood pressure medications (particularly prazosin), fluid producing medications (diuretics), tranquillisers, lithium and some depression-treating drugs (tricyclic antidepressants).

A **fistula** (abnormal opening) between the bladder and vagina may be caused by a very difficult childbirth, particularly in poorer countries. These poor women constantly dribble urine through their vagina.

OTHER CAUSES OF URINARY INCONTINENCE MAY INCLUDE:

- surgery to the pelvis and genitals (e.g. hysterectomy)

- stroke (cerebrovascular accident)

- loss of consciousness

- epileptic fit

- damage to the brain (e.g. cerebral palsy, tumour, Parkinson's disease)

- senility or dementia (e.g. Alzheimer disease)

- tumours or stones in the bladder

- pelvic injury

- multiple sclerosis

- injury to the spinal cord (e.g. paraplegia or quadriplegia)

- poorly controlled diabetes mellitus

- diabetes insipidus (disease of the pituitary gland in the brain).

Rarer causes include severe allergy reactions affecting the genitals, psychiatric disorders (e.g. severe depression) and birth abnormalities of the bladder structure.

INVESTIGATION

X-rays of the bladder and kidneys, and cystoscopy (looking into the bladder through a thin tube) can be used to investigate the cause of the incontinence. Sometimes videourodynamics, a procedure in which the passing of urine is watched, measured and X-rayed, is performed.

Incontinence is not a disease but a symptom, and the responsible disease needs to be diagnosed before any treatment can start.

TREATMENT

The main way to treat incontinence is to treat any identifiable cause (e.g. infection). Unfortunately, particularly in older women, this may be impractical.

Surgery may be performed to tighten the muscles of the pelvic floor and improve the angle between the bladder and the opening into the urethra. This is a common operation in middle-aged women who have completed their families.

Medications play only a very small role in the treatment of urinary incontinence that has an anatomical cause, but drugs such as pitressin may be tried.

In many cases it is necessary for a catheter to be inserted or urine-absorbing panty pads to be worn. These are very practical and if changed regularly, do not smell or cause discomfort.

In men, a penile sheath can be used instead of a catheter.

BED WETTING

Bed wetting is a medical problem that makes businessmen dread overnight trips to a conference, causes marriages to break up, stops teenagers from spending the night at a friend's, and drives the mothers of some children to desperation.

The medical term for bed wetting is enuresis.

CAUSES

Normally, urine is retained in the bladder by the contraction of a ring-shaped bundle of muscle that surrounds the bladder opening. When one wishes to pass urine, this ring of muscle relaxes, and the muscles in the wall of the bladder and around the abdominal cavity contract to squirt the urine out in a steady stream.

Those who are bed wetters tend to sleep very deeply, and during the deepest phases of this sleep, when all the main muscles of the body are totally relaxed, the sphincter ring muscle that retains the urine in the bladder also relaxes. Because there is no associated contraction of the muscles in the bladder wall or elsewhere, the urine just dribbles out slowly in the night, not in a hard stream.

Many children may be three or four years old before bladder control is obtained.

The first step is to **investigate** the patient to exclude any cause for bed wetting. Chronic urine infections, structural abnormalities of the bladder and other rarer conditions may cause a weakness or excessive irritability of the bladder. These problems must be excluded by urine tests and X-rays.

In children, lifestyle stresses (e.g. family break up, moving home, hospital admission), social pressures (e.g. poverty, overcrowding, lack of privacy) and excessively strict toilet training may cause psychological barriers to bladder control. Mental subnormality may make it impossible for a child to learn the reasons for bladder control.

Other uncommon possible causes include diabetes mellitus (lack of insulin production in the pancreas), diabetes insipidus, epilepsy, paraplegia, Bartter syndrome (inherited disorder that causes short stature, thirst, frequent passing of urine and muscle weakness), spina bifida (congenital damage to the spinal cord) or a fracture of the pelvis.

A number of very rare brain disorders may also cause enuresis.

Premature treatment of bed wetting can cause
significant psychological problems.

TREATMENT
There are several steps in any treatment regime for this condition, but they should not be started before five years of age. They include:

- restrict **fluids** for three hours before bedtime, take child to the toilet during the night, and establish a reward system for dry nights.

- a bed wetting **alarm** that consists of a moisture-sensitive pad that is placed under the patient, a battery and an alarm. When it becomes wet from the first small dribble of urine, it sounds the alarm, the patient is woken, and can empty the bladder before returning to sleep. After a few weeks use, most people learn to waken before the alarm.

- the medication amitriptyline (**Tryptanol**) is taken every night to alter the type of sleep. Over a few weeks, the dosage is slowly lowered and hopefully, the bad sleep habits and bed wetting do not return.

- **desmopressin** nasal spray at bed time acts on the pituitary gland in the brain, and this instructs the kidney to reduce the amount of urine produced during the night.

- psychotherapy in the most resistant cases.

Please remember that treatment before five years of age can cause permanent sleep disturbances in a child, but there are no serious long-term medical consequences from bed wetting.

Incontinence of Faeces
Incontinence of faeces is the inability to prevent the escape of faecal matter through the anus resulting in anything from slight staining of the underwear to total loss of the bowel contents on an irregular basis.

CAUSES
Severe **diarrhoea** can be an obvious and embarrassing cause of incontinence of faeces (soiling), due to the massive amounts of hard-to-control fluid present in the lower bowel.

The inability to control the passing of faeces may be due to **psychological** or psychiatric conditions, particularly in the elderly. A loss of inhibitions associated with a dementia (e.g. Alzheimer disease) is a common cause, while psychiatric patients may use it as an attention-seeking device.

In children, **behavioural** disorders or emotional stress may be responsible.

Soiling may be due to damage to the brain (e.g. a stroke, cerebral palsy) or the nerves supplying the muscle ring around the anus (e.g. paraplegia, fractured pelvis).

In advanced **pregnancy** the pressure on the lower bowel from the growing baby may make control of faeces difficult. Damage to the anus from a difficult birth may be a temporary or, very rarely, a permanent cause of faecal incontinence. Surgery can be performed to control the problem in these cases.

Any surgery to the anus, for problems as diverse as piles and cancer, may be responsible for loss of control.

A greatly dilated lower bowel (**megacolon**) may cause large amounts of hard faeces to collect just inside the anus, and remain for a long time, while watery faeces flows around the outside of this faecal mass in the bowel, to leak out through the anus.

No one over sixty should ever trust a fart.

TREATMENT

The treatment of faecal incontinence is again initially tackled by treating any identifiable cause.

The next step is to modify the diet to reduce the production of gas and to make the faeces firmer. Medications may also be used for this purpose, and interestingly, fibre supplements that are used for constipation may also be used for loose motions to give them more form.

Sometimes medications to slow over-active bowels may be used, but the alternating use of laxatives and antidiarrhoea medications is not appropriate. Regular nappy changes may often be the only solution.

CURIOSITY

Extract from a 1797 medical text book:

'An India rubber bottle, properly fashioned and applied, is best for the incontinence of urine. It is an affliction I have never seen cured'.

INDIGESTION

Indigestion can be any problem in dealing with the food that is eaten, from burping and heartburn to nausea and abdominal pain that is aggravated by eating.

You can look after yourself and avoid indigestion by sensible eating habits, eating slowly and taking a sip of liquid between each mouthful.

BURPING

Burping is bringing up air or gas from the stomach into the mouth. That air has to get into the stomach in the first place to be burped, and in the vast majority of cases, it gets in by being swallowed.

People who **eat quickly** tend to swallow air with their food. If a person is nervous, before an exam or interview etc., they may swallow more often as a sign of **anxiety** and take in extra air. Drinking **fizzy liquids** such as lemonade or beer will also take gas into the stomach. If small amounts of gas are swallowed, it will move on into the gut to be absorbed or passed through the anus as flatus. Otherwise excess gas tries to escape by going up and out through the mouth.

Smoking and alcohol slacken the lower oesophageal sphincter allowing the reflux of acid.

This is not as easy as it seems because there is a muscular valve (lower oesophageal sphincter) at the top of the stomach that stops the food and acid in the stomach from running back up the gullet into the mouth with bending or lying down. Only when sufficient pressure builds up, or the person can relax the muscular valve themselves, can the air escape, causing the often unexpected and embarrassing explosion. When the gas escapes, it may take small amounts of acid and food with it, causing heartburn or nausea at the same time.

A **hiatus hernia** occurs when part of the stomach pushes up through the diaphragm (the sheet of muscle that separates the chest and abdominal cavities) into the chest. The lower oesophageal sphincter that prevents stomach acid from coming back up into the oesophagus then fails to work effectively, allowing reflux oesophagitis to occur very easily.

The excess amounts of acid present in the stomach of patients with a peptic ulcer may also damage the muscle ring at the lower end of the oesophagus, and increase the amount of burping.

DYSPEPSIA

Belly pains that are made worse by eating are referred to as **dyspepsia**.

The stomach contains very concentrated hydrochloric acid that is used to digest food. Extra amounts are secreted when food is eaten, or even the smell of food may trigger acid secretion. The stomach is lined with a thick mucus that protects it from being digested by the acid it contains. **Gastritis** is an inflammation of the stomach caused by the mucus lining becoming too thin, or excessive acid secretion. Upper belly pain, often made worse after eating, and burping, are the most common symptoms. If the acid succeeds in damaging the stomach or small intestine, a peptic ulcer will develop, and pain may become more constant.

Severe **anxiety**, and physical or emotional stress, may increase acid production and cause gastritis or inflammation of the first part of the small intestine (the duodenum).

If stomach acid runs up into the unprotected gullet (oesophagus), particularly after eating a large meal, intense burning pain will be felt behind the breast bone, and a bitter taste and burping may be experienced. This is **reflux oesophagitis**.

Cholecystitis is an inflammation or infection of the gall bladder, usually caused by gall stones that have formed within it. In most cases it causes pain and indigestion, particularly after eating a fatty meal, but if the gall bladder becomes very swollen it may obstruct the bile duct to prevent bilirubin from leaving the liver to cause jaundice (yellow skin).

Other causes of dyspepsia include pancreatitis (damage to the pancreas by infection, gall stones, alcoholism or a cancer), irritable bowel syndrome, cancer of the stomach and food allergies.

Some **medications** (e.g. nonsteroidal anti-inflammatory drugs used for arthritis) may also irritate the stomach.

HEARTBURN

Heartburn is a form of indigestion which causes a burning pain behind the breast bone in the centre of he chest. It is often associated with burping and a bitter taste at the back of the throat. The cause is a leakage of concentrated hydrochloric acid from the stomach up into the gullet (oesophagus) which runs from the back of the throat, down through the chest to the stomach. The stomach is lined with a thick layer of acid-resistant mucus, but the oesophagus lacks this protection, and any stomach acid entering it causes burning pain.

Common simple **causes** include over-eating, rapid eating, excess alcohol consumption and advanced pregnancy (pressure of the enlarged womb causes acid to be forced up into the oesophagus from the stomach). Smoking can be an aggravating factor in all causes of heartburn.

More serious causes include inflammation of the oesophagus from acid repeatedly coming up from the stomach (reflux oesophagitis) and a hiatus hernia (part of the stomach slips up into the chest cavity).

Sometimes a peptic ulcer (ulceration of the stomach from excess acid production) or, rarely, a cancer of the stomach or oesophagus may cause heartburn.

A number of serious conditions may cause pain in the chest that can be mistaken for heartburn. A heart attack is the most common of these, but a blood clot in the

HEARTBURN

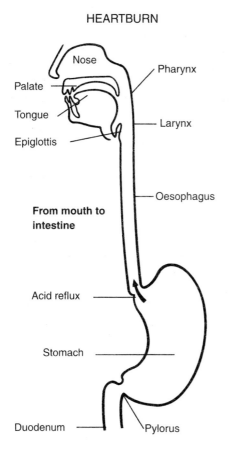

Nose
Pharynx
Palate
Tongue
Larynx
Epiglottis

Oesophagus

From mouth to intestine

Acid reflux

Stomach

Duodenum
Pylorus

lungs, angina, (reduced blood supply to the heart) and inflammation of the membrane around the heart (pericarditis) may also be responsible. As a result, any heartburn that does not respond rapidly to simple medications (e.g. antacids) must be checked by a doctor.

Chest pain may also be angina or a heart attack, and not indigestion, so must not be ignored.

HEARTBURN IN PREGNANCY

Indigestion or heartburn affects about half of all pregnant women because during pregnancy the lower oesophageal sphincter that closes off the upper part of the stomach from the oesophagus (gullet) loosens and allows digestive juices from the stomach to flow back up the oesophagus and irritate it. In late pregnancy the enlarging uterus presses on the stomach and aggravates the condition.

Heartburn can be very uncomfortable but is not harmful. Symptoms may be reduced by eating small, frequent meals, so that there is never too much food present but always enough to absorb the stomach acid. Antacids can usually be taken safely at most stages of pregnancy, and may be used to relieve more severe symptoms. The problem disappears when the baby is born.

REFLUX OESOPHAGITIS

Reflux oesophagitis (gastro-oesophageal reflux disease – GORD) is the back-flow of acid from the stomach up through a normally closed muscle ring (lower oesophageal sphincter) into the lower end of the oesophagus (gullet). It most commonly occurs in babies and overweight elderly men.

Some infants have a defect or temporary weakness in the muscle ring at the bottom of the oesophagus.

IN ADULTS, REFLUX OESOPHAGITIS MAY BE CAUSED BY:

• obesity

• smoking

- over-eating

- hiatus hernia

- rapid eating

- excess alcohol

- stress

- anxiety

- poor posture

These causes may result in the excessive production of acid in the stomach and/or slackness in the muscle ring at the lower end of the oesophagus.

Infants with reflux are in pain, with crying and irritability the main symptoms.

Adults experience a burning sensation behind the breast bone (heartburn), a bitter taste on the back of the tongue and burping as gas escapes easily from the stomach. It is often worse at night after a large meal when the patient is lying down. If attacks are regular, ulcers may develop.

Complications include scarring and narrowing of the lower end of the oesophagus to the point where it may be difficult to swallow food (Barrett syndrome), severe bleeding from ulcers in the oesophagus, and cancer of the oesophagus.

A bitter taste at the back of the mouth is called waterbrash,
and is characteristic of acid reflux.

The reflux can be proved by gastroscopy or a barium meal X-ray.

Most children will grow out of the problem, but to ease the symptoms, position the child with head elevated while feeding, give small frequent thickened feeds, burp the baby regularly, loosen the nappy before feeds and do not allow the child to lie flat after a feed. If not adequately helped, preventive medication is given as a mixture.

Management in adults involves weight loss, raising the head of the bed, having the main meal in the middle of the day, avoiding bending and heavy lifting, stopping smoking and reducing alcohol. Antacids to reduce the acid concentration in the stomach, and medication to empty the stomach faster (e.g. prokinetic agents such as cisapride) and reduce acid production (e.g. H2 receptor antagonists and proton pump inhibitors) can be taken. In resistant cases is it necessary to resort to quite major surgery (e.g. fundoplication).

TREATMENTS
ANTACIDS
Drugs that neutralise acid in the stomach are antacids. A very large number of these medications are available without prescription as both mixtures and tablets.

Sometimes they cause problems with the absorption of other medications if taken at the same time. They often contain multiple ingredients including aluminium hydroxide, magnesium hydroxide, and simethicone.

Antacids are available at supermarkets, and H2 receptor antagonists without a prescription from chemists.

H2 RECEPTOR ANTAGONISTS

Peptic ulcers and reflux have caused belly pains for millennia, and were poorly treated until a significant advance in medication occurred in the late 1970s with the introduction of **cimetidine**, the first of the H2 receptor antagonists.

These drugs are distantly related to antihistamines and act to cure ulcers of the stomach, duodenum and oesophagus by reducing the amount of acid secreted into the stomach. This also enables them to control reflux oesophagitis (heartburn), which may accompany a hiatus hernia, and inflammation of the stomach (gastritis) caused by excess acid. Treatment is usually rapidly effective, but must be continued for weeks or months to prevent relapses. This class of medication is now being replaced by the more potent proton pump inhibitors.

Examples of drugs in this class include cimetidine (Tagamet), famotidine (Pepcidine), nizatadine (Tazac) and ranitidine (Zantac).

Side effects are usually minimal, but may include occasional headache, diarrhoea, rash, breast enlargement in men, dizziness and tiredness. Cimetidine can sometimes interact with other drugs that control epilepsy and blood clotting.

Cimetidine has sometimes been used to treat cases of multiple skin warts with some success, but the mode of action is unknown.

PROTON PUMP INHIBITORS

This very effective class of medications was introduced in 1991, and has revolutionised the treatment of more resistant peptic ulcers and reflux oesophagitis. Proton pump inhibitors are usually prescribed when the presence of an ulcer or reflux is strongly suspected on clinical grounds, or after a gastroscopy proves the presence of an ulcer or reflux. They act by inhibiting the activity of the enzyme in the stomach lining that is responsible for acid production.

Examples include lansoprazole (Zoton), omeprazole (Losec), esomeprazole (Nexium), rabeprazole (Pariet) and pantoprazole sodium (Somac). Their side effects are minimal, but they must be used with care in pregnancy.

CURIOSITY
Extract from an 1831 medical text book:
'In the form of snuff, tobacco has not infrequently been found to produce indigestion'.

INFERTILITY

Fertility is the joint property of a man and a woman, and infertility may be due to factors in either, or between them. Couples should look after themselves by not planning too strictly, relaxing and letting nature take its course, but if a pregnancy does not develop after twelve months of 'normal marital endeavour' (as older text books so politely described sex), seek expert medical advice.

For a pregnancy to occur, an egg must be released from one of a woman's ovaries, move into the Fallopian tube, and down that towards the uterus. At the same time, sperm released during ejaculation by a man must move from the vagina through the cervix and uterus and into a Fallopian tube which contains a recently released egg. One sperm and an egg must then fuse together, start dividing into a multi-celled structure, and implant into the lining of the woman's uterus, where it can obtain nutrition from the mother and continue to grow.

About 15 per cent of couples fail to conceive after at
least 12 months of 'normal marital endeavour'.

JOINT CAUSES

If **sex** is **infrequent**, then it may occur at times when the woman is not ovulating (releasing an egg). Conception can occur in a woman on only five or six days a month, so if sex occurs only once a month, those vital days may be missed. This is actually a quite common cause of apparent infertility in this busy modern society where both potential parents may work, are stressed and over-tired. Occasionally, poor sexual technique, with ejaculation near the outside of the vagina, may be a problem.

Extremely fit athletes of both sexes who **exercise** very vigorously may have their fertility affected as sperm counts drop and ovulation fails to occur.

Diseases of the pituitary gland in the brain, hypothyroidism (an under-active thyroid gland in the neck), poorly controlled diabetes mellitus and a deficiency of vital minerals (e.g. zinc) may also be responsible for infertility in both sexes.

It takes two to tango and make a baby.

MALE INFERTILTIY

Male infertility is far easier to **investigate** than female, so the male is often checked first by being asked to provide a fresh sample of ejaculated semen for analysis in a laboratory. If this shows that the sperm are alive and healthy, and the joint factors above are absent, then investigation of the woman can commence. An abnormal sample of semen will result in extensive detailed investigations to determine the cause of the abnormality.

CAUSES

If a man is **impotent** (unable to sustain an erect penis) then obviously successful intercourse is not possible.

OTHER CAUSES OF INFERTILITY DUE TO THE MALE MAY INCLUDE:

- regularly wearing of tight clothing while exercising (e.g. bike pants) that keeps the testes against the warm flesh in the groin and overheats them

- premature ejaculation (the man ejaculates before penetration of the vagina)

- surgery to the prostate gland that causes impotence or retrograde ejaculation

- damage to the testes (e.g. torsion of both testes, injury)

- undescended testes

- failure of the testes to develop normally

- bacterial or viral infection to the testes that results in reduced sperm production

- inflammation of the testes with a mumps infection

- tumours or cancer of the testes

- irradiation of the testes

Genetic diseases, such as Klinefelter syndrome, will result in poorly functioning testes.

When he enters a new relationship, it is not unknown for a man to deliberately forget, or subconsciously repress the memory, that he has previously had a vasectomy, and the discovery of this during a physical examination may prove embarrassing to both parties.

Because it is easier, men are usually investigated before women.

SEMEN TEST

The purpose of a semen test is to determine the health of a man's sperm if he and his partner are having difficulty in conceiving a child. The man will ejaculate a sperm sample into a sterile container, which will be sent to a laboratory and examined to establish the number of sperm, whether they are normal, and if they are able to swim sufficiently strongly to make their way to the woman's Fallopian tubes to fertilise an egg. The semen sample must reach the laboratory as soon as possible after ejaculation. The man should not ejaculate for three days before the test.

Semen tests are also performed about six weeks after a vasectomy to ensure that the operation has been a success and the man is infertile.

They may also be useful to diagnose the bacteria causing an infection of the prostate gland or epididymis (sperm draining tubules at the back of the testicle).

FEMAILE INFERTILITY

Investigation of female infertility varies from relatively old-fashioned but simple methods such as keeping accurate temperature charts, to regular blood tests of hormone levels, specialised X-rays, and surgical examination of the ovaries using a laparoscope (tube into the belly).

FEMALE REPRODUCTIVE SYSTEM

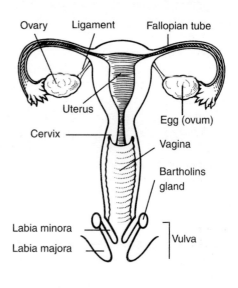

CAUSES

Vaginismus is the term used for a strong spasm of the muscles in the vagina that prevents the penis from entering. It usually results from anxiety or stress related to sex, lack of privacy, inadequate foreplay, sexual inhibitions due to a puritanical background, pain or discomfort associated with sex, or other psychological problems.

The cervix may be damaged by **surgery** for cancer or severe **infection**, or injured by an object placed in the vagina. The resultant scarring may prevent the passage of sperm.

There is no evidence that early or prolonged use of the contraceptive pill alters long-term fertility.

Endometriosis is a sinister disease, which is due to cells that normally line the inside of the uterus becoming displaced and moving through the fallopian tubes to settle around the ovary, in the tubes themselves or on other organs in the belly. In these abnormal positions they proliferate, and when a menstrual period occurs, they bleed as though they were still in the uterus. This results in pain, adhesions, damage to the organs they are attached to and infertility.

Rarely, a woman may be **allergic** to, and develop antibodies against, her partner's sperm, which are rejected and destroyed. Sperm from another man are not normally affected.

Other causes of female infertility may include:

- abnormalities of the uterus due to poor development

- fibroids (hard lumps in the wall of the uterus)

- polyps in the uterus

- infections of the Fallopian tubes (salpingitis)

- cancer or tumours in the ovaries

- ovarian cysts

- the polycystic ovarian syndrome (Stein-Leventhal syndrome)

- hydrosalpinx (blockage of the Fallopian tubes with fluid from persistent inflammation)

- Turner syndrome (born with only one X chromosome)

- Asherman syndrome (complication of surgically clearing out the uterus after a miscarriage or for heavy bleeding after childbirth).

TREATMENT
ARTIFICIAL CONCEPTION
In recent times, techniques have been developed to enable conception to be carried out artificially without the need for the act of intercourse. At its simplest level, this is called artificial insemination and involves male sperm being deposited into the woman, usually by means of a syringe. This may be undertaken when the woman's partner is infertile and the couple decide to have a child technically fathered by another man with whom the woman does not wish to have intercourse.

In vitro fertilisation (IVF) takes place outside the human body and was first successfully carried out in England in 1978.

'In vitro' means in glass, i.e. outside the body.

In IVF, an egg (ovum) is removed from the ovary of a woman at a precise time that is determined by hormones that are given to her in order to stimulate ovulation (production of an ovum or egg). The egg is removed under general anaesthetic in a process known as laparoscopy, in which two tubes, each about 1cm in diameter and 20–30cm long, are put into the abdominal cavity through small cuts on the surface of the abdomen. One cut may be placed in the umbilicus to minimise scarring. The gynaecologist looks through one telescope tube, and through the other operates to remove the egg.

The egg(s) obtained are placed in a special nutrient solution in a test tube or flat glass dish. To this is added sperm from the woman's partner, or if the partner is infertile, another donor's sperm may be used (AID – artificial insemination by donor). The eggs are examined under a microscope, and any eggs that are fertilised are then placed into the woman's uterus (womb) using a fine tube that is passed through the vagina and cervix into the uterus. From this position, it is hoped that the fertilised egg(s) (embryos) will implant into the wall of the uterus and grow into a baby (or babies). The success rate with any one IVF procedure is only about 25 per cent, but in a series of procedures, success rates in excess of 70 per cent have been achieved.

There are a number of other variations on this procedure that may be used.

The **success** rate for all procedures to achieve artificial conception reduces rapidly after the age of 40, and unfortunately very few women are successful over the age of 45, although techniques to help these women are improving all the time.

> *By using every technique available, only three per cent*
> *of couples are left completely infertile.*

GIFT

Another technique to overcome infertility in women is GIFT (gamete intra-Fallopian transfer). A gamete is a technical name for an ovum (egg) or a sperm. In this procedure, the egg is obtained in the same way as for in vitro fertilisation (IVF – see above), but it is then placed into the woman's Fallopian tube along with a quantity of the partner's or donor's sperm, and fertilisation occurs in the biologically normal place – the Fallopian tube. The fertilised egg then migrates down to the uterus in the normal manner for implantation. The GIFT technique is only useful in women who have a normal Fallopian tube and a disease-free pelvis. Its success rate is about 35 per cent for each procedure.

INTRACYTOPLASMIC SPERM INJECTION

Intracytoplasmic sperm injection (ICSI) is the direct injection under a microscope of a sperm into an ova (egg) in order to the fertilise the egg and artificially create a fertile cell that will develop into an embryo.

CLOMIPHENE

Clomiphene (Clomid) is a medication used to stimulate ovulation in infertile women. It must be taken cyclically as directed by a doctor, and often for many months before success occurs. Side effects may include hot flushes, bloating, belly pain and multiple pregnancies. It should not be used in women with liver disease.

CURIOSITY

The first child born after IVF, Louise Brown, was conceived using a technique developed by English gynaecologist Patrick Steptoe in 1978.

INFLUENZA

L ook after yourself by having an influenza (flu) vaccine every year from age 18 onwards, or earlier if you have a significant respiratory illness (e.g. asthma). Although there is always an uncomfortable week or two after being infected, flu may be fatal in some people and cause significant organ damage in others.

Influenza (the flu or grippe) is a debilitating generalised viral infection caused by one of the more than 80 known strains of the influenza virus. It spreads by microscopic droplets in a cough or sneeze from one person to another.

The various flu virus strains are named after the
places where they were first isolated.

SYMPTOMS
Muscular aches and pains, overwhelming tiredness, fever, headache, cough, runny nose, stuffed sinuses, painful throat and nausea are the main symptoms. It can be a very serious disease, but deaths are now rare except in the elderly and debilitated.

DIAGNOSIS
The diagnosis of influenza, and the specific form present, can be confirmed by a blood test that detects a specific immunoglobulin antibody. The test is not routinely performed as it does not change the treatment and often serves no useful clinical purpose.

TREATMENT
Rest and time, aspirin, anti-inflammatory drugs and medications to help the phlegm and cough are given. A light nutritious diet that contains minimal fat and a reasonable fluid intake are sensible.

Influenza can now be cured, but only if the antiviral medication (zanamivir or oseltamivir) is given within the first 36 hours of symptoms developing.

Zanamivir is an antiviral used as an inhaler twice a day for five days to treat influenza. It must be used with caution in asthma, but may be used in pregnancy. Side effects are minimal, but unusually dizziness, diarrhoea, a wheeze and headache may occur. It was released in 1999 as the first medication for the treatment of influenza, and was developed in Australia.

Oseltamivir is an antiviral tablet used for the treatment of influenza. One capsule is taken twice a day for five days, starting within 48 hours of onset of symptoms. It should be used with caution in pregnancy and breast feeding, and is not for use in children under 12 years. Use with care with significant kidney disease. Common side effects may include nausea and vomiting, while less commonly, sleeplessness, diarrhoea and dizziness may occur. It was released in 2001.

Flu can now be cured, but the treatment is expensive
and must be started as soon as symptoms appear.

PREVENTION

Influenza can be prevented by an annual **vaccination** in autumn which gives more than 80 per cent protection from contracting the infection, but only for one year, as the formulation varies every year to match the strains of flu virus present in the community. Two injections a month apart are required for a first vaccination if under 18 years of age. It is not designed to be used in pregnancy, but no adverse effects are expected if a vaccination given inadvertently. It may be used in breast feeding, but is used in children only if specifically indicated. Do not have a flu vaccine if suffering from Guillain-Barré syndrome, AIDS, a high fever or if allergic to eggs, poultry products, neomycin, polymyxin or gentamicin. Side effects may include local discomfort and redness at the injection site and, uncommonly, fever and muscle pain.

One influenza vaccine gives good limited protection, but the protection increases further with subsequent doses. It should be given to everyone over 65 years, those with debilitating illness and chronic diseases (e.g. of the lung, heart, kidneys etc.), patients undergoing immunotherapy, all health and medical personnel and anyone who wishes to avoid catching the flu that season.

Unfortunately the vaccine does not prevent the common cold, and many people who complain that their flu shot has not worked are suffering from a cold caused by yet another group of viruses.

Amantadine tablets will prevent some forms of flu while they are being taken.

Secondary bacterial infections of the throat, sinuses, lungs and ears may occur as a complication of influenza, and these can be treated with antibiotics.

PROGNOSIS

Influenza normally lasts for seven to ten days, and the vast majority of patients recover without complications, although it may be fatal in the elderly, debilitated and if a more virulent strain appears.

Influenza was originally a disease of pigs and ducks that passed to humans
only after these animals were domesticated 7000 years ago.

BIRD FLU

Bird flu (avian influenza) has been in the news more in recent years. It's a virus that affects all types of birds, but particularly ducks and chickens kept in close confinement. There are at least 15 different types of this virus, with the most common being types H5N1 and H7N7. It normally spreads from one bird to another through contamination of the uninfected bird by the urine, faeces, sputum or vomitus of an affected bird. It is common in all species of wild water birds, in which it is not a serious problem, but it has become a problem in Asia where birds tend to be kept closely confined in unhygienic conditions near humans.

There is a vaccination available for birds, but its effectiveness is questionable. It may prevent the vaccinated bird from being affected by the virus, but the vaccinated bird may still pass the virus on to an unvaccinated one, so the vaccine may not limit the spread of the disease while masking its presence and symptoms. The usual treatment is destruction of any flock that contains affected birds.

In uncommon situations, the virus can spread from birds to humans (but so far, not from one human to another), where it causes a particularly severe and frequently fatal form of influenza.

In humans the incubation period is three to ten days, and the symptoms are the same as a severe case of normal influenza. The treatment of bird flu in humans is the same as the normal forms of influenza.

CURIOSITY

Influenza was once thought to be due to 'influences in the atmosphere', thus giving its name.

More people died in 1919 from the worldwide flu pandemic than in the immediately preceding World War I, and most of the deaths occurred (for a still unknown reason) in young, fit adults.

INSOMNIA

Insomnia is an inability to sleep; either a difficulty in getting to sleep, waking repeatedly or for prolonged periods, or early morning waking (EMW) after initially falling asleep. Sleep is as essential for the normal functioning of the human body as food and drink, so it important that you look after yourself by looking after the amount and quality of sleep that you have.

Doctors do not completely understand why we need sleep, but they do understand what happens when we are asleep.

TYPES OF SLEEP

There are two main types of sleep – **deep** sleep and **REM** sleep. REM stands for rapid eye movements, and several times a night, the level of sleep lightens, and while the eyelids remain closed, the eyes themselves move around rapidly. It is during this stage of sleep that dreams occur, and it is the more valuable form of sleep. If a volunteer is observed and woken every time they starts REM sleep, they will remain tired and irritable and obtain little benefit from the sleep. REM sleep does not start until an hour or so after first falling asleep, and long periods of deep sleep occur between each episode.

Unfortunately, many sleeping tablets induce deep sleep but tend to prevent REM sleep, so that people using them do not benefit from their sleep as much as those who sleep naturally. This is one of the reasons that doctors are reluctant to use sleeping tablets until all other avenues have been explored.

Someone deprived of sleep for just 24 hours functions at the level of someone who has a blood alcohol level of 0.05 (illegal to drive).

SLEEP REQUIREMENTS

The amount of sleep needed varies dramatically from one person to another. Some require only three or four hours a day; most require seven or eight hours; others may need ten hours. As we **age**, our sleep needs change too. An infant requires 16 or more hours of sleep a day; in middle age, eight hours is normal; but the elderly need only five or six hours sleep.

The problem here is that older people may have less to occupy their days, and so look forward to the escape of eight hours sleep every night, but find they cannot obtain it because their bodies do not require that much. This is further exacerbated by the low activity levels of many elderly people, and any midday naps they take. As a result, some elderly people seek help in obtaining extra sleep from their doctors by means of sleeping pills. This is not true insomnia, merely a desire for extra sleep, above what is biologically necessary.

CAUSES
There are, of course, those who genuinely cannot get to sleep for a variety of reasons, and 15 per cent of the population fall into this category.

SPECIFIC CAUSES OF INSOMNIA INCLUDE:

- stress and anxiety (including post-traumatic stress disorder)

- pain

- depression (particularly early morning waking)

- menopause and its associated hormonal fluctuations

- snoring and associated sleep apnoea (stopping breathing in sleep)

- restless legs syndrome

- Cushing syndrome (over-production of, or excessive medication with, cortisone).

Numerous **drugs**, both illegal and prescribed, may cause sleeplessness. Examples include alcohol, caffeine, marijuana, cocaine, slimming pills and pseudoephedrine (Sudafed) for runny noses.

There are many things other than medication that can be done to ease the problem.

INVESTIGATIONS
Sleep studies are performed mainly on patients with respiratory problems during sleep (e.g. sleep apnoea, snoring), but also sometimes on patients with neurological problems and insomnia. Obstructive sleep apnoea is diagnosed by having various instruments attached and a series of measurements made throughout the night while the patient is sleeping – electrodes on the head to establish sleep states, special bands around the chest and abdomen to detect movement, a sensor to detect air flow at the nose and mouth, and an oximeter on the finger or ear to detect oxygen levels in the blood.

TREATMENT

THE SIMPLE STEPS THAT ANYONE CAN USE TO AID SLEEP INCLUDE:

- Bed is for sleep and sex only, not for watching television or reading.

- Go to bed when you feel tired, not when the clock tells you to.

- Do not lie down or nap during the day.

- Do not have a clock in the bedroom.

- Avoid exercise immediately before bed. Take time to wind down before going to bed.

- Avoid drinks containing caffeine such as tea, coffee or cola. Caffeine is a stimulant.

- Do not smoke before going to bed.

- Relax by having a long warm bath and/or a warm milk drink before going to bed.

- Lose weight if you are obese. A slight weight loss can significantly improve sleep.

- Avoid eating a full meal immediately before bed time. Give your food time to settle.

- If you cannot sleep once in bed, get up and read a book or watch television for half an hour before returning to bed. Never lie in bed tossing and turning.

- Learn to relax by attending specific relaxation classes, which your doctor may recommend. Follow up by listening to relaxation tapes.

- Instead of counting sheep or worrying about your problems, focus your mind on a pleasant incident in your past (such as a holiday, journey or party) and remember the whole event slowly in intricate detail from beginning to end.

- Remember that the harder you try to fall asleep, the less likely you are to succeed, so relax!

If all else fails, and sleep is still impossible, a doctor can prescribe medications that can be taken ideally for a short time only, to relieve the problem.

Medication is the worst way to get to sleep,
and should only be used as a last resort.

Antihistamines (e.g. promethazine – Phenergan) are very useful and safe medications to help sleeplessness, and they can be purchased without a prescription. They may cause a dry mouth as a side effect, and can have the added benefits of drying up a dripping nose and stopping any itches from insect bites.

Sedatives and **hypnotics** are overlapping groups of drugs that induce sleep (hypnotics), or reduce bodily awareness and activity (sedatives). Most sleeping pills are very safe provided they are taken in the recommended manner, but if used constantly for many weeks or months, patients may become dependent upon them.

The greatest problem with the use of sleeping pills is that they are taken unnecessarily, particularly by elderly people who do not need large amounts of sleep. The pills are better taken intermittently when really needed, when they will work far more effectively. Care must be exercised when taking hypnotics in the evening so that the patient is not still affected by the sedation the following morning.

Examples of sedatives include flunitrazepam (Hypnodorm, Rohypnol), nitrazepam (Mogadon), temazepam (Normison), triazolam (Halcion), zolpidem (Stilnox) and zopiclone (Imovane).

Side effects may include confusion and reduced alertness, and they may cause dependence or addiction if taken regularly. They must be used with caution in pregnancy and glaucoma, and should not be given to infants. Lower doses are required in the in elderly.

SLEEP PROBLEMS IN BABIES
More than half of all parents experience problems with their baby's sleep pattern between six and 12 months of age. These problems may include difficulty in getting to sleep, frequent night waking, and failing to return to sleep after waking. They are often the result of a behaviour the child has learned, and rarely due to any underlying medical problem.

Strategies to change the behaviour of these babies is successful in the vast majority if correctly applied, but this may take up to three weeks of persistence in applying a consistent form of behaviour. Sedative medications should very rarely be used under 12 months of age, and, even in older children, should be used with great caution.

Different babies need different amounts of sleep, and what is appropriate in one child is not necessarily what is appropriate in another. Nine out of ten babies under 12 months will need a daytime nap, and some need two. These naps may vary from 15 minutes to two hours in length between six and 12 months of age.

A child may be put down to sleep at any convenient time between 6 pm and 10 pm or even later, but this time will become a long-term habit. Babies may take up to half an hour to fall asleep, and most then sleep for more than ten hours, but most also wake at least once during the night.

Waking during the night is very common, but is only a problem when the baby is unable to fall asleep again without a parent's assistance. This problem can be worsened by the way in which the baby is put to sleep initially, as this is the way the child expects to return to sleep after waking, so that if a baby normally falls asleep in a parent's arms, or while being rocked, that is the way in which they will expect to return to sleep after waking.

> *Babies are creatures of habit in all their activities.*
> *Encourage good sleeping habits as early as possible.*

A baby who becomes used to falling asleep with a **dummy** in its mouth may be unable to return to sleep if the dummy falls out during the night. Tie the dummy to a short ribbon and attach this to the clothing collar. When the baby wakes and starts to cry for the dummy, run the infant's hand from the collar down the ribbon to the dummy and let them reinsert it themselves. Most children learn this trick by eight months of age.

It may become necessary to teach the child to fall asleep on its own. When starting a new scheme to teach a baby to sleep, start by changing the sleep environment by altering the position of the cot in the room, and installing (or removing) a night light. The baby should be put in the cot while awake, and then allowed to fall asleep.

IF THE BABY CRIES, THIS CAN BE DEALT WITH IN THREE WAYS:

- -

- leaving the child alone to cry itself to sleep. Very tiring on the nerves and may lead to an insecure child.

- controlled crying. This means comforting the child when it starts crying, but during the night, extending the time between each comfort session. As soon as the child settles, it should be left alone immediately and allowed to fall asleep by itself. If crying starts again, return after an increased time to comfort it again. On subsequent nights the times between each comfort are slowly extended further.

- allowing the child, in its cot, to fall asleep while a parent lies beside the cot. Initially the parent may be actually touching the child gently with a hand, but gradually, night by night, the parent moves further and further away, and eventually out of the room.

Spending a week or three changing a child's sleep habits will be very tiring for the parents, and possibly stressful in the short-term for the child, but in the long-term, everyone will benefit.

After one year of age sleep problems steadily decrease, but even at three years of age, one in 20 children wake during the night.

CURIOSITY

Fatal familial insomnia is an extraordinary and very rare inherited disease resulting from the destruction of the thalamus (part of the brain) by a prion (self-replicating protein) that is transmitted from one generation to the next. Symptoms start in middle or late life, and patients have a total inability to sleep for months on end, disturbances to hormone secreting glands, difficulty in speaking, muscle spasms, tremor, poor coordination, increased reflexes, hallucinations and mild dementia. No treatment is available, and the condition leads inevitably to death within a year or two of onset.

ITCH

Everyone experiences itchy skin (pruritus) at some time or another, but in most cases it settles rapidly and easily. Look after yourself by driving to the doctor for help, rather than being driven to distraction, if a persistent itch develops.

CAUSES

There are scores of different conditions which may be responsible for an itch that may arise in the skin itself due to infections or infestations, result from liver diseases, or may arise from other organs in the body.

Over-cleaning the skin with **soap** removes the oil that is necessary for the health of the body's surface, and causes the skin to dry out and become itchy. Soaps and skin cleansers may also cause a mild allergy reaction in the skin that is itchy.

Urticaria (**hives**) is an allergy reaction in skin that causes marked swelling in patches across the affected area, which is also red and itchy. Any one of several trillion substances, from plants, animals or chemicals, may be responsible.

Bites from **insects** (e.g. mosquitoes, sand flies, fleas) or spiders may cause a red itchy spot or patch on the skin.

Never, never, never scratch an itch, it will only damage the skin and make the itch worse.

Fibreglass (e.g. in ceiling insulation) and other irritants can act on the skin to cause microscopic damage, redness and itching.

Heat rash (miliaria) is a skin reaction of the arms, trunk and groin that occurs in hot, humid climates, and more commonly in overweight people due to the blocking of over-active sweat ducts. It causes a burning, itching, red, slightly bumpy rash that is eased by cool lotions.

Atopic **eczema** occurs almost exclusively in children and young adults. It is a skin reaction that may be triggered by changes in climate or diet, stress or fibres in clothing, and there is a genetic predisposition. The rash occurs in areas where the skin folds in upon itself (e.g. groin, arm pits, inside elbows and eyelids), and is more common in winter and urban areas. The rash is extremely itchy, and any blisters that form are rapidly destroyed by scratching which changes the appearance of the eczema, so that it appears as red, scaly, grazed skin.

Contact **dermatitis** is very common. The skin is red, itchy, swollen, burning and may be blistered in an area that has come into contact with a substance to which the patient has reacted. After a few days, the area may become crusted, weeping and infected with bacteria. Substances that a person has used or touched regularly for many years without any adverse effect may suddenly sensitise them, and cause a reaction. This is particularly common in the workplace (e.g. solvents, dyes, rubber, inks) and with cosmetics.

Scabies is an infestation (not an infection) that occurs when a tiny insect called *Sarcoptes scabiei* burrows under the skin to create tracks that can be 1cm or more in length. These burrows and the tissue around them become red, itchy and inflamed. It is caught by close contact with someone who already has the disease. The most common areas for it to settle are the fingers, palms, heels, groin and wrists; but it can spread across the entire body.

Both bacterial (**impetigo**) and fungal (**tinea**) infections of the skin may cause an itch.

Severe **lice** infestations may cause a mild itching from the bites on the skin or scalp.

OTHER SKIN CAUSES FOR AN ITCH MAY INCLUDE:

- seborrhoeic dermatitis (excess oil on the skin)

- psoriasis (plaques of red, itchy, scaly skin)

- intertrigo (due to heat, sweat and friction)

- Grover disease (triggered by heat and sweat)

- pressure areas on the skin

- pityriasis rosea (dark red, scaling, slightly raised, oval-shaped patches appear)

- lichen simplex (persistent dermatitis that is thought to be a form of nerve rash)

- ichthyosis (inherited condition in which the skin lacks oil glands)

- dermatitis herpetiformis (sensitivity to gluten, which is found in many cereals)

- lichen planus (causes small, shiny, flat-topped growths that may join to form a plaque)

- stasis dermatitis (develops in areas of the body that are not drained of blood, particularly the feet of disabled and elderly people)

- pemphigoid (large, fluid-filled blisters on widespread areas of the body).

LESS COMMON CAUSES FOR AN ITCH MAY INCLUDE:

- bilharzia (microscopic animal that enters into the body by burrowing through the skin)

- other infestations by microscopic animals (e.g. hookworm, hydatid, echinococcus)

- viral infection of the liver (hepatitis A and B)

- cholecystitis (inflammation or infection of the gall bladder)

- cirrhosis (damaged liver)

- jaundice (liver damage)

- under-active thyroid gland (hypothyroidism)

- poorly controlled diabetes

- severe emotional upsets or stress may cause a nerve rash (neurodermatitis)

- fixed drug eruption (adverse reaction to a drug)

- itchy upper arm syndrome (severe itch but no rash)

- Fox-Fordyce disease (itchy armpits in women)

- uraemia (kidney failure)

- polyarteritis nodosa (an inflammation of arteries)

- haemochromatosis (excess iron in the body)

- Sjögren syndrome (an autoimmune disease)

- AIDS

- many different cancers and leukaemia.

Some **medications** may cause an allergy reaction to give red, itchy skin, or may cause an itch without any associated rash.

There are many other possible causes of itchy skin.

Never, never, never scratch an itch, it will
only damage the skin and make the itch worse.

ANAL ITCH

An itchy anus is a relatively common problem, and most people will experience it at some time due to sweating, friction, uncomfortable underwear, irritating soaps or after episodes of diarrhoea.

Pruritus ani is a common condition that results in a persistently itchy anus caused by the patient themselves. For one of the reasons above or below, the anus becomes itchy. The patient then scratches the area (sometimes while asleep) to irritate the delicate skin around the anus. The damaged skin then becomes itchier, leading to more scratching and then more itching – a vicious cycle. This can only be treated by never scratching the anus, not using soap on the area, never scratching, soothing creams, never scratching, loose underwear, never scratching, washing the area with plain water if sweaty, never scratching, dabbing rather than wiping with toilet paper after passing a motion, never scratching, using mild steroid creams in severe cases and never scratching (get the idea?).

Piles (haemorrhoids) and an anal fissure may also cause an anal itch.

Numerous **infections** of the bowel, anus and adjacent skin may cause an anal itch. Examples include thrush (a fungal infection), worms (many different types, but thread worms most common in developed countries), molluscum contagiosum (virus that causes tiny blisters), gonorrhoea and syphilis (bacterial infection transmitted by anal sex) and condylomata accuminata (sexually transmitted warts).

Any condition of the bowel that causes **diarrhoea** may also cause anal itching. Examples include gastroenteritis (a viral infection), Crohn disease (inflammation and thickening of a section of intestine) and diverticulitis (inflammation of small outpocketings in the large intestine).

Skin diseases that cause itching anywhere on the body may also occur around the anus. Various types of dermatitis, eczema and psoriasis (associated with red scaly plaques) are examples.

Other possible causes of an itchy anus include intertrigo, polyps or skin tags around the anus, poorly controlled or undiagnosed diabetes, and poor personal hygiene.

Never, never, never scratch an itch, it will
only damage the skin and make the itch worse.

GENITAL ITCH

The genitals (penis and scrotum in the male, vulva and vagina in the female) may become itchy for similar, or totally different reasons in males and females.

Any skin condition that causes itching can also affect the genital skin. Common examples are eczema, reactive dermatitis and psoriasis.

Excessive **sweating** in an area that is usually well covered and constricted by clothing is a common cause of skin irritation and itching. The damaged skin can then become infected by fungi and/or bacteria to cause a painful, oozing rash. Prevention is better than cure, and regular washing of the area when sweaty, loose clothing and cotton underwear (nylon may look sexy, but is not good for skin) can all help.

Other causes common to both sexes include an **allergy** reaction (e.g. to soaps, clothing, antiperspirants, toiletries, perfumes, contraceptive creams, lubricants etc.), infestation of the pubic hair (e.g. with scabies, lice or crabs), genital herpes, genital warts (caused by the human papilloma virus) and poorly controlled diabetes (due to excessive sweating and superficial infections of the affected skin by fungi and bacteria).

Psychiatric conditions, including **depression**, may often include itching of the more private parts of the body as one of their symptoms. This may be because the mind becomes focussed inwards, magnifying minor irritations, and excluding the outside world.

Conditions that may cause genital itching in **women** include thrush (fungal infection of the vagina), vaginal infections by bacteria or parasites (e.g. Trichomonas), excessive natural vaginal secretions (leucorrhoea often due to excess oestrogen), infection of the bladder (cystitis), urinary incontinence (urine can irritate the genital skin), cancer of the vulva (may first be noted as a hard area of itchy skin), and a lack of oestrogen in older women after the menopause can cause the vagina to become dry and itchy. The burning vulva syndrome is a rare condition that causes exquisite tenderness and itching of the vulva, but its cause is unknown.

In **men** a genital itch may be due to fungal and bacterial infections under the foreskin of the penis, venereal diseases that cause a penile discharge (e.g. gonorrhoea, chlamydia) and, rarely, cancer of the penis.

Never, never, never scratch an itch, it will only damage the skin and make the itch worse (have you got the message?).

NIPPLE ITCH

Itchy nipples are a relatively common problem. Women with small breasts may go without a bra and their nipples are irritated by clothing moving across them, or a loose-fitting bra may constantly move across the nipple irritating it. Other causes include synthetic materials in a bra, allergies to soaps, perfumes and washing powders, and fungal infections such as thrush (common in breast feeding mothers).

Padding a bra may help small breasted women, and an adhesive dressing over the nipple can give quick relief.

TREATMENT

Treating any identifiable cause is the first step, but in many cases this is not possible, and so anti-itch medications are necessary.

The best first aid for an irresistible itch is **ice**. Never scratch an itch – merely put an ice pack (frozen peas work well) on the itchy area, and the itch will subside. Methylated spirits is another quick trick, as the evaporation of the alcohol cools the area, but don't do this if the skin is broken as the alcohol will cause stinging. If neither are available, firm constant **pressure** on the itchy area sometimes eases the problem.

The next step is simple anti-itch **creams** and lotions such as calamine lotion, papain, bufexamac and aluminium sulphate (Stingose). The bath additive pine oil (e.g. Pinetarsol) can help a widespread itch (e.g. chickenpox). Lanolin can be used on dry skin.

Antihistamine tablets and mixtures are very useful if the itch is due to an allergy (e.g. hives), but less effective in other cases.

Steroid creams will settle down inflammation, and therefore itching, particularly in eczema and dermatitis, but also for insect bites, and can be applied regularly to unbroken skin.

As a last resort, steroid tablets (e.g. prednisone) or injections can be given to relieve intense distressing itching.

CURIOSITY

The itchy upper arm syndrome (brachioradialis pruritus) is a real disease despite its descriptive name, and is an abnormal response of the skin to long-term sun damage and the constant release of the irritating substance histamine from allergy (mast) cells in the affected skin. Patients with chronic sun damage to their skin may develop intense itching and burning on the outer surface of the arm that is worse in summer, but have no apparent rash. Very strong steroid creams or ointments can be tried, but the condition is generally resistant to treatment.

LIGHTHEADEDNESS

W e have all experienced lightheadedness at some time, even if it only after a rough sea trip or excess alcohol. Look after yourself by making sure that any unexplained episode of lightheadedness is properly investigated.

CAUSES

The vague feeling of lightheadedness is commonly associated with an excessive intake of **alcohol**, illegal **drugs** (e.g. marijuana, heroin) or adverse effects of some **medications** (e.g. tranquillisers, narcotics, sedatives, antihistamines).

Overdoses of other medications, particularly those that affect heart function and lower blood pressure, may also be responsible.

Dizziness and disorientation after a rapid ride on a side show amusement, rough boat trip (sea sickness) or other causes of **motion sickness**, persistent stress and anxiety, and a prolonged lack of sleep are other causes.

Numerous medical conditions may also be responsible for this unpleasant sensation.

Any severe **infection** by a bacteria or virus, and its associated fever, may result in both lightheadedness and dizziness.

Poor **circulation** of blood to the brain due to hardening of the arteries with cholesterol deposits (atherosclerosis) will make it difficult for the brain to receive an adequate blood supply, particularly when the patient changes from lying to sitting, or sitting to standing, and gravity drains blood from the head to the feet (postural hypotension). Elderly people are usually affected, and must ensure that they move gradually from one position to another.

*A noise that makes you rise from sleep suddenly can make
you lightheaded, as the rapid unexpected change in
position causes blood to rush from the head to the legs.*

OTHER CAUSES OF LIGHTHEADEDNESS INCLUDE:

- migraines (often associated with visual symptoms and headache)

- a lack of food and poor nutrition

- disorientation and confusion (due to dementia, deafness or poor vision)

- hyperventilation (very rapid shallow breathing)

- transient ischaemic attacks (temporary blockage of a small artery in the brain)

- psychiatric conditions (particularly those that cause excitement or over-activity)

- arthritis or spondylosis of the neck

- disturbances of the balance mechanism in the inner ear (e.g. infection, glue ear)

- Ménière's disease (dizziness, deafness and ringing in ears)

- inner ear tumour.

CURIOSITY

The head is not light at all. It is actually the heaviest and densest part of the body due to the large amount of bone in the skull and jaw.

LYMPH NODES

L ymph nodes can act as warning signs for a problem in the body, in the same way as red lights on the car dashboard indicate a problem in the vehicle. Look after yourself by noting changes in lymph nodes such as pain, increasing size and redness. In the same way as you would go to a mechanic if red lights persisted, if lymph node problems persist or worsen, take your body to a doctor for the cause to be diagnosed.

ANATOMY

The lymphatic system regulates **tissue fluid** throughout the body. For example if you injure your knee, the surrounding tissues will swell up with excess fluid. This fluid will be removed and returned to circulation by the lymphatic system.

All the cells in the body are surrounded by fluid. This fluid is constantly fed with oxygen and nutrients from the bloodstream. As well as being topped up, fluid must be constantly removed, otherwise it would accumulate in the tissues. Some of it is removed through the bloodstream and some through the **lymphatic system**. This consists of minute lymphatic capillaries (very narrow vessels with very thin walls) leading into progressively larger lymphatic vessels, or channels, which eventually unite to form two big ducts emptying into veins at the base of the neck – returning the fluid to the bloodstream. The lymphatic system thus complements the circulatory system.

The tissue fluid that is filtered into the lymphatic capillaries is called lymph. It is a colourless liquid not unlike blood plasma in its consistency and appearance, although it has a slightly different chemical composition. There are special lymph vessels in the small intestine to absorb fat after a fatty meal. These are called lacteals, because their fluid has a milky appearance.

When patients refer to sore glands, they are actually talking about inflamed lymph nodes, which are not glands at all.

All along the lymphatic vessels are tiny **lymph nodes** (often incorrectly called glands). Lymph nodes are collections of infection-fighting white cells that filter out bacteria, viruses and other organisms, and abnormal cells (e.g. cancer cells), from the organs whose waste products they drain. These tiny, bead-like structures also produce white blood cells and antibodies. They are concentrated around the neck, in the arm pits, groin and in the membrane (mesentery) that loosely connects the intestine to the back wall of the abdomen. They may become noticeably painful and swollen during an infection.

Unlike the circulatory system, which includes the heart, there is no pump to keep lymph moving through the lymphatic system. Therefore, frequent valves exist to stop the fluid flowing backwards and the circulation of lymph is maintained by intermittent pressure on the lymph ducts from breathing, muscle contractions and body movement.

The lymphatic network also includes three large glands – the **tonsils**, the **spleen** and the **thymus**. Each of these consists of lymphatic tissue and produces antibodies and white blood cells to fight infection. In particular, the tonsils act as a barrier to infections entering through the mouth. The thymus is present in the lower neck of children but shrinks after puberty. The spleen is a gland in the abdomen.

TONSILS

The tonsils are located at either side of the pharynx at the back of the mouth. They are made of a large number of infection-fighting white cells, and are the main protector from infection of the throat and airways. In children they are almost invariably enlarged, as children are building up their immunity to many bacteria and viruses as they develop one respiratory or throat and nose infection after another.

Infections of the tonsils themselves are relatively common, but most viral infections settle with time, and bacterial infections (tonsillitis) can be settled by appropriate antibiotics. If the tonsils become repeatedly infected they may be surgically removed.

In 1950, 20 times more tonsils were removed than in 2000 due to the better availability of antibiotics.

SPLEEN

The spleen is the largest and most sophisticated gland in the human body. It is a soft dark red organ that weighs about 100g and is roughly the same size as a clenched fist. Shaped rather like an inverted pudding bowl, it is in the abdominal cavity tucked under the lower ribs on the left side.

THE SPLEEN HAS THREE MAIN FUNCTIONS:

- it filters blood, removing damaged cells and extracting and storing reusable elements such as iron from these cells.

- it stores antibodies developed by the body during an infection, so that when a similar infection occurs in the future the antibodies can be called into play quickly.

- it helps to produce from stem cells, along with bone marrow, new red and white blood cells. White cells fight infection and red cells transport oxygen.

The most frequent reason for medical attention is that the spleen is damaged in an accident. If the chest is squashed in an accident, the spleen may be pierced by a rib or ruptured by the pressure. Because it consists of a very large number of blood vessels, it bleeds freely, and the blood loss into the abdomen may be life-threatening. It is difficult to repair surgically because it is a bit like trying to sew up sponge rubber – the stitches tear out very easily and every stitch hole bleeds. It is therefore sometimes necessary to remove it to save the victim's life. The removal of the spleen has remarkably little effect on an adult, because the bone marrow can take over most of its functions. In babies, the situation is rather different, as the spleen is essential for the early formation of blood cells, and it is removed from children only if there is no alternative.

If the spleen becomes overactive, it may destroy blood cells too rapidly so that the person becomes severely anaemic, susceptible to infection, and bleeds and bruises excessively.

Some early anatomists thought the tiny piece of unusual tissue behind the breastbone that forms the thymus was the location of the soul.

THYMUS

The thymus in the adult is a small irregular strip of glandular tissue that lies behind the upper part of the breastbone (sternum) and extends up into the front of the neck. In a child it is proportionally much larger and more important. It reaches its maximum size of about 30g at puberty.

The thymus plays a major role in the development and maintenance of the immune system. It produces specific types of white cells (B and T cells) that are vital in allowing the body to become immune to infection. It also secretes a hormone that maintains the competence of the cells it produces.

If the thymus fails to develop or is removed, the patient will be unable to fight off infection or cancer effectively. Excess activity of the gland can cause the disease myasthenia gravis.

INVESTIGATIONS

LYMPH NODE BIOPSY

A lymph node biopsy is a procedure in which a lymph node is removed and analysed for abnormalities. It may give information about certain infections or about one of the cancers attacking the lymphatic system, including the spleen, such as Hodgkin's disease.

To remove a lymph node, the area of skin over the node is anaesthetised and then cut so that access can be gained to the node, which then is removed. The cut is then stitched with one or two stitches. The procedure takes about 15–30 minutes and is not painful, although, as with any cut, the area will be sore for a day or so. A child may be given a general anaesthetic.

BLOOD TESTS

A simple blood test, such as a full blood count, can give a great deal of explanation as to the possible causes of an enlarged or painful lymph node, as this blood test measures and compares the number of different cells present in blood, and can indicate the presence of everything from infection and allergy to cancer and anaemia.

ENLARGED AND/OR PAINFUL LYMPH NODES

The term **lymphadenopathy** refers to any disease affecting the lymph nodes, while **adenitis** is an infection or inflammation of the lymph nodes.

CAUSES

Any **infection**, bacterial or viral, may result in the draining nodes becoming enlarged, red and painful. For example, if a finger is infected, the lymph nodes in the arm pit may become involved, while a throat infection will cause swelling and pain in neck nodes. The patient develops a fever and feels ill. An untreated infection may cause the lymph node to break down into an abscess.

Some infections are more likely to cause swollen painful lymph nodes than others. These include **glandular fever** (infectious mononucleosis), measles, brucellosis (caught by meat workers), septicaemia (blood infection), tuberculosis (TB), toxoplasmosis (carried by cats), cat scratch disease, and the cytomegalovirus (with fever, joint pain and large liver). The sexually transmitted diseases syphilis, gonorrhoea and AIDS are other possible causes.

Parasites may enter the blood stream and infest lymph nodes. These are very uncommon in developed countries, but in poorer tropical countries diseases such as filariasis (elephantiasis) and trypanosomiasis may occur. The bacterial infections lymphogranuloma venereum (sexually transmitted disease with large lymph nodes in groin), tularaemia (infection of rats) and plague (black death with pus oozing nodes in armpits and groin) are also mainly limited to these countries.

Lyme disease is an infection passed from mice and deer to man by tics. It is common in North America, but rare elsewhere. It causes a spreading rash, fever, chills, muscle pains, headache, arthritis and enlarged lymph nodes.

All lymph nodes that cause discomfort must be examined by a doctor as the adenitis may be due to a cancer.

Lymphangitis is a bacterial infection or inflammation of the lymph ducts under the skin that drain waste products from tissues back to the heart. It often starts from a skin wound and *Streptococcus* and *Staphylococcus aureus* are the most common bacteria involved. The usual symptom is a red, tender streak running under the skin, usually along an arm or leg, and narrowing as it approaches the body. Other symptoms may include enlarged and tender lymph nodes and a fever. Ulceration may occur at the site of the skin injury, or over-infected lymph nodes, if left untreated.

OTHER CAUSES OF LYMPH NODE PAIN OR ENLARGEMENT MAY INCLUDE:

- cancer which may spread (metastasise) from its original organ along the lymph ducts to the nearby lymph nodes

- leukaemia

- Hodgkin's disease and lymphomas (cancer starting in the lymph nodes)

- immunisation (e.g. for cholera and typhoid) may cause a temporary reaction in nearby lymph nodes

- some drugs (e.g. phenytoin for epilepsy) may have enlarged lymph nodes as a side effect.

- systemic lupus erythematosus (an autoimmune disease in which the body inappropriately rejects some of its own tissue)

- serum sickness (a reaction to receiving a blood transfusion or other blood products)

- chronic fatigue syndrome

- AIDS

- Felty syndrome (a complication of rheumatoid arthritis).

TREATMENT
Blood tests may be performed to identify serious infections, or in cases where cancer is suspected. The white cell count is elevated on blood tests when infection is present.

If the infection is bacterial, the treatment is antibiotics. Viral infections, such as mumps and glandular fever, will need to run their course, with rest and painkillers the only treatment. Most bacterial infections settle well with antibiotics.

Cancerous lymph nodes need to be surgically removed. The prognosis varies depending on the cancer type.

LYMPHOEDEMA
Lymphoedema is a common complication of surgery when lymph channels are disrupted by the removal of lymph nodes in the arm pit or groin because of breast or other cancers. The lymphatic fluid is unable to return to the circulation normally and accumulates in the limb. The limb becomes very swollen, tense and sore. In severe cases the arm is rock-hard and three times its normal size, and ulceration and infection of the skin and deeper tissues in the affected limb may occur. The Stewart-Treves syndrome (form of cancer developing in a limb affected by lymphoedema) is another complication.

Lymphoedema is a very difficult problem to **treat**. Elevation, exercises, pressure bandages and a plastic sleeve that envelopes the arm and is rhythmically inflated by a machine can be tried. The severity varies dramatically from one patient to another, with only a partial relationship to the severity of the surgery. It often persists for many years before gradually subsiding as new lymph channels are formed.

CURIOSITY
Whipple's disease is a rare disorder of the lymphatic system caused by obstruction of the lymphatic ducts draining the small intestine and a persistent bacterial infection of the gut. Patients develop joint and belly pain, diarrhoea, weight loss and a slight fever. They may also have increased pigmentation of the skin and enlarged lymph nodes. A faeces examination shows the presence of excess fat, and small bowel X-rays are abnormal. The diagnosis is confirmed by a biopsy of the small intestine. There is no cure, but most cases are controlled by long-term antibiotics (e.g. sulphas).

MASTURBATION

Masturbation is any form of genital sexual stimulation by oneself. Everyone, both men and women, masturbates, especially during adolescence and at times of their lives when they do not have a sexual partner. Men masturbate by rubbing the penis or otherwise stimulating this organ.

In women, a dildo (artificial penis) or finger are inserted in the vagina, or the clitoris is stimulated.

Anyone who says they have never masturbated is a liar.

Some religions have frowned on the practice and insisted on their adherents regarding it as sinful. Dire threats have sometimes been made that unpleasant physical consequences such as blindness will result. This is nonsense.

Masturbation is harmless, and if it provides pleasure and sexual relief it is quite reasonable to engage in it.

CURIOSITY

Froteurism is achieving sexual arousal by rubbing against another person.

Masturbation was referred to as onanism, from the biblical figure Onan, who 'allowed his seed to fall upon the ground'.

Extract from an 1850 medical text: 'Self-pollution (masturbation) will cause epilepsy, softening of the brain, insanity and moral imbecility. The victim must be put in a straightjacket with his hands tied behind to prevent the inevitable consequences of speedy insanity and death'.

MEMORY

Your own identity is tied up in your memory – you are your memory – and so a loss of memory is a frightening and distressing development. Look after yourself by understanding the process of memory and the possible causes for problems.

EXPLANATION

Memory is the most complex and least understood function of the brain. It requires several steps including **acquisition** of information, **storage**, and **recall**.

Memory is stored in the brain in three forms – immediate, short-term and long-term.

Immediate memory lasts about half a minute and can store between five and ten items. It is very susceptible to distraction and requires concentration. Doctors test this by asking a patient to remember and repeat four numbers backwards.

The **short-term memory** lasts from a few minutes to hours, and has a much larger storage capacity than immediate memory. After this time it is sorted so that important memories are placed in the long-term section of the brain, while other less important memories fade as they are gradually discarded. Doctors test this form of memory by asking the patient to repeat a list of three or four objects after several minutes.

Long-term memory lasts weeks to a lifetime, and contains knowledge, personal experiences and social interactions. Long-term memory requires the production of new proteins and new connections between nerve cells (neurons) in the brain.

MEMORY CAN BE FURTHER SUBDIVIDED INTO:

- reference memory (previous experiences)

- episodic memory (information about a specific place and/or time)

- working memory (updates of old memory by current experiences)

- semantic memory (unchanging facts of everyday life)

- explicit memory (detailed facts about past experiences)

- procedural memory (learned skills).

Memory is extraordinary in many ways. Sometimes you cannot think of your best friend's name, or remember what you had for breakfast, let alone recollect the name of a famous person or a well-known place when suddenly called upon to do so. But, if you pick up a book that you read ten years ago, within a page or two, and sometimes a few sentences, you will realise that you have read the book and usually recollect its plot. The same phenomenon can occur with a piece of music, a film or even a painting or photograph.

Nominal aphasia is the inability to name a person who is familiar to you. It can occur at anytime, but usually when you unexpectedly have to introduce two of your good friends to each other.

The exact nature of memory, and its location, is still a matter of debate amongst physiologists, but long-term memory probably involves patterns of nerve connections throughout the brain rather than only one area.

MEMORY DISTURBANCE
Memory disturbance is different to memory loss (amnesia).

Dementia is caused by degeneration of the brain in old age, and is associated with abnormal thought processes, poor memory and hallucinations.

Alzheimer disease (see page 279), is one of the most common forms of dementia and memory loss in the elderly.

The female sex hormone, oestrogen, has an effect upon every cell in the body, not just the breasts, uterus and other reproductive organs. During and after the **menopause**, the levels of oestrogen fluctuate irregularly, and then it disappears altogether. A lack of oestrogen will have effects on the brain that include memory disturbances. Hormone replacement therapy can correct the problem.

The **organic brain syndrome** is a result of severe emotional disturbance (e.g. horror, fear) and causes memory disturbances, disorientation, poor logic and behavioural changes. Drug use, epilepsy, cancer outside the head and severe infections may also trigger this syndrome.

Some illegal **drugs** (e.g. heroin, marijuana) and prescribed narcotics and sedatives may affect memory. Long-term alcoholism may cause memory disturbances.

Alcohol abuse is by far the most common cause of memory disturbance.

MEMORY LOSS
A loss of existing memories (amnesia) may be temporary or permanent. Causes may include:

- alcohol intoxication (will result in loss of memory during the time of intoxication)

- abuse of illegal drugs (e.g. LSD, marijuana, heroin)

- any injury to the brain

- stroke (cerebrovascular accident)

- bleeding into the brain

- brain tumour

- brain abscess

- infection (encephalitis, meningitis)

- convulsion (e.g. due to epilepsy)

- hysteria associated with severe shocks or stress

- post-traumatic stress syndrome

- psychiatric conditions (e.g. fugue states)

- high fever (may result in amnesia for the period of the fever)

- dramatic changes to the blood chemistry (e.g. low blood sugar and salt levels)

- exposure to extreme cold (hypothermia)

- oxygen deprivation (e.g. near drowning)

- Wernicke's encephalopathy (Korsakoff syndrome – a permanent form of brain damage caused by a lack of vitamin B1 and alcoholism).

The brain is surrounded by a supportive fluid (cerebrospinal fluid – CSF), and there are interconnected cavities within the brain that also contain CSF. If there is too much CSF produced, or an insufficient amount is absorbed, the pressure of this fluid in and around the brain will gradually increase (**hydrocephalus**). The resultant pressure on the brain will affect its function and result in headaches, personality changes, reduced intelligence, memory loss and convulsions.

ALZHEIMER DISEASE

Alzheimer disease (second childhood or senile dementia) used to be called second childhood, or the patient was described as eccentric. Today it is recognised as the most common form of dementia in the elderly, but it may start as early as the mid-fifties.

Alzheimer disease is named after the Wroclaw (Poland) neurologist Alois Alzheimer, who was born in 1864, and first described the disease.

The cause is a faster than normal loss of nerve cells in the brain, the exact cause of which is unknown, but studies suggest specific genes may predispose a person to the disease, and there is a familial tendency (runs in families from one generation to the next).

Initially it **causes** loss of recent memory, loss of initiative, reduced physical activity, confusion and loss of orientation (confused about place and time), then progresses to loss of speech, difficulty in swallowing which causes drooling, stiff muscles, incontinence of both faeces and urine, a bedridden state and eventually the patient is totally unaware of themselves or anything that is happening around them. Some patients may not deteriorate for some time, then drop to a lower level of activity quite suddenly. Admission to a nursing home or hospital is eventually necessary.

Reduced brain volume and wasting may show on a CT scan, but the diagnosis is primarily a clinical one made by a doctor after excluding all other forms of dementia by blood tests, X-rays, electroencephalogram (EEG) and sometimes taking a sample of the spinal fluid. The progress of the disease can be followed by tests of skill, general knowledge, simple maths, etc.

Medication is useful for restlessness and insomnia, and a number of medications are now being used to slow the progression of the disease. In women, hormone replacement therapy after menopause reduces the incidence of Alzheimer disease, and slows its progress. Visits by the family general practitioner, physiotherapists, occupational therapists, home nursing care and health visitors are the main forms of management. Many claims have been made for various herbal remedies, but none have proved to be beneficial.

There is no cure, and treatments are aimed at keeping the patient content. From diagnosis to death takes seven years on average.

CURIOSITY

Prosopognasia is the inability to recognise faces that should be familiar. The usual causes are a stroke or brain tumour, but there are many other possibilities.

MENINGITIS

It is critical in looking after yourself and your family to be aware of the early signs of the different forms of meningitis, and be able to differentiate them from other symptoms, so that urgent medical attention can be sought when necessary.

The brain and spinal cord are surrounded, supported and protected by three layers of fibrous connective tissue known as the meninges. These are called, from the outside to the inside, the dura mater, arachnoid mater and pia mater. The cerebrospinal fluid circulates in the space between the arachnoid and pia mater.

An infection or inflammation of the meninges is known as meningitis.

INVESTIGATION

The diagnosis of both types of meningitis is confirmed by taking a sample of cerebrospinal fluid from the lower end of the spine (which is an extension of the brain) in a process known as a **spinal tap**, and examining it under a microscope for the presence of certain cells, and it can be cultured to find the responsible bacteria. Blood tests also show abnormalities.

VIRAL MENINGITIS

Viral (**aseptic**) meningitis is a relatively benign condition that may be caught by close contact with someone who has a viral infection, or it may be a complication of diseases such as mumps, glandular fever and herpes.

The **symptoms** include a fever, headache, nausea and vomiting, tiredness and sometimes muscle weakness or paralysis, and neck stiffness may be present.

No specific **treatment** or prevention available, but bed rest, good nursing and paracetamol, and sometimes medication for vomiting is prescribed. It is rare for there to be any after-effects and patients usually recover in one or two weeks.

Two types of bacterial meningitis can be prevented by vaccination,
but there is no protection against the milder viral infections.

BACTERIAL MENINGITIS

Bacterial (**septic**) meningitis is caught from people who are carriers of the bacteria, but the victims are usually weak, ill, under stress or have their ability to resist infection reduced in some way. There are many different bacteria that may be responsible. The most common form of bacterial meningitis is caused by *Haemophilus influenzae B* (HiB), while the most serious is meningococcal meningitis (caused by *Neisseria meningitidis*).

It is a much more serious condition than viral meningitis, with the severity and symptoms varying depending upon which type of bacteria is responsible.

Common **symptoms** include severe headaches, vomiting, confusion and high fevers. Patients become delirious, unconscious and may convulse. Neck stiffness is quite obvious, and patients may lie with their neck constantly extended as though they are looking up.

Complications include permanent deafness in one or both ears, damage to different parts of the brain, heart or kidney damage, arthritis and the excess production of cerebrospinal fluid which can put pressure on the brain (hydrocephalus). The worst complication is intravascular coagulation, which involves the blood clotting within the arteries and blocking them.

The **treatment** of septic meningitis involves antibiotics in high doses, usually by injection or a continuous drip into a vein, and patients always require hospitalisation. Patients can deteriorate very rapidly and most deaths occur within the first 24 hours. The overall mortality rate is about 20 per cent, although it is higher in children and with the Meningococcal form.

MENINGOCOCCAL MENINGITIS

Meningococcal meningitis is an uncommon, serious form of bacterial meningitis affecting both the meninges and blood stream (septicaemia). Sporadic outbreaks occur worldwide, usually in winter, but up to 40 per cent of the population carry the responsible bacteria in their nose and throat without any symptoms. Infection is more common in closed communities such as military camps and boarding schools. It affects about one person in every 100,000 every year.

The **cause** is the bacteria *Neisseria meningitidis*, which occurs in five common strains (forms), and several dozen uncommon strains. It is spread by sputum and phlegm in coughs and sneezes.

Symptoms include a high fever, severe headache, vomiting, neck and back stiffness, limb pains, confusion, convulsions and a rapidly spreading bruise-like rash that starts on the arms and legs. In terminal stages the patient becomes delirious, and goes into a coma. Rarely, abscesses may form in the brain, and pneumonia may develop.

There are many different strains of Neisseria meningitidis
that can cause meningococcal meningitis, and the vaccine
only protects against some of the most serious ones.

Cultures of blood and/or spinal fluid from the lower back are taken before **treatment** is started and can confirm the presence of the responsible bacteria, then penicillin, or more potent antibiotics, are given by injection as soon as the diagnosis is suspected. The patient should be admitted to hospital for confirmation of the diagnosis, and continuation of antibiotics given through a drip into a vein. Life support in an intensive care unit may be necessary. The infection may be rapidly progressive causing death within hours, but overall 80 to 90 per cent of all cases survive, with only 5 per cent of survivors developing long-term consequences such as epilepsy.

A **vaccine** is available against a couple of strains of the bacteria, and can be given to infants, and is now part of most routine vaccination schedules.

HAEMOPHILUS INFLUENZAE B INFECTION

Haemophilus influenzae B (**HiB**) is a bacterial infection that causes meningitis or epiglottitis in children, and in adults may affect numerous organs. It is spread by close contact and can cause infections in any age group, but is far more serious in children.

IN CHILDREN IT MAY CAUSE:

- **Meningitis** that results in a fever, irritability, lethargy, seizures and coma. The onset of meningitis may be so rapid that the child may be permanently affected (e.g. by deafness, learning difficulties and other forms of brain damage) before any treatment can work.

- **Epiglottitis** which is a life-threatening infection of a piece of cartilage at the back of the throat that may swell and block the airways.

In adults it may cause a serious form of **pneumonia** and less serious types of throat infection, sinusitis, middle ear infection, bronchitis, joint infection, skin infection, heart infection and meningitis. Adults with reduced immunity (e.g. with AIDS) may have the same serious infections as children.

> *The long-term consequences of Haemophilus meningitis can be seriously disabling, but vaccination is now routine in children.*

Infections in adults can be readily **treated** with appropriate antibiotics (usually as tablets), with minimal long-term complications. In children far more potent antibiotics are needed, and they must be given by injection. The swollen epiglottis (piece of cartilage at the back of the throat) may choke the child before the antibiotics can work, so urgent hospitalisation and intubation (placing a tube into the throat to permit breathing) is essential.

Good recovery occurs if the infection is diagnosed and treated early, but permanent damage or death are possible in children if treatment delayed.

A **vaccine** for infants has been available since 1993 to prevent HiB infections. It is given as three or four doses, two months apart, starting at two months of age. It is not recommended for use in adults, but is unlikely to cause problems if given accidentally. Common side effects may include redness and soreness at the injection site, while unusual effects may include irritability, tiredness, sleeplessness, diarrhoea and a rash. It should be used with caution in fever, acute infection or immune system problems. It must not be injected into a vein.

LISTERIOSIS

Listeriosis is a rare form of meningitis in newborn babies caused by the bacteria *Listeria monocytogenes* which can be caught from contaminated food, particularly soft cheeses (e.g. brie) and salads.

In adults and children, the bacteria usually causes no **symptoms** and is harmless, but if a pregnant woman is infected, the bacteria may spread through her bloodstream to the placenta and foetus, where it may cause widespread infection, miscarriage, or death of the foetus and a stillbirth.

Antibiotics can be used in newborn infants, but they are often not successful. **Treatment** is more successful if started during pregnancy, but the infection is rarely detected before the infant is born. Infants that survive birth suffer from a form of septicaemia (blood infection) that soon progresses to a meningitis that is frequently fatal.

CURIOSITY

The singular of meninges is meninx, a word that means membrane in Latin.

MENOPAUSE

M others teach their daughters all about periods and procreation, but nobody teaches *them* about what happens when it all stops. Look after yourself by learning as much as possible about the menopause, its cause, effects, consequences and management.

Menopause has only been a fact of life for most women in the last century or two. Prior to this, the majority of women did not live long enough to reach menopause, many dying in their forties from the complications of childbirth.

Once a woman passes her menopause, her ovaries will no longer produce eggs, her monthly periods will cease, and no more female hormones will be manufactured.

WHEN

The process usually **occurs** gradually over several years, between the early forties and the mid-fifties, but it may occur as early as 35 or as late as 58. It is therefore not unusual for a woman to spend more of her life after the menopause (or change of life) than she spends being fertile, but this does not mean that she loses her femininity. Many women treat the end of their periods as a blessing and lead very active lives (active sexually as well as physically and mentally) for many years afterwards.

The menopause was called 'the climacteric' until the 1950s.

WHAT

The unpleasant part of the menopause is the change from one stage to another, when the hormones go crazy, the headaches and hot flushes take over, and depression occurs. The first **symptoms** are usually an irregularity in the frequency and nature of the periods, and the gradual disappearance may be the only symptom in 25 per cent of women. About 50 per cent have other symptoms that cause discomfort, and the remaining 25 per cent go through severe and very distressing symptoms.

Other symptoms can include bloating and associated headaches and irritability as excess fluid collects in the brain, breasts and pelvis; hot flushes when hormone surges rush through the bloodstream after excess amounts are released by the ovaries; abdominal cramps caused by spasms of the uterine muscles; and depression which can be a reaction to the changes in the body, a fear of ageing or a direct effect of the hormones on the brain.

The menopause is a natural event, and psychologically most women take it in their stride as simply another stage of life, but it is wrong to dismiss the unpleasant physical symptoms without seeking medical assistance. Doctors find the biggest problem to be the failure of their patients to tell them exactly what they are feeling and what effects the menopause is having on them. The first step in treating someone with menopausal symptoms is explanation. If they know why something is happening, it often makes the problem more bearable.

WHY
The sex hormones are controlled by the brain and released from the **ovaries** into the bloodstream on regular signals from the **pituitary gland**, which sits underneath the centre of the brain. Once in the blood, these hormones have an effect on every part of the body, but more particularly the uterus, vagina, breasts and pubic areas. It is these hormones that make the breasts grow in a teenage girl, give the woman regular periods as their levels change during the month, and cause hair to grow in the groin and armpits.

For an unknown reason, once a woman reaches an age somewhere between the early forties and early fifties, the brain breaks rhythm in sending the messages to the ovaries. The signals become irregular – sometimes too strong, at other times too weak. The ovaries respond by putting out the sex hormones in varying levels, and this causes side effects for the owner of those ovaries.

INVESTIGATION
Doctors can perform **blood tests** to determine relative hormone levels and tell a woman if she is through the change of life or not. These tests are very difficult to interpret if the woman is taking hormone replacement therapy or the contraceptive pill.

Menopause cannot be cured, because it is a natural occurrence, not a disease.

MANAGEMENT
Doctors can relieve most of the symptoms of the menopause, and ease a woman's passage through this change of life.

Sex **hormone replacement therapy** (HRT – see separate entry in this book) is the main stay of treatment. The hormones can be taken constantly after the change has finished, but during the menopause they are usually taken cyclically. One hormone (oestrogen) is taken for three weeks per month, and a different one (progestogen) is added in for the last ten to 14 days. This maintains a near-normal hormonal balance, and the woman will keep having periods, while underneath the artificial hormones, her natural menopause is occurring, so that when the tablets are stopped after a year or two, the menopausal symptoms will have gone. Hormones may also be given as skin patches, vaginal cream and by injection.

After the menopause, women may continue the hormones to prevent osteoporosis, skin thinning, Alzheimer disease and slow ageing. Taking combined oestrogen and progestogen hormone replacement for longer than five years slightly increases the risk of breast cancer, although it slightly decreases the risk of some other cancers.

Sometimes symptoms can be controlled individually. Fluid tablets can help bloating and headaches, and other agents can help uterine cramps and heavy bleeding. Depression can be treated with specific medications.

Help is available, and there is no need for any woman to suffer as she changes from one stage of her life to another.

CONTRACEPTION

An obvious problem faced by a woman passing through the menopause is when to stop using contraceptives. As a rule of thumb, doctors advise that contraception should be continued for six months after the last period, or for a year if the woman is under 50. Taking the contraceptive pill may actually mask many of the menopausal symptoms and cause the periods to continue. It may be necessary to use another form of contraception to determine whether the woman has gone through the menopause.

ANDROPAUSE

The **male menopause** (andropause) is a natural event that occurs in all men. After the andropause no male hormones are manufactured in the testes, the testes no longer produce sperm, and the man is infertile.

Yes, men do have a menopause, but one or two decades later than women, and with far fewer symptoms.

The male sex hormone (**testosterone**) is released from the testes into the blood in response to signals from the pituitary gland, which sits underneath the centre of the brain. These hormones effect every part of the body, but more particularly the penis, scrotum and body hair production. For an unknown reason, once a man reaches an age somewhere between the late sixties and late seventies, the pituitary gland stops sending messages to the testes, which results in the symptoms of the andropause.

The man experiences the gradual onset of a loss of interest in sex (low libido), difficulty in maintaining or achieving an erection of the penis, a lack of ejaculation during sex, thinning of body and pubic hair, and shrinking of the testicles. Osteoporosis may occur, particularly if there is a family history, or the andropause occurs at an early age. These symptoms are far more subtle, and far less distressing than those that occur in the female menopause.

Blood tests can determine the levels of testosterone and the stimulating hormone released by the pituitary gland.

No treatment is normally necessary as it is a normal part of the ageing process, but if the andropause occurs earlier than normal, or following an injury or surgery to the testes or pituitary gland, testosterone supplements may be given by tablet, injection or implant.

CURIOSITY

Extract from an 1891 book on women's health discussing the menopause:

'The perturbations in the general system which occur at this time are of a character so profound as to be wholly inexplicable'.

MIGRAINE

Migraine is a form of headache that is usually associated with other significant symptoms. Migraines may occur once in a person's life, or three times a week; may cause a relatively mild head pain, or may totally disable the patient. Look after yourself by preventing your migraines, and having a good strategy in place to deal with a migraine if one occurs.

EXPLANATION

CAUSE

Migraines are caused by the contraction of an artery in the brain, which may give the patient an unusual sensation and warning of an attack (**aura**), followed within a few seconds or minutes by an overdilation of the artery. Excess blood passes to the part of the brain that the artery supplies and it is unable to function properly.

The patient feels intense pressure, pain and other symptoms. The artery dilation may occur for no apparent reason, or be triggered by certain foods, anxiety and stress, hormonal changes, allergies, loud noises or flashing lights. The frequency and severity of migraines tends to decrease with age – an initial attack over the age of 40 is unusual, and they may cease in old age.

When they close their eyes, people usually see swirls and smooth grey patterns, but patients with a migraine see multicoloured zigzag patterns and light flashes.

EFFECTS

The **symptoms** vary dramatically from one patient to another, depending on the part of the brain involved. As well as intense head pain, most patients suffer nausea and vomiting, and loud noises or bright lights aggravate the pain. Other symptoms may include partial blindness, personality changes, loss of hearing, noises in the ears, paralysis, numbness, and violence. Migraines are rarely serious, but a patient may be disabled for some hours or days.

DIAGNOSIS

There are no specific diagnostic **tests**, but doctors can sometimes diagnose a migraine by its visual pattern. If the patient closes their eyes, patterns can be seen on the back of the eyelids, which are actually the random activity of the nerves in the light-sensitive retina at the back of the eye and in the visual centre of the brain. In normal people, a swirling smooth pattern will be seen, but a patient with a migraine will see flashes of light, bright colours and jagged patterns.

TREATMENT

Migraines may be prevented by regular medication, or treated when they occur.

Many different drugs can be taken regularly to **prevent** migraines including propranolol, methysergide, clonidine, sodium valproate, ketoprofen and pizotifen. It is often a matter of trial and error to find the most effective one.

Migraines should be treated as rapidly as possible after their onset.
Every hour of delay makes treatment more difficult.

The longer a migraine has been present, the more difficult it is to **treat**. They can be rapidly cured in most patients by nose sprays, tablets or injections containing naratriptan, sumatriptan or zolmitriptan. The more often these medications are used, the more effective they become. Other treatments include tablets which may be placed under the tongue or swallowed (e.g. ergotamine, isometheptene), or normal pain killers (e.g. paracetamol, aspirin), antihistamines, mild sedatives and anti-vomiting medications (e.g. promethazine). Strong narcotic pain killers should be avoided if possible. Resting in a cool, dark room is also helpful.

Most cases can be prevented or effectively treated, but a small number are resistant to all medications.

PIZOTIFEN

Pizotifen (Sandomigran) is a tablet used for the prevention of migraine. One to nine 0.5 mg tablets are taken a day in one or more doses. It should be used with caution in pregnancy, breast feeding and children, and not used at all if suffering from glaucoma or difficulty in passing urine.

Pizotifen has no effect on acute migraine attacks.

Common **side effects** include sedation and increased appetite, while unusual ones may include dizziness, dry mouth, constipation, nervousness in children, swelling of tissues, headache, rash, muscle aches, tingling sensation and impotence.

Increased sedation occurs if pizotifen is taken with alcohol, sedatives, hypnotics and antihistamines. It is an older but widely-used medication, and large doses are often necessary. Increase the dosage slowly though.

PROPRANOLOL

High blood pressure, migraine, irregular heartbeat, stage fright, prevention of heart attack, exam nerves, angina, over-active thyroid gland and tremors – all these diseases can be controlled, or treated, by the amazingly versatile betablocker drug, propranolol. It is available on prescription in tablet form.

Beta receptors are present on certain nerves in the body, and blocking the action of these nerves with betablockers such as propranolol produces the desired effects. Because it can control a fine tremor and anxiety about performance, this drug is banned in the Olympic and Commonwealth games, as it would give athletes such as archers and shooters an unfair advantage.

Betablockers are generally very safe medications. **Side effects** may include low blood pressure, slow heart rate, cold hands and feet, nightmares, stuffy nose and impotence. It must not be used in asthmatics as it can trigger an asthma attack, and care must be used when giving it to diabetics.

If a migraine occurs more than once a month,
prevention is better than treatment.

ERGOTAMINES

Acute migraine attacks can be treated by the use of painkillers and sedatives, or the use of specific drugs that deal with the over-dilated arteries that cause migraine. The ergotamines is one class of drugs that works in this way. Some are combined with other medications and painkillers to improve their effect. All must be used as soon as a migraine attack starts, and they may cause significant side effects in some people. They may also interact with other drugs, and are available as tablets (for both swallowing and dissolving under the tongue), suppositories (anal use), and injections.

This class of drugs was the mainstay of migraine treatment for many years, but has now been superseded in many cases by the newer 5HT receptor agonists.

Examples include dihydroergotamine (Dihydergot) and ergotamine (Ergodryl). **Side effects** may include nausea, diarrhoea, pins and needles and chest pain. They should not be used in pregnancy, heart or liver disease.

5HT RECEPTOR AGONISTS

The 5-hydroxy tryptamine receptor agonists are a class of drugs introduced in the early 1990s that acts to rapidly treat migraines and cluster headaches by acting on specific receptors in brain arteries, causing the over-dilated arteries that cause migraines, to constrict. They are available as tablets, injections and nose sprays.

Examples of medications in this class include naratriptan (Naramig), sumatriptan (Imigran) and zolmitriptan (Zomig).

Side effects may include chest pain, tingling, flushing, dizziness, weakness and fatigue. They should be used with caution in pregnancy, and not in heart disease or after a stroke.

CURIOSITY

The term migraine comes from a corruption of the Greek phrase for half a head, as migraines tend to occur on one side of the head.

MISCARRIAGE

Women contemplating pregnancy need to look after themselves in every possible way, including understanding the possibility of the most devastating and common complication of early pregnancy, a miscarriage.

EXPLANATION

Any abnormal vaginal bleeding that occurs away from the normal menstrual period, may be caused by a very early miscarriage.

A miscarriage (spontaneous abortion) is always most upsetting to the parents, particularly if the woman has had difficulty in falling pregnant in the first place. A miscarriage usually starts with a slight vaginal bleed, then period-type cramps low in the abdomen. The bleeding becomes heavier, and eventually clots and tissue may pass.

A miscarriage occurs when a pregnancy fails to progress, due to the death of the foetus, or a developmental abnormality in the foetus or placenta.

If the baby is lost before 20 weeks, it is considered to be a miscarriage. After 20 weeks, doctors consider it to be a premature birth, although the chances of the baby surviving if born before 28 weeks are very slim. Most miscarriages occur in the first twelve weeks of pregnancy, and many occur so early that the woman may not even know that she has been pregnant and may dismiss the problem as an abnormal period.

Most miscarriages are nature's way of removing a tissue
growth that would never develop into a normal baby.

CAUSE

In more than half the cases, the miscarriage occurs because there is no baby developing. What develops in the womb can be considered to be just placenta, without the presence of a foetus (a **blighted ovum** is the less-than-pleasant technical term). There is obviously no point in continuing with this type of pregnancy, and the body rejects the growth in a miscarriage.

Some women do not secrete sufficient **hormones** from their ovaries to sustain a pregnancy, and this can also result in a miscarriage. These women can be given additional hormones in subsequent pregnancies to prevent a recurrence of the problem.

Malformations of the uterus are another, though rarer, cause. This problem may be surgically corrected to prevent the cervix from opening prematurely, or to remove fibrous growths that may be distorting the womb.

There are dozens of other reasons for a miscarriage, including **stress** (both mental and physical), other **diseases** of the mother (e.g. diabetes, infections), **injuries**, and **drugs** taken in early pregnancy. Each case has to be considered individually.

INCIDENCE

Miscarriages are far more common than most women realise. Up to **15 per cent** of diagnosed pregnancies, and possibly 50 per cent of all pregnancies, fail to reach 20 weeks. There is virtually no treatment for a threatened miscarriage except strict rest, sedatives and pain relievers. If the body has decided to reject the foetus, medical science is normally helpless to prevent it.

MANAGEMENT

Once a miscarriage is inevitable, doctors usually perform a simple operation (**dilation and curettage**) to clean out the womb, and ready it as soon as possible for the next pregnancy.

Heavy bleeding that may lead to anaemia, infections in the uterus, and the retention of some tissue in the uterus are the most common complications. Retained tissue may make it difficult for a further pregnancy to occur.

In most cases, there is no reason why a subsequent pregnancy should not be successful. It is only if a woman has two miscarriages in succession that doctors become concerned, and investigate the situation further.

*There is no treatment that will prevent a miscarriage
from occurring once it has commenced.*

DILATION AND CURETTAGE

A curette is actually a sharp-edged spoon used by surgeons to clean out the inside of any small cavity within the body (e.g. an abscess). The name of this surgical instrument is now often applied by gynaecologists to the actual operation of cleaning out the contents of the womb (uterus), which is one of the most common surgical procedures.

The uterus is a thick muscular sac, lined with special cells that rapidly multiply during the month to accept any pregnancy that may occur. If no pregnancy develops, the lining of cells breaks away, and causes bleeding that a woman recognises as her monthly menstrual period. If this delicate process is affected by one or more of several diseases and fails to operate correctly, many different complications can occur. A dilation and curettage can be used to both diagnose and cure many of these problems.

The **procedure** only takes ten minutes, but will involve a visit to hospital, and a brief general anaesthetic. Once the patient is asleep, the doctor will use an instrument to look into the vagina. Through this, the opening into the uterus (the cervix) can be seen. This is normally closed, and a series of successively larger smooth rods are slid through the cervix to gradually dilate it. For this reason the operation is called a dilation and curettage (D & C).

Once the cervix is wide enough, a small curette is passed into the uterus, and is scraped along the inside of the uterus in sweeping motions to remove all the cells and tissue inside the womb. These are collected for later examination under a microscope by a pathologist.

It is normal to perform a D & C after a miscarriage. When a miscarriage occurs, some unwanted tissue may be left behind, and it is necessary for this to be removed to prevent any infection in the uterus and allow another pregnancy to start.

Other than a slight ache low down in the abdomen, similar to a period cramp, there are no after-effects from a curette. Complications are rare, and the menstrual periods usually start again three to six weeks after the operation.

CURIOSITY

Although 15 per cent of diagnosed pregnancies end as a miscarriage, it is believed that a further 15 per cent of pregnancies end as an abnormal menstrual period before the woman suspects that she is pregnant.

MOUTH ULCERS

Mouth ulcers are common, painful and annoying. Look after yourself by understanding the cause of these pests, and learn how to deal with them yourself. Only rarely is a doctor's advice necessary.

By far the most common form are the aphthous ulcers which everyone experiences every few months or so. They are caused by an imbalance between the bacteria, viruses and fungi which normally inhabit the mouth.

Every individual's proportions of these normally harmless germs is different, but those in the mouth of sexual partners are almost identical. The balance is one that suits each person, but if that balance is disturbed by an additional infection, emotional or physical stress, or an injury, the brew of germs may start to attack the lining of the mouth to cause an ulcer.

These are easily **treated** by non-prescription antiseptic and pain-killing mouth washes, paints and gels (e.g. those containing choline salicylate or triamcinolone). Vitamin B and folic acid supplements may also be beneficial, and in resistant cases pastes that contain steroids and antibiotics can be prescribed.

Your boss, through work stress, may cause your mouth ulcers.

OTHER **CAUSES** MAY INCLUDE:

- injury to the moist mucous membrane lining the mouth (e.g. from very hot foods or drinks, sharp objects, biting the inside of the cheek, poorly fitting false teeth, dental procedures)

- infections of the skin (e.g. chickenpox, glandular fever, shingles, hand foot mouth disease, tuberculosis)

- food sensitivities and allergies

- cancer in the mouth

- leukaemia

- Behçet syndrome (recurrent mouth and gum ulcers, genital ulcers, eye inflammation, arthritis and brain damage).

Medications used to treat cancer (cytotoxics) are notorious for causing mouth ulcers. Antibiotics may also upset the normal balance of germs to create the problem.

CURIOSITY

The bacteria, viruses and fungi in the mouth are essential for good health, as they aid in the digestion of food and keep the crevices of the tongue clear of debris. Yoghurt has a good mixture of these and can be used after a course of antibiotics to restore a normal balance.

MUSCLE CRAMPS

There are many different causes for the many different types of muscle cramp that may occur anywhere in the body. You can look after yourself by ensuring an adequate intake of fluids when exercising and not over-straining muscles by excessive premature exercise.

COMMON CAUSES
Night-time cramps of the calf and foot muscles are very common and suffered by nearly everyone at some time. Patients experience a sudden, painful spasm of the muscles in the calf muscles, or of muscles elsewhere in the body. Although far more common at night and in the legs, they may occur at any time and in any muscle. Their cause is a build-up of waste products in the muscles, usually after exercise, but sometimes after a prolonged period of inactivity (e.g. a long air flight). Pregnant women are particularly prone to these cramps. Prevention involves having plenty of fluids, particularly tonic water that contains quinine, or taking quinine tablets.

Vigorous exercise may cause microscopic **tears** to muscles, particularly in the legs, and they may go into spasm during the exercise or soon afterwards. A similar effect may be responsible for the repetitive strain injury (RSI) of typists and pianists when overuse of muscles causes damage and spasm.

Compression of **nerves** as they leave the spinal cord through small holes between the vertebrae in the back may result in inappropriate stimulation of the nerves and contractions of the muscles they supply.

Rapid shallow breathing (**hyperventilation**) reduces the amount of carbon dioxide in the blood, which becomes more alkaline (raises the pH). Small muscles in the hand are sensitive to this change in the blood to the point that they go into spasm, with the wrist bent and fingers and thumb bunched together and pointed towards the wrist. This is known as tetany (totally different to the disease tetanus) and can be cured by getting the patient to breathe into a paper bag for a few minutes while they slow down their breathing with repeated reassurance. Hyperventilation may start after a shock, surprise, injury or vigourous exercise. A low level of blood calcium due to diseases of the parathyroid glands in the neck, may cause the same effect.

Severe diarrhoea (e.g. cholera), kidney failure or an overdose of fluid tablets (diuretics) may cause very low levels of **salt** in the body. Salt is an essential substance for the effective function of nerves and muscles, and very low levels will result in inappropriate nerve stimulation and muscle spasm.

UNCOMMON CAUSES

Tetanus and hypothyroidism (under-active thyroid gland) may also cause muscle cramps.

Many **medications** (e.g. phenothiazines used for psychiatric conditions), particularly in overdose, may cause muscle spasms. The poison strychnine acts by causing painful muscle spasms that affect the heart.

Tonic water or bitter lemon drunk after exercise may
help night cramps as these drinks contain quinine.

TREATMENT

Night-time leg cramps may be treated by stretching the affected muscles by standing on the balls of the feet to ease the spasm. Prevention is better than cure, and taking adequate amounts of fluid during and after exercise prevents dehydration. If this is insufficient, medications (e.g. quinine) can be prescribed to be taken after sport to prevent the cramps.

The treatment of other types of muscle cramps will depend on their cause.

If no specific cause can be found, or the cause cannot be treated, muscle relaxants such as diazepam (Valium) and baclofen (Lioresal) may be used to ease the spasm.

CURIOSITY

Period cramps suffered by women are also a form of muscle cramp, as the uterus is made of very strong muscle that is used every month to expel the lining of the uterus as a period, and a few times in a lifetime to expel a baby during labour. The muscles of the uterus are some of the strongest in the body, but only rarely used to their maximum capacity.

NAILS

octors can learn an enormous amount about a person's health by examining their nails, as many diseases, both past and present, may alter the normal nail characteristics.

Look after yourself by looking after your nails, as they can protect the fingers and toes if well-cared for, or cause considerable pain and discomfort if bitten, torn or cut too short.

ANATOMY

Nails consist of dead cells, and the visible hard part is composed of the same protein (keratin) that makes up hair.

Nails form a kind of armour plating for the sensitive and vulnerable ends of the fingers and toes. They lie over the nail bed. At the bottom of the nail bed is an overlapping fold of skin topped by the cuticle. The nail bed has a very good blood supply, and it is this, together with the fact that the nail is thin (barely 0.5mm thick) and transparent, which gives nails their pinkish colour. At its base the nail becomes denser and the blood supply less generous, giving rise to the white half-moon, technically called a lunula.

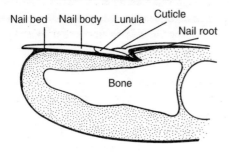

NAIL CROSS SECTION

Nail bed   Nail body   Lunula   Cuticle   Nail root   Bone

Hidden under the fold of skin at the base of the nail is the root from which the nail grows. The growth is continuous in finger nails and takes place at the rate of 3 to 4cm a year – considerably slower than hair which grows at three or four times this rate. Nail growth is quickest in early adulthood and slowest in infancy and old age. The right thumbnail in right-handed people usually grows faster than the other nails and similarly the left thumbnail in left-handed people – possibly because usage leads to increased blood supply. Fingernails grow more quickly than toe nails – by about four times. Nails usually grow more quickly in summer than in winter.

Good quality nails = good quality health.

Nail **growth** also depends on nutrition and general state of health. Poor health will lead to discoloured, dry and cracked nails. Any period of ill-health will sometimes be shown by transverse ridges in the nails, because the illness will have slowed nail growth for a time.

Nails are extremely porous and can absorb 100 times as much water as an equivalent amount of skin. This causes them to swell and, although they dry out fairly efficiently and resume their normal shape, if the process is repeated too often they may split and become painful.

DISCOLOURED NAILS
BLACK
A black nail may be due to injury to the nail and its bed that causes bleeding under the nail (subungal haematoma). The blood may initially appear red, but will slowly turn black in colour. A melanoma is the most serious form of skin cancer, and in rare cases it may develop under the nails to form a black patch. A benign (non-cancerous) blue naevus (really a very dark blue) may be confused with a melanoma in this position. Some bacterial and fungal infections under the nail may give a blackish appearance to the nail.

BROWN
Brown nails may be caused by nicotine staining of the nails of heavy smokers, chemicals that interact with the nails (e.g. in laboratory and process workers), uraemia (advanced kidney failure), Addison's disease (failure of the adrenal glands), and poisoning by mercury or silver salts.

*Brown nails due to nicotine stains from heavy smoking
are slowly becoming an historic abnormality.*

YELLOW
Yellow nails may be due to jaundice (liver failure from hepatitis, gall stones etc.), fungal infections (onychomycosis) of the nails, lymphoedema (build up of waste products in an arm or leg due to a blockage of the lymph ducts), and the antibiotic tetracycline that, if taken for a long period, may cause yellow discolouration of the nails, teeth and bones of children.

BLUE
If insufficient oxygen enters the blood, usually because of lung or heart disease, the blood will become a bluer colour than normal, and a blue tinge will appear on the lips, under the nails, and, in severe cases, on other thin skinned areas of the body. Other causes of blue nails include Wilson's disease (excess deposition of copper in tissues) and the medications mepacrine, chloroquine and amodiaquine (all used for prevention and treatment of malaria), which may cause blue discolouration of the nails as a side effect.

WHITE
White patches under one or more nails may be due to lifting the nail from its bed, the skin disease psoriasis (the nails are also pitted), fungal infections under the

nail, a lack of albumin in the blood (often associated with poor nutrition), severe heart or liver disease, low body temperature, kidney failure, arsenic poisoning, or a side effect of medications used to treat cancer (cytotoxics).

RED
Red nails may be due to blood collecting under the nail from an injury, and exposure of a hand or foot to cold will increase the microcirculation and redden the nail bed. The white half moons at the base of the nails may become red with congestive heart failure.

GREEN
Infections under the nail caused by the bacteria Pseudomonas or the fungi Aspergillus and Candida may give a dark green tinge to the affected nail.

NAIL PAIN
The most obvious cause of nail pain is an **injury** to the nail, or more precisely, the sensitive nail bed over which the nail slides as it grows. The nail itself has no sensation. Lifting the nail from the nail bed or injuring the nail so that bleeding occurs under it (e.g. accidentally hitting it with a hammer) are both very painful. If blood accumulates under the nail, it should be released as soon as possible to both relieve pain and give the nail a chance to reattach to the nail bed.

Other common causes of nail pain include an **ingrown** nail, when one leading corner of the nail grows into the adjacent flesh (often caused by tearing the nail rather than cutting, or tight shoes); and **infections** of the nail bed (a paronychia), which require antibiotic and anti-inflammatory treatment, and sometimes minor surgery to lance an abscess.

Less common causes include a herpes virus infection around the edge of the nail (a whitlow), and tumours or cancers (e.g. melanoma) under the nail.

NAIL INFECTION
A **paronychia** is an infection of the nail bed (pink tissue under a nail) and surrounding tissues caused by an ingrown nail, damage to the side and base of the nail from habitually picking at the area, working in water, working with chemicals (e.g. detergents and soaps), dermatitis, and gardening, when particles of dirt may be pushed between nail and skin.

A red, tender, painful swelling develops at the side and base of the nail.

Treatment involves applying antibiotic ointment to the infected skin around the nail, taking antibiotic tablets, and, if an abscess is present, having it lanced to drain pus. If not treated, infected tissue can break down to form an abscess, which may damage the nail bed and cause the nail to come off. Most settle quickly with treatment.

Nail analysis centuries after death can diagnose
the presence of poisons such as arsenic.

NAIL ABNORMALITIES

PITS IN NAIL

Small isolated or joined pits on the surface of one nail may be due to a persistent **infection** at the base of the nail (paronychia).

If several nails are involved it may be due to **eczema** on the adjacent finger or toe skin.

If most nails are affected, the skin disease **psoriasis** may be a cause.

Strangely, patients with alopecia areata (patchy hair loss on the scalp) may also have pitted finger nails.

If every nail is affected, it may be an inherited trait.

RIDGES ALONG NAILS

The development of multiple ridges along the length of the nail is a common phenomenon in **elderly** people. This is due to reduced blood supply to the finger tips, and other generalised diseases such as rheumatoid arthritis, diabetes and other causes of damage to small arteries may also be responsible. The skin disease lichen planus is an unusual cause. A single ridge in a particular nail may be caused by a tiny cyst or tumour in the nail bed or base of the nail.

RIDGES ACROSS NAILS

Multiple ridges across one or a small number of nails may be due to a persistent **infection** at the base of the nail (paronychia) or **eczema** on the adjacent skin. If most nails are affected by cross ridges, a generalised condition will be responsible. Examples include Raynaud disease (excessive spasm of arteries due to cold), carpal tunnel syndrome (constriction of arteries and nerves in the wrist), a deficiency of protein in the diet and persistently wet nails (e.g. from dish washing).

Women who have very painful and heavy **periods** may develop a small ridge across most nails every month.

Some people develop a habit of pulling back the quick at the base of the nail. This will damage the nail growth to cause cross ridging of the affected nails.

A single cross ridge (Beau's line) on most nails may occur after an episode of severe physical **stress**, major illness or significant emotional upset, during which time nail growth may slow temporarily.

ROUNDED NAIL

Clubbing of the fingers is a term used in medicine to describe swelling of the tissue immediately behind the fingernails so that the groove between the nail and flesh disappears, and becomes raised and rounded. The nail is also markedly rounded and raised. It is a phenomenon that is often looked for by doctors as a sign of serious disease, but rarely noted by patients.

Clubbing is caused by over-growth of the soft tissue and underlying bone at the tip of the fingers due to a lack of oxygen in the blood, while the actual amount of blood reaching the area is increased.

Long-standing diseases of the **lungs**, **heart**, or, less commonly, the **bowel**, are the cause of clubbing. It is not specific as to the type of disease in these organs, but common examples include emphysema (usually caused by smoking), tuberculosis, bronchiectasis (damage to the tubes in the lung leading to repeated infection), asbestosis and cancer in the lungs; abnormal valves, holes in the heart and abnormal blood vessels in the heart; and regional enteritis (inflammation of part of the intestine) and Crohn's disease (thickening and ulceration of part of the wall of the small and/or large intestine) in the gut.

Less common causes include cystic fibrosis (which causes thick secretions in the lungs and bowel) and sarcoidosis (infiltration of abnormal tissue into the lungs and other organs).

Some people are born with clubbing of the fingers, and in others it is a family trait, passing from one generation to the next. In both these situations, it is not significant medically.

Brittle nails may be due to excessive dampness, detergents, iron deficiency, diabetes, excessive use of nail polish remover or a lack of vitamins A, B6 or C.

THICK NAIL

If the nail is thicker than normal, a severe **fungal** infection of the nail bed is by far the most common cause. These infections have been notoriously difficult to treat, but in recent years a number of expensive lacquers and tablets have been developed that, if used for a long period of time, will completely cure the problem, and remove the embarrassment of ugly nails.

Other causes of nail thickening include the skin diseases psoriasis and lichen planus.

Rarely, it may be a congenital defect of nail development.

UNDER-DEVELOPED NAIL

A number of unusual conditions may cause most nails to be poorly developed or even absent. These include the Fong syndrome (poorly developed or defective nails and knee caps), Coffin-Siris syndrome (excess body hair, mental retardation and coarse facial features), foetal alcohol syndrome (caused by the mother drinking excessive amounts of alcohol during pregnancy) and Goltz syndrome (scar-like areas of thin skin on the scalp, thighs and sides of the belly).

NAIL INJURY

A **subungal haematoma** (nail bruise) is a collection of blood under a finger or toe nail. They are caused by an injury to the nail, and result in a very painful nail that is black in colour and loose on its bed.

Blood can be released from under a nail using the following simple trick. Partially unbend a metal paper clip so that one end is at right angles to the folded part. Heat the end in a flame (e.g. candle) until it is red hot. Apply the end to the nail over the blood collection. The paper clip will burn through the nail to form a hole through which the blood can escape. No pain will be felt by the patient until the hot tip penetrates the nail, at which point a small burn will be felt, and the paper clip can be immediately removed.

This results in immediate relief of pain, but the nail is usually lost as a new nail grows out underneath old one.

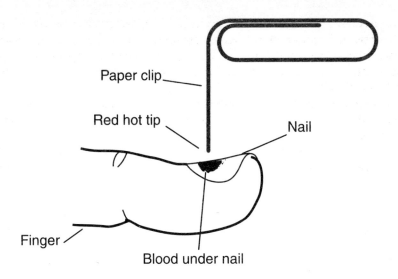

Paper clip

Red hot tip

Nail

Finger

Blood under nail

INGROWN NAIL

An ingrown toenail occurs with penetration of the tip of the nail edge into the flesh at the side of the nail, most commonly on the big toe. The nail has usually been torn, or cut too short, or shoes are too tight. This allows the skin at the end of the toe to override the end of the nail, so that when the nail grows, the corner of the nail cuts into the flesh and causes damage, pain and infection in the affected flesh beside the nail.

The infection is treated with antibiotic ointments and tablets, while the ingrown corner of the nail must be allowed to break free of the skin by avoiding shoes and pulling the flesh away from the ingrowing nail corner with tape or regular massage. If this is unsuccessful, one of a number of minor operations may be necessary.

The most common operations involve cutting away the excess flesh that is growing over the nail, or cutting away a wedge of the nail, nail bed and tissue beside the nail (a wedge resection) to permanently narrow the nail. Surgery usually cures an ingrown toenail.

High heels with narrow toes are a common cause of ingrown nails.

WEDGE RESECTION OF NAIL

The **Zadek procedure** (wedge resection) is one of the more radical methods of curing an ingrown toenail, but will result in a permanent cure of the problem in most cases, although there may be a recurrence in about ten per cent of patients. It is only performed if the nail is significantly ingrown, or previous procedures have been unsuccessful. The aim of the operation is to permanently narrow the nail by one-quarter to one-third of its width.

After cleaning the toe with an antiseptic solution, the patient will be given an anaesthetic injection into either side of the base of the toe. There is then a five to ten minute wait for the anaesthetic to be effective. Sometimes a third injection is given into the end of the toe after this time.

A tourniquet (often a broad rubber band) is then placed around the base of the toe, it is again cleaned with antiseptic, and draped with a sterile dressing. The operation is then performed. The patient may feel pulling and tugging, but no pain should be felt. If pain is experienced, the patient should tell the doctor, and more anaesthetic will be given.

During the procedure a cut is made from the flesh behind the base of the nail, through the entire length of the nail. A second cut is made around the outside edge of the nail to curve around and meet the first cut at both ends. These cuts are deepened to meet in the flesh beneath the nail, and a wedge of nail and flesh is removed. Part of the nail bed behind the base of the nail is also removed in the wedge.

ZADEK PROCEDURE

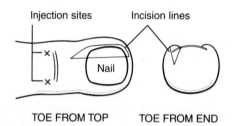

Injection sites   Incision lines

Nail

TOE FROM TOP   TOE FROM END

In most cases, the defect in the nail is then sewn up with stitches through both the flesh and the nail, the tourniquet is removed, and a firm dressing is applied. It is necessary to return to have a lighter dressing applied after one day, and to have the stitches removed after ten days.

When the anaesthetic wears off after about 90 minutes, there will be considerable discomfort in the toe due to the depth of the incision and the pressure from the bandage. The doctor will give the patient pain killing tablets to take as necessary for the next 24 hours. After the dressing is changed the next day, much of the pain will ease, and paracetamol is all that is normally needed for the next couple of days.

Bleeding from the wound into the dressing is common in the first few hours. Additional bandaging may be added to the original dressing if necessary. Keeping the foot elevated will prevent both bleeding and pain. The patient should not walk any more than is absolutely necessary for the first day, and shoes should not be worn until after the stitches are removed. Sandals, thongs and open-toed shoes that do not put pressure on the wound are appropriate.

If you have had other procedures to correct ingrown toenails that have failed, a wedge resection is the way to go.

The wound should be kept clean, dry, covered and elevated as much as possible until the sutures are removed. The patient may shower briefly, remove the dressing after showering, pat the toe completely dry, then apply a clean dry dressing. The patient must not swim or take a bath unless the toe is kept out of the water. A soggy wound is more likely to get infected and heal poorly.

An immediate complication may be excessive bleeding from the wound, and this may require further suturing or dressing. Infection is an uncommon possibility that may occur one or more days after the procedure. If there is a foul ooze, smell, increasing pain or redness in the toe, the patient should return to the doctor for antibiotic treatment.

A long-term complication may be the growth of a spicule of nail from the damaged nail bed. This can grow out parallel to the existing nail, or may grow into the flesh at an angle to cause pain and infection. If this occurs, a further operation may be necessary.

In some cases the remaining nail may be distorted without growing into the flesh again, and may not be as cosmetically attractive as the patient may desire, although still pain free.

CURIOSITY

The Fong, or nail-patella, syndrome is a congenital abnormality of fingernails and toenails, and the knee cap. Children with this syndrome have gross nail defects, small or absent knee caps, bony outgrowths of the pelvic bone, elbow joint abnormalities and kidney failure may occur. Excess protein is found in the urine, and X-rays show bony abnormalities. Plastic and orthopaedic surgery is performed, but patients have persistent knee problems and premature arthritis.

NOSE BLEED

Everyone has a bloody nose (medically known as epistaxis) at some time. It can be one of the most annoying, embarrassing and distressing symptoms, but fortunately the vast majority of cases have no serious cause. Look after yourself by knowing how to deal with a nose bleed without a doctor's help.

NOSE ANATOMY

Air is breathed in through the nostrils (the openings to the nose), and then passes into the pharynx (throat) and down the larynx and trachea to the lungs. The nose warms the air to blood temperature and moistens it so that it will not harm the delicate tissues of the lungs.

The part of the nose we can see consists of cartilage and bone covered with skin. Behind it is the internal nose consisting of two nasal cavities divided by a septum, which is also made up of cartilage and bone. The septum has three curled bones called turbinates attached to it that swirl the air around as it moves through the nose to improve the efficiency of the warming and moisturising process.

CROSS SECTION OF MOUTH AND NOSE

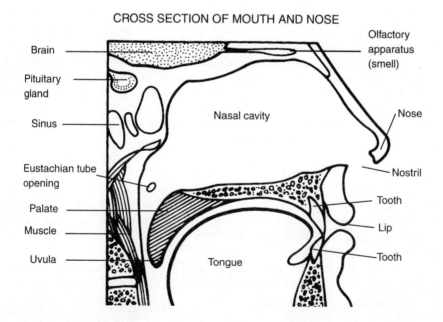

The main functions of the nose are to warm,
moisturise and filter the air entering the lungs.

As well as providing a passage for air, one of the main functions of the nose and pharynx is to **filter** air and trap infections before they reach the lungs – hence the frequency of coughs and colds and other minor upper respiratory ailments which, although tiresome, are preferable to serious lung diseases such as pneumonia.

The nose begins this filtering process very efficiently with its lining of tiny hairs, called cilia, which trap particles of foreign matter. The hairs at the front of the nose are bigger and coarser than those at the back, so that large particles such as grit and dirt are caught before they get very far. Smaller particles which manage to find their way through the front hairs will usually come to grief in the finer hairs at the back. Once particles such as dust and bacteria are trapped, a sneeze will expel them, or they cling to the mucous membrane lining the nose, which itself has bacteria-destroying properties, and are moved by the waving of the hairs down to the throat and on to the stomach where they are processed by the digestive system. Alternatively they may be expelled in the mucus by coughing. Particularly harmful substances cause a sneeze and expel the irritant at the beginning. The reason it is better to breathe through the nose than the mouth is that the nose is much more effective at dealing with foreign matter and bacteria.

A healthy adult produces about a litre of **mucus** in a day. If an infection takes hold, this amount will increase substantially to cope with the extra load involved in ridding the infection from the body – hence the blocked or runny nose of a cold.

During a cold, the nose can produce more than three litres of mucus a day.

Surrounding the nasal cavities are air spaces opening into the bones of the skull through small gaps. These are the nasal sinuses. Matching pairs of sinuses exist in the forehead, the cheeks and the front and back of the nose itself. The sinuses do not seem to fulfil any specific respiratory function but rather exist to lighten the skull and add resonance to the voice. They enlarge significantly at puberty and so are a factor in the size and shape of the face. Despite their apparent lack of usefulness, the sinuses are very vulnerable to infection.

The nose is also the organ of smell. Odour receptors are situated in the roof of the nasal passages and these communicate with the brain.

CAUSES OF NOSE BLEED

If the moist nose-lining membrane **dries out** because of a hot dry climate, high altitude, viral or bacterial infections, it will crack and the tiny arteries under it will suddenly start bleeding quite profusely. If the drying occurs further back in the nose, the arteries on the turbinates may bleed, and most of the blood will go down the back of the throat rather than out the nose.

If the nostril lining is damaged by an **injury** such as picking the nose or a blow, bleeding may also occur. A severe blow to the nose may fracture the bone, and this almost invariably causes bleeding.

High blood pressure may increase the risk of a nose bleed, but other causes are usually also present.

Polyps, tumours and, very rarely, cancer in the nostril may bleed unpredictably.

Children often place **foreign objects** in the nose, and they may be difficult to see without proper instruments. A foreign body should always be suspected as a cause of a nose bleed in children and adults with subnormal mentality.

All causes of abnormal bleeding may be responsible for nose bleeds. Examples include a lack of cells (platelets) or substances necessary for normal clotting (e.g. haemophilia), and medications that are used to reduce the risk of blood clots (e.g. aspirin, warfarin).

Leukaemia is a rare cause of abnormal and excessive bleeding.

If recurrent nose bleeds occur, investigations must be undertaken to determine its cause.

Painting the inside the nose with a cotton bud dipped in Vaseline can prevent the lining from drying, cracking and bleeding.

TREATMENT

In order to stop a nose bleed, the patient should sit (not lie) still and hold the nostrils firmly without letting go for **ten minutes**. Ice applied to the nose will also help. If bleeding continues after repeating the above three times, medical attention is necessary to find and treat the cause of the bleeding (e.g. cauterising the bleeding point with heat, removing a nasal polyp).

A Foley catheter (normally used to drain the bladder) can be inserted into the nose and then the balloon at the end of the tube can be inflated to stop an intractable nose bleed.

Very rarely, repeated severe nose bleeds may cause anaemia, but most cases of epistaxis settle quickly with appropriate treatment.

CURIOSITY

Extract from a 1797 medical text:

'A discharge of blood from the nose often cures dizziness, headache, a phrenzy [sic] and even epilepsy'.

OBESITY

I n Roman times, a beautiful woman was considered to be well proportioned and rounded in the style of Venus de Milo (plus arms of course!).

During the Renaissance, voluptuous females of Junoesque proportions were appreciated.

Today the tall, skinny, anorexic fashion model is considered to be in vogue.

It is possible that those overweight by today's standards were merely born in the wrong era!

Two centuries ago the average person walked 12 kilometres a day, getting adequate exercise and burning off excess weight. As a result, obesity was a sign of wealth, as the person did not need to walk long distances for work, or had access to a carriage rather than a horse (horse riding also uses energy).

One of the most important ways in which you can look after yourself, your health and longevity is by maintaining your weight within the healthy range.

INCIDENCE

Up to 40 per cent of people in developed countries are overweight, but only five per cent are considered to be obese by medical standards. Obesity is medically defined as being more than 40 per cent over the ideal weight for sex, height and age. Men tend to develop '**apple**' obesity (fat around the middle of the body) while women are '**pears**' (fat deposits around the buttocks). The 'apple' form has a far higher risk of heart complications.

Those whose weight is within 20 per cent of their recommended weight have little to fear health-wise. Those who exceed this limit are more likely to develop strokes, heart disease, diabetes, arthritis and liver disease.

The 'French paradox' is that a nation of people who eat a lot of animal fats (e.g. paté) have a lower than average incidence of heart disease. This is explained by their regular but moderate (in most cases) use of wine throughout life.

BODY MASS INDEX

The body mass index (BMI) is a guide to obesity that is simple to apply, but does not take account of body shape, muscle bulk and fitness. Most elite athletes, particularly those in strength sports such as wrestling and throwing, have a very high BMI.

The BMI is calculated by the formula:
  weight in kilograms/height in metres squared

A person weighing 70kg and with a height of 1.7m would have a BMI of:
  $70/1.7^2 = 24.3$

which is satisfactory.

With a weight of 80kg, the same person has a much higher BMI, thus:
  $80/1.7^2 = 27.7$

which is overweight.

BMI ranges and their interpretations are:
  Under 20   Underweight
  20-25   Healthy weight
  25-29   Overweight
  29-35   Obese
  Over 35   Severe obesity

WAIST-HIP RATIO

Another measure of obesity is the ratio between the circumference of the waist at the umbilicus and the hips. In men a waist-hip ratio of greater than 1.0 indicates an increased risk from obesity, while in women a ratio of greater than 0.8 (i.e. the waist should be no more than 80 per cent of the hip circumference) is a risk.

> *In Western society, poor people are more likely to be obese than wealthy. The reverse is true in developing countries.*

CAUSES

THE CAUSES OF OBESITY CAN BE SIMPLY LISTED (IN ORDER OF IMPORTANCE) AS:

• inherited tendency

• too much food eaten

• too little exercise

• metabolic (body chemistry) disorders.

LIFESTYLE

The vast majority of cases of obesity are due to **excessive food** and **physical inactivity**, but if your parents were obese, your chances of also being obese are greatly increased. Some people have very efficient bodies (like a fuel-efficient car), and require remarkably little energy in the form of food to remain healthy and active. If the amount of energy used (calories/kilojoules) in exercise and normal body function exceeds the amount of energy taken in as food and drink, the person will always lose weight. If the reverse is true, weight will increase. It should be remembered that calories and kilojoules are a measure of the energy content of food, and not the fat content.

MEDICAL PROBLEMS

Diseases which may cause weight gain include hypothyroidism (an under-active thyroid gland in the neck), congestive cardiac failure (a damaged heart that slows down and is unable to beat effectively) and Cushing syndrome (over-production of steroids in the body, or taking large doses of cortisone).

Middle-age spread occurs as the metabolic rate of the body (the rate at which all organs in the body function) slows with age, at the same time that exercise levels tend to reduce, and food intake increases with more leisure and security. Many women gain weight after the menopause due to a slowing of the body's metabolic rate when oestrogen levels drop. This effect may be slowed by hormone replacement therapy.

The floppy eyelid syndrome is a persistent drooping of the upper eyelid. Obesity and the deposition of excess fat in the eyelid is the usual cause.

OTHER METABOLIC CAUSES OF OBESITY MAY INCLUDE:

- disorders of the pituitary gland under the brain (caused by a tumour, cancer, stroke, infection, injury or other disease)

- poorly controlled insulin-dependent diabetes

- Prader-Willi syndrome (chromosomal defect)

- syndrome X (cause of difficult to control high blood pressure)

- Stein-Leventhal syndrome (multiple cysts in the ovaries)

- Fröhlich syndrome (late onset of puberty, thin wrinkled skin, scanty body hair)

- Laurence-Moon-Biedl syndrome (night blindness, mental retardation, obesity, small genitals and sometimes extra fingers or toes).

Some **medications** may have weight gain and increased appetite as an unwanted side effect. Examples include steroids, tricyclic antidepressants (for depression) and thioridazine (used in psychiatry).

WEIGHT GAIN

Weight gain (or loss) is really a function of energy (calories or kilojoules) in and energy out. If the **energy in exceeds energy out**, weight will increase, as food is merely a form of energy for our bodies, in the same way that petrol is the energy source for a car. The fact that eating is pleasurable is a problem that mankind has yet to solve, leading to the present epidemic of obesity. If a person wishes to lose weight, they have to alter the equation by decreasing energy in (food), and/or increasing energy out (exercise).

There are a number of disease which can affect this balance, but still do not alter the basic equation. Part of the energy output goes to maintaining the basic operations of the body, such as breathing, heart beat, digestion etc. This is the metabolic rate, and this rate varies from one person to the next. If the metabolic rate is high, the person needs more energy (food) to maintain it, and is unlikely to gain weight. If the metabolic rate is low, the reverse is true. Diseases which slow the metabolic rate can therefore affect weight by reducing the energy (food) needs of the body.

When shopping, always park as far as possible
from the shops, and walk to them briskly.

BASAL METABOLIC RATE

The basal metabolic rate (BMR) is the minimum amount of **energy** that must be used to keep the essential bodily activities functioning. These activities include the heart beat, breathing, body temperature, liver and brain function, intestinal activity and digestion. The BMR varies between individuals, and is to some extent inherited.

Those with a naturally high BMR tend to remain thin despite high food intake, while the reverse is also true. The BMR uses far more energy (and therefore burns more fat) than even the most vigorous exercise.

The BMR is controlled by the brain through the thyroid gland and the hormone thyroxine.

EFFECTS

IF THOSE WHO ARE MEDICALLY OVERWEIGHT REDUCE THEIR WEIGHT BY JUST TEN PER CENT, THEY WILL:

- reduce blood pressure by 10 to 20mm

- reduce the symptoms of angina by 90 per cent

- reduce the bad forms of cholesterol in their blood

- reduce the risk of developing diabetes by 50 per cent

- reduce the risk of death from heart disease, diabetes and cancer by more than 20 per cent

- improve the quality and quantity of sleep

- reduce daytime drowsiness

- increase sexual desire and activity

- improve overall assessment of health by more than 20 per cent

Weight loss is never constant, but occurs in a series of steps.

MANAGEMENT

Obese men and women tend to spend an incredible amount of money in their attempts to become thin by buying special foods and medicines. The cheapest and most effective way to lose weight is to spend less, by buying less food, particularly less of the expensive processed foods. If you find your willpower is lacking, or the craving for rich foods becomes unbearable, doctors can prescribe tablets that are designed to reduce your appetite (anorectics). These drugs are expensive, and should not be used for long periods, but they are effective.

The metabolic cases of obesity must have the underlying condition treated, and not the obesity itself.

Skip the lift and take the stairs instead.

LIFESTYLE CHANGES

Those who are serious about losing weight should follow the plan below. It is effective, and not expensive. It is inappropriate to spend more money to lose weight, as a correct diet is actually cheaper as less food is required, and the food purchased should be fresh rather than processed.

WEIGHT LOSS DIET

- EAT ONLY THREE TIMES A DAY.
  Never eat between, before or after your normal meals. Drink only water, black tea/coffee or diet drinks if thirsty.

- EAT THE RIGHT FOODS.
  Eat a balanced selection of the correct foods. This means that those foods with low kilojoule values, selected from all food groups (fruit, vegetables, meats, cereals) are the only ones to eat. Do not stick to one food group for long periods of time, as this can seriously upset the body's metabolism. Tables of relative food values are readily obtainable from doctors. For example, avocado is very rich in kilojoules, cucumber is low.

- EXERCISE DAILY
  Exercise to the point where you are hot, sweaty and breathless. If you are over 40, you should check with your doctor to determine what level of exercise is appropriate. 400 kilojoules (100 calories) will be used by walking briskly for 20 minutes, swimming for ten minutes, or running flat out for seven minutes.

- IF NECESSARY, EAT LESS.
  If you are not losing weight at the rate of 1kg per week, averaged over a month, you need to eat less!

- KEEP GOING
  Continue until you reach your target weight, and continue dieting to maintain that weight.

Park the car further and further away from work every day.

ANORECTICS

Anorectic drugs are used to reduce appetite. These drugs do not reduce weight but act as an aid to controlling appetite while the patient complies with a strictly controlled diet. They are available in tablet and capsule form only. Anorectics should not be used for long periods, as dependence can occur. Some are stimulants, which may cause insomnia if used in the evening, and are used illegally by long-distance drivers and others who wish to remain awake for long periods of time. They should not be mixed with alcohol, and their use during pregnancy is controversial. Many drugs in this class have been removed from the market in recent years because of abuse, interactions and side effects.

Examples include diethylpropion and phentermine (Duromine).

ORLISTAT

Orlistat (**Xenical**) is a drug introduced in 2000 to treat significant obesity. It acts by preventing the absorption of fat from the intestine.

Common side effects include diarrhoea (worse if fat eaten), flatulence, liquid faeces and headache.

It should be used with caution in pregnancy and children, with peptic ulcers, psychiatric disturbances, adhesions in the belly, kidney stones and serious heart, liver and kidney disease.

Patients should not take it if they are breast feeding, suffering from pancreatitis or some types of gall bladder disease, or are normal or underweight.

SIBUTRAMINE

Sibutramine (**Reductil**) is a medication that was released in 2002, which acts on the brain to reduce appetite. A weight reduction of five per cent can be expected in three months in most patients. It cannot be used by patients who are on some antidepressants and patients with heart disease or high blood pressure. Blood pressure must be monitored regularly, and the medication is quite expensive. There are many other groups who should not use this medication, including those over 65 years. Its use should be carefully discussed with a doctor.

Avoid all between-meal snacks, they are almost invariably high in fat and sugar.

GASTRIC BANDING

Gastric banding is a **surgical technique** to aid in weight loss in the severely obese.

Using a laparoscopic technique, an inflatable band (with the trade name Lap-Band) is tightened around the stomach to create a smaller pouch for the reception of food. The band controls the flow of food from the small pouch into the rest of the stomach and intestine. The patient feels comfortably full with a small amount of food, and because of the slow emptying, the patient will continue to feel full for several hours after eating, thus reducing the urge to eat between meals. Appropriate follow-up of the patient after the procedure is essential.

The size of the opening between the two halves of the stomach created by the band can be adjusted after the operation without additional surgery, depending on the patient's reactions and results. This is done by inserting a needle through the skin into a reservoir of fluid (usually saline) that controls the tension in the inflatable circular band. X-rays such as a barium meal are normally performed before and after any inflation.

In cases with complications such as vomiting, obstruction and oesophageal enlargement, it is possible to completely deflate the system, opening up the stomach. In the following weeks it is possible to gradually inflate the system again.

Weight loss and diet must be carefully monitored indefinitely after the application of a gastric band.

After the procedure, patients can usually eat less than a quarter of a normal sized meal without causing discomfort or nausea. Most patients lose over a third of their excess weight over the next three years.

Surgery to produce weight loss is a serious undertaking, and each patient should clearly understand what the proposed operation involves.

GASTROPLASTY

Gastroplasty is a surgical procedure on the stomach to alter its shape. It is used in the treatment of obesity and is usually performed by a line of staples being inserted through the stomach wall to reduce the amount of food the stomach can hold.

The only person who can lose weight for you is you.
It is not up to anyone else to make you lose weight.

RESULTS

The long-term **success** rate for those who are truly obese and try to lose weight is very discouraging. Most have yo-yo weights which fluctuate up and down over the years by 20kg or more as they try different diets and exercise programs. This weight fluctuation can be more harmful than staying fat. Overall, less than one in 20 of obese people manage to return to within normal weight limits and stay there for more than five years.

If you do manage to stay on a diet for about five years, and maintain your weight constantly within the desired range, the body will adapt to its new shape, and the metabolic rate may also adjust, so that you may suddenly find after years of dieting that you can relax a little, and still maintain the new weight.

CURIOSITY

The Pickwickian syndrome is named after the extraordinarily obese Dickens character, and is a complication of being seriously obese that usually occurs in women. Patients have significant shortness of breath, gross obesity, tiredness, blue skin (cyanosis), shallow breathing, cor pulmonale (high blood pressure in lungs), high blood pressure (hypertension) and heart failure. Pneumonia and other serious infections are common. The prognosis is poor unless the patient succeeds in losing a large amount of weight.

OSTEOPOROSIS

L ooking after yourself and avoiding osteoporosis is a matter of choosing the right parents, being male (both options, although being totally out of our control, are still important), eating the right foods, exercising regularly and not smoking.

DESCRIPTION

Osteoporosis is a common bone condition affecting one quarter of women over the age of 50, in which the basic constituent of bone, calcium, drops to a dangerously low level, and the bones soften and may bend, break or collapse.

Most patients do not know they have osteoporosis until they fracture a bone (particularly the hip or a vertebra) with minimal injury, or on a routine X-ray their bones are seen to be more transparent than normal. Deformity of the back, severe arthritis, and neuralgia caused by the collapsing bones pinching nerves, can occur in due course.

CALCIUM

Calcium (Ca) is a mineral that makes up the main part of the structure of bones. Two per cent of the weight of the body is due to calcium, with half in the bones and half in solution in the blood and other bodily fluids. The level of calcium in the bones and blood is controlled by two hormones, parathormone (which raises blood calcium) and calcitonin (which lowers blood calcium) which are produced in the parathyroid glands in the neck. Calcium is essential for the production of many enzymes, in muscle contraction, and electrical conduction in nerves, as well as bone structure.

The absorption of calcium from the gut is dependent on vitamin D, which is obtained in the diet and by sun irradiation of cholesterol in the skin.

Women who eat a high calcium diet before menopause build up their calcium stores and are less likely to suffer from osteoporosis after the menopause.

CALCIUM IS FOUND IN NUMEROUS FOOD GROUPS BUT PREDOMINANTLY IN:

- all dairy food (particularly cheese)

- sardines

- shellfish, beans

- nuts

- tripe.

Adults require up to 800mg of calcium, and children and pregnant women up to 1400mg a day.

The structure of bones is being constantly renewed, and a lack of calcium over many years leads to a gradual deterioration in bone strength. Once women reach the menopause, the drop in hormone levels accelerates the loss of calcium from bones. It may be hereditary and is more common in petite, small-boned women.

INVESTIGATION
DENSITOMETRY
The density of bone can be ascertained from the amount of mineral contained in it. **Dual photon densitometry** is a type of bone scan that is able to measure the mineral content of bone and is a way of diagnosing the onset of osteoporosis, or thinning of the bones.

The patient lies on a bed with a very mild source of radiation under it, and a long-armed scanner then moves slowly down the body emitting photon beams which can determine the density of the tissue they are passing through. The procedure takes about half an hour and is completely painless. A screening test may involve only checking the density of the bone in the forearm.

Densitometry cannot necessarily predict osteoporosis in normal people but is very useful for high-risk subjects or people who already have signs of osteoporosis, so that remedial treatment such as biphosphonate drugs, hormone replacement therapy and calcium supplements can be administered.

DEXA
Dual-energy X-ray absorptiometry (DXA or DEXA) is a more sophisticated system than dual photon densitometry to measure bone density and diagnose osteoporosis.

A focussed beam of X-rays with two frequency peaks (dual energy) is passed through a bone and its surrounding tissues as a special X-ray machine moves along a limb or the back. A complex computer program is used to calculate the amount of X-ray energy absorbed by the bone compared to the surrounding tissue and normal bone, to give a result that effectively measures the bone mineral density. The mineral present is primarily calcium. This figure is a measure of the severity of any osteoporosis that may be present.

Different DXA machines give different results and cannot be compared one with another unless identically calibrated.

Many cases of osteoporosis are first detected on a
plain X-ray of the body taken for other reasons.

PREVENTION

LIFESTYLE

Prevention involves adding **calcium** to the diet before menopause, and by taking calcium supplements and hormone replacement therapy after menopause. Regular **exercise** is important, as the minor stresses on the bones keep them stronger.

Other factors that can help are reducing the intake of coffee and alcohol, and stopping smoking. Control is good once the condition is diagnosed, but reversal of existing damage is difficult.

In more serious cases, sophisticated, very effective medications (e.g. alendronate, risedronate, disodium etidronate) that force calcium into bones to strengthen them may be prescribed to be taken regularly for several years.

ALENDRONATE

Alendronate (**Fosamax**) is a tablet that can be taken in low doses daily, or high doses weekly, to prevent osteoporosis and Paget disease. It is a potent and effective medication for osteoporosis that was introduced in 1996. Once a week doses (70mg) introduced in 2001 have dramatically increased ease of use. Patients should use it with caution in cases of recent peptic ulcer and kidney damage. Calcium and vitamin D levels must be monitored, and do not take any other medications within two hours. Do not take at all if suffering from an active peptic ulcer.

Common **side effects** may include nausea, vomiting and indigestion, while less common ones may be ulceration of oesophagus and stomach, mouth ulcers, peptic ulcers, muscle pain and headaches. Stop the medication and consult a doctor if vomiting of blood or black motions occur.

Alendronate interacts with calcium supplements, antacids, biphosphonates and aspirin, and may affect almost any medication taken by mouth.

DISODIUM ETIDRONATE

Disodium etidronate (**Didronel**) is a tablet used daily for the prevention of osteoporosis. It is often combined with calcium in the one tablet. It is not for use in pregnancy, breast feeding or children. Use it with caution in cases of peptic ulcer, inflamed bowel and kidney stones, and do not take if suffering from osteomalacia or bone cancer. The diet must contain adequate calcium and vitamin D.

Common **side effects** may include diarrhoea and nausea, while less commonly bone pain and bleeding from the bowel may occur. It may interact with antacids, vitamin and mineral supplements and high calcium foods (e.g. cheese, sardines).

RISEDRONATE

Risedronate (**Actonel**) is a tablet used for the management of osteoporosis introduced in 2001 as a new way of preventing vertebral fractures and subsequent curvature of the spine in older women. It must only be taken with plain water, 30 to 60 minutes before the first food of the day. The patient must be upright when taking medication, and must not lie down for 30 minutes. The tablet must not be chewed, sucked or broken.

It is not designed to be used in pregnancy, breast feeding or children. Use it with caution in cases of kidney disease, oesophageal ulceration and peptic ulcers, and do not take it if suffering from low blood calcium or if unable to sit upright or stand for 30 minutes after taking the tablet. Food and beverages interfere with the absorption of risedronate. Calcium and vitamin D supplements may be necessary.

Common **side effects** may include belly and muscle pain, while unusual side effects may include mouth, eye and bowel inflammation. Liver damage is a rare complication.

Risedronate interacts with antacids, aspirin, NSAIDs, other drugs used to treat osteoporosis and some minerals (e.g. iron, magnesium).

CURIOSITY

Women who have an early menopause are more likely to develop osteoporosis than those whose menopause occurs later in life.

OVERDOSE

A n overdose of medication may be taken accidentally (e.g. a child, confused elderly person) or deliberately as a suicide attempt.

There are ways to prevent both situations and look after yourself and your family by having child-proof medication cabinets, dosette boxes for the elderly, and seeking help from a doctor rather than considering suicide. Unfortunately suicide is sometimes an almost spontaneous act, and may have minimal warning signs.

SYMPTOMS
A person who has taken an overdose of drugs may feel faint, slur their speech, have convulsions and gasp for breath. They will generally have a rapid, weak pulse and they may be unconscious.

Try to find out **what** drug has been taken and whether it has been swallowed, inhaled or injected. If you can find any containers, syringes or ampoules, send them to the hospital with the victim. If the victim has vomited, try to collect a sample.

A medication does not have to be on prescription to be dangerous.
Paracetamol is one of the most dangerous medications in overdose.

FIRST AID
The appropriate first aid by the person discovering the overdose may be lifesaving. Some medications are far more dangerous than others when taken in excess.

For virtually all medication overdosages, the first aid treatment is to administer **charcoal** to neutralise the medication. Charcoal tablets and solutions are readily available from chemists without a prescription, and should be included in any home medicine chest. If charcoal is not available and there will be some delay in obtaining medical attention, it is preferable to induce **vomiting** rather than allow the medication to be absorbed. Do not induce vomiting unless you are sure it is appropriate.

Vomiting should NOT be induced if the patient is unconscious or otherwise liable to inhale any vomitus.

Charcoal should be given at any time after the overdose being taken. Induction of vomiting is most beneficial within 30 minutes of the overdose being taken, but even up to two hours later it may be beneficial. Many medications cause vomiting as part of their overdose effects, but by this time, the drug has already been absorbed and the vomiting is unlikely to reduce the effects of the drug significantly.

Vomiting can be induced by giving ipecacuanha syrup and water, by giving soapy water to drink, by applying pressure to the upper belly or by putting a finger down the back of the persons throat (be careful not to be bitten, particularly if patient is likely to convulse). The patient should be lying on their side with the neck extended, or sitting up and leaning over to avoid inhaling vomitus.

Always make sure you really know the emergency phone number in your country. People have been known to phone incorrect numbers they have become familiar with through television.

Carers should seek **medical advice** as soon as possible, and sometimes urgent medical attention must be obtained by phoning the emergency number for immediate attendance by an ambulance.

If the victim is unconscious, place them on their side in the recovery position (see separate entry under 'unconsciousness' in this book) and continue to monitor breathing and pulse until help arrives. If breathing or the heart stops, carry out the ABC (airway, breathing, circulation) of first aid and give mouth-to-mouth resuscitation and/or cardiopulmonary resuscitation as required.

CURIOSITY

All substances are dangerous in overdose. Even water, if taken in sufficient quantities, can cause disruption to the biochemistry of the body, and some vitamins may be very dangerous in overdose.

PALPITATIONS

Palpitations are an excessively rapid and strong heartbeat that may be irregular. To look after yourself, make sure that the cause of any episode of palpitations is determined.

CAUSE

Palpitations occur in everyone with **exercise**, anxiety, stress, **pain** or a fright, but usually settle quite quickly.

Heavy **smoking**, **caffeine** in cola drinks, tea or coffee, excess **alcohol**, food sensitivities and some food preservatives and colourings may trigger palpitations.

Pregnant women generally have a faster heart rate, and **hormonal** surges may trigger brief episodes of palpitations.

Any palpitation that does not have an obvious
cause must be checked by a doctor.

Bacterial and viral **infections**, or any other disease that causes a fever, will cause an increased heart rate while the fever is present.

Paroxysmal atrial tachycardia (PAT) is a very common condition, particularly in women. For no apparent reason, but sometimes because of hormonal changes during the menstrual cycle and menopause, the heart will start beating rapidly, usually at double its normal rate. This harmless but distressing condition may last for a few seconds or several hours before settling spontaneously.

OTHER CAUSES MAY INCLUDE:

- a heart attack (myocardial infarct)

- atrial fibrillation (irregular heart beat due to heart damage)

- ectopic beats (occasional extra normal beat)

- anaemia

- infections of the heart (endocarditis, myocarditis)

- inflammation of the heart muscle

- over-active thyroid gland (hyperthyroidism)

- reflux oesophagitis

- phaeochromocytoma (black-celled tumour of the adrenal glands)

- da Costa syndrome (a psychiatric disturbance).

Medications such as salbutamol (Ventolin – for asthma), glyceryl trinitrate (Anginine – for heart pain), terbutaline (Bricanyl – for asthma), aminophylline (for lung conditions) and imipramine (for depression) may have palpitations as a side effect.

The incidence of palpitations increases with age.

MISSED HEARTBEAT

Occasional **dropped beats** are very common in older people and are no cause for concern.

If the dropped beats are more frequent (say one in every five), then it is necessary for tests such as an electrocardiogram (ECG) to be done to determine the cause. Even in this situation, there may be no serious problem. The occasional extra heartbeat fits into this category also.

Stress, alcohol, smoking and exercise are common causes of dropped or extra beats. More serious diseases may also be responsible, such as high blood pressure, rheumatic heart disease and as an after-effect of a heart attack.

TREATMENT

No treatment for palpitations can be given until the cause is determined, and it is the cause that is treated, not the palpitations themselves. There are many effective medications available, the most common belonging to the betablocker class (e.g. propranolol, atenolol), and calcium channel blockers (e.g. verapamil).

CURIOSITY

The da Costa syndrome is a heart function abnormality that is also known as the effort syndrome. It is characterised by persistent palpitations that are triggered by anxiety, exercise or stress, but have no other sinister underlying cause. An ECG (electrocardiograph) shows a rapid heart rate but no other abnormality, and the blood pressure shows a high systolic and low diastolic reading (wide pulse pressure). The syndrome is resistant to psychiatric care and betablocker medications are used to successfully control the symptoms, but cure is difficult.

PELVIC PAIN

Many pelvic pains have simple explanations, particularly in women, and do not require medical attention, but it is important to look after yourself by seeking medical advice for any pelvic pain that is severe, worsens or persists.

ANATOMY

The pelvis is a basin-shaped group of bones that support the lower end of the abdominal cavity and contain the rectum, loops of small intestine, the bladder, and, in women, the uterus and ovaries.

At the back of the basin is the sacrum, which is really five fused vertebrae. The top of the sacrum supports the spinal column and its vertebrae.

The sides of the pelvis are formed by the iliac bones, which can be felt as the arch of bone above the hip. We sit on a very thick arch of bone called the ischium. The front of the pelvis is formed by the pubic bone. These three bones fuse together as fixed joints where there is no movement. At the point where the three bones meet is the socket (acetabulum) for the hip joint.

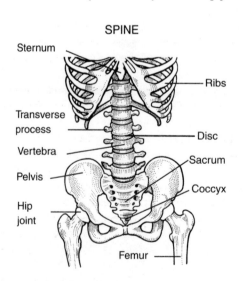

Pain in the pelvis or lower abdomen (hypogastrium) may come from any of the organs in the pelvis including the last part of the large bowel (rectum), bladder, vagina, uterus, ovaries, Fallopian tubes, prostate gland, testes or lymph nodes.

CAUSES

Painful **periods**, and the associated spasms and cramps of the uterus are a common cause of pelvic pain on a regular basis. The intrauterine contraceptive device (IUD) may aggravate these period pains.

Similar cramping pains to those of a period may be felt before and during a **miscarriage** of pregnancy.

An **ectopic pregnancy** is the development of a growing foetus in the Fallopian tubes instead of the uterus. The tube becomes swollen and sensitive, and pain during deep sex may be noticed some days before other painful symptoms develop.

Fibroids are hard balls of fibrous tissue that form in the muscular wall of the uterus, often after pregnancy. They can distort the shape of the uterus to cause pain when the uterus contracts during a menstrual period or orgasm.

Cysts may form on a regular basis in an ovary because of errors in the release of ova (eggs) every month. When **ovarian cysts** leak or burst they release a fluid that is very irritating and causes inflammation and pain.

Any persistent pelvic pain that cannot be properly explained
(e.g. period cramps) must be checked by a doctor.

OTHER **GYNAECOLOGICAL** CAUSES OF PELVIC PAIN INCLUDE:
- salpingitis (infection of the Fallopian tubes)

- endometriosis

- retrograde menstruation (menstrual blood goes up a Fallopian tube and into the pelvic cavity)

- ovarian torsion (twisting of an ovary on the stalk of tissue that supplies blood and nerves)

- cancer of an ovary

- pelvic congestion syndrome (associated with fluid retention in the pelvis).

IN **MEN**, PELVIC PAIN MAY BE DUE TO:
- prostatitis (bacterial infection of the prostate)

- torsion of the testis (the testicle twists around and cuts off the blood vessels that supply it).

CAUSES OF PELVIC PAIN AFFECTING BOTH SEXES INCLUDE:
- severe constipation

- hernia (inguinal or femoral)

- cystitis (bladder infection)

- bladder stones

- diverticular disease (formation of numerous small outpocketings of the large gut)

- irritable bowel syndrome

- ulcerative colitis (lining of the large intestine becomes ulcerated and bleeds)

- adhesions

- appendicitis

- peritonitis (infection of the lining the belly cavity).

PELVIC LUMP

A doctor may feel an abnormal lump or mass in the pelvis while feeling the lower abdomen or doing an internal examination through the vagina or anus. Occasionally patients discover such a lump themselves.

Lumps in the pelvis may come from the last part of the large bowel (rectum), bladder, vagina, uterus, ovaries, Fallopian tubes or lymph nodes.

Cancer of any of the organs in the pelvis listed above may be responsible for a lump. There is usually accompanying pain, tenderness and abnormal function of the organ (e.g. bleeding and abnormal bowel function in bowel cancer).

Pregnancy is a certain cause of an enlarging mass in the pelvis, and some women have presented to doctors after finding it, without being aware that they are pregnant.

The only way to effectively examine the pelvis is through the anus or vagina.

OTHER **GYNAECOLOGICAL** CAUSES OF A PELVIC LUMP INCLUDE:

- ectopic pregnancy (development of a foetus in the Fallopian tubes instead of the uterus)

- fibroids (hard balls of fibrous tissue that form in the muscular wall of the uterus)

- endometriosis

- pelvic inflammatory disease (generalised infection of the organs in the pelvis)

- ovarian cysts (sometimes of enormous size)

- hydrosalpinx (a severely inflamed Fallopian tube that swells with fluid).

OTHER CAUSES OF A MASS IN THE PELVIS INCLUDE:

- severe constipation

- abscess in the pelvis

- lymphoma (cancer of the lymph nodes)

- very rarely an abnormally positioned kidney.

CURIOSITY

Between the base of the penis and the anus in men, and the back of the vagina and anus in women, there is a slight thickened ridge of the skin called the raphe. This is caused by the joining of the two halves of the body at an early point in the development of the embryo.

PERIOD PROBLEMS

Women should look after themselves by ensuring that their monthly menstrual period does not interfere with their lifestyle. If the period is not doing what she wants it to, there is no longer any need for most women to suffer, as doctors now have an enormous range of treatments available to control the menstrual cycle in a user-friendly way.

EXPLANATION

Once a month, just after a woman releases the egg (at ovulation) from her ovary, the lining (endometrium) of the womb (uterus) is at its peak to allow the embedding of a fertilised egg.

If pregnancy does not occur, the endometrium starts to deteriorate as the hormones that sustain it in peak condition alter. After a few days, the lining breaks down completely, sloughs off the wall of the uterus, and is washed away by the blood released from the arteries that supplied it in a process known as menstruation. Contractions of the uterus help remove the debris.

After three to five days, the bleeding stops, and a new lining starts to develop ready for the next month's ovulation.

SCHEMATIC REPRESENTATION OF HORMONE CHANGES DURING MENSTRUAL CYCLE

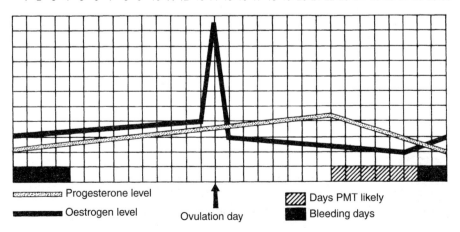

1 2 3 4 5 6 7 8 9 10 11 12 13 14 15 16 17 18 19 20 21 22 23 24 25 26 27 28 29 30

Progesterone level

Oestrogen level

Ovulation day

Days PMT likely

Bleeding days

FAILURE OF MENSTRUAL PERIODS TO START

Normally, a young woman starts her menstrual periods with **puberty** between 11 and 14 years of age, but there are some who commence early and later, without any subsequent problems. If a girl fails to start her periods by the age of 16, investigation is appropriate. If the breasts have not developed, and there is no sign of pubic hair by the age of 14, investigation may be commenced earlier.

A number of uncommon medical conditions may be responsible for the problem, which is medically known as primary amenorrhoea.

In some girls, the **hymen** completely covers the vaginal opening and has no hole, so that menstrual blood accumulates in the vagina with no way to escape. The periods are occurring, but no blood appears.

The hypothalamus is the part of the brain that controls the pituitary gland at the base of the brain. The pituitary gland in turn controls all other glands in the body, including the ovaries. If there is damage to the **hypothalamus** or **pituitary gland** from a tumour, cancer, abscess, infection, poor blood supply or other disease, the appropriate signals may not be received by the ovary to activate its production of the sex hormone oestrogen, which is essential for the transformation of a girl into a woman at puberty.

The **ovaries** may not develop normally in some girls due to a birth defect, or chromosomal abnormalities such as Turner syndrome.

Congenital adrenal hyperplasia (**adrenogenital syndrome**) affects the adrenal glands that sit on top of each kidney, and stimulates them to produce abnormal steroids in the body, which affect sexual development.

Tumours may develop in the ovaries, or very rarely in other tissue, that produce inappropriate levels of the male sex hormone **testosterone**, which blocks the effect of any oestrogen that may be produced.

Every woman between 15 and 50 whose periods stop
is considered to be pregnant until proved otherwise.

LACK OF MENSTRUAL PERIOD

Women expect their menstrual periods to occur regularly every month, and become concerned when this does not happen. The obvious causes for periods to stop are **pregnancy** and **menopause**.

Breast feeding will delay the return of regular menstrual periods. There are also a number of medical conditions which may be responsible.

The oral **contraceptive pill** may cause menstrual periods to become lighter and lighter until they disappear completely. Some women take the pill constantly, without a monthly break off the pill or taking sugar tablets, and stop their periods for the sake of convenience. This practice is completely safe and causes no long-term harm.

OTHER COMMON REASONS FOR PERIODS TO STOP INCLUDE:

- significant emotional trauma (e.g. loss of job, death in family)

- physical stress (e.g. vigorous athletic training)

- serious illness (e.g. major infection)

- poor nutrition (e.g. lack of food, vomiting and diarrhoea)

- significant weight loss as a result of deliberate dieting

- cancer almost anywhere in the body

- psychiatric disturbance (e.g. anorexia nervosa)

*Amenorrhoea is a lack of menstrual periods, while
oligomenorrhoea is infrequent menstruation.*

UNCOMMON CAUSES FOR THE PERIODS TO FAIL INCLUDE:

- tumours, cysts or cancer in an ovary that affect the production of oestrogen

- a lack of thyroxine (hypothyroidism)

- Asherman syndrome (damaged lining of uterus after curettage)

- Addison's disease (failure of the adrenal glands)

- Stein-Leventhal syndrome (multiple cysts in the ovaries)

HEAVY MENSTRUAL PERIODS

Excessive blood loss during a menstrual period (flooding) is uncomfortable, distressing and may lead to **anaemia** and other health problems.

In most women it is a **constitutional problem**, in that there is no specific disease or condition causing the problem but it is the way that their body deals with the monthly hormonal changes. In a few cases though, there is an underlying medical problem. This is more likely if the periods have changed to become heavier over a few months.

The **menopause** occurs in the late forties and early fifties in most women. Instead of cycling smoothly and evenly through the monthly changes, sex hormone (oestrogen and progestogen) levels start to change suddenly, irregularly and inappropriately. This causes the symptoms of menopause, which include irregular menstrual periods that can vary from very light to very heavy, hot flushes, headaches, irritability, personality changes, breast tenderness, tiredness and pelvic discomfort.

Inappropriately high levels of **oestrogen** being prescribed for hormone replacement therapy may cause heavy periods.

Psychological disturbances (e.g. severe stress, shock or anxiety) may affect oestrogen production and irregular heavy periods may follow.

Intrauterine contraceptive devices (**IUD**) may irritate the lining of the uterus to cause heavier and more painful periods in some women.

OTHER CAUSES OF MENORRHAGIA INCLUDE:

- fibroids (hard balls of fibrous tissue that form in the muscular wall of the uterus)

- cysts in an ovary

- ulcers and erosions of the cervix (opening of the uterus into the vagina)

- endometriosis (abnormal deposits in the pelvis of tissue from inside the uterus)

- a miscarriage (may cause abnormal bleeding before a woman is knows she is pregnant)

- ectopic pregnancy (foetus in the Fallopian tubes instead of the uterus)

- salpingitis (infection of the Fallopian tubes)

- hypothyroidism (an under-active thyroid gland)

- Stein-Leventhal syndrome (multiple cysts in the ovaries affect their function)

- thrombocytopenia (blood clotting disorder).

Tumours, polyps or cancers of the uterus or cervix may cause irregular heavy bleeding, which may not be related to the menstrual cycle, but be caused by direct bleeding from the growth.

The technical term for heavy periods is menorrhagia,
and for painful periods is dysmenorrhoea.

PAINFUL MENSTRUAL PERIODS

In more than eight out of ten cases, there is no serious cause for painful periods. Although distressing, they are merely the way in which a woman, and her uterus, copes with menstruation.

The uterus mainly consists of powerful muscle fibres, which should only come into use during the delivery of a baby, and, to a minor extent, when blood and the unused lining of the uterus is expelled in the monthly menstrual period. Period pain is usually caused by excessive spasms of these muscles in the uterus, but sometimes may be due to other medical problems.

During the **menopause**, the natural sex hormones produced by the ovaries may be produced irregularly and in greater quantities, leading to an increased build-up of the uterine lining during the month, or excessive stimulation of the uterine muscles during a period.

An intrauterine contraceptive device (**IUD**) may irritate the uterus to trigger more powerful contractions than usual.

Salpingitis (infection of the Fallopian tubes), often by sexually transmitted diseases, may result in the tubes becoming blocked and painful. Pelvic inflammatory disease is a more widespread infection of the organs within the pelvis. During a period, contractions of the uterus may irritate these infected organs to cause pain.

Endometriosis is a disease in which the cells that normally line the inside of the uterus become displaced, and move through the Fallopian tubes to settle around the ovary, in the tubes themselves, or on other organs in the belly. In these abnormal positions they proliferate, and when a menstrual period occurs, they bleed as though they were still in the uterus. This results in pain, adhesions, damage to the organs they are attached to, and infertility.

Fibroids are hard balls of fibrous tissue that form in the muscular wall of the uterus, often after pregnancy. They can distort the shape of the uterus to cause pain when the uterus contracts during a period or orgasm.

The uterus is normally bent forwards at about 60° to the vagina. In some women, the uterus is straighter, or bent backwards (**retroverted**). These women seem to suffer from more painful periods.

Other causes of dysmenorrhoea include a prolapse of the uterus (uterus slips down into the vagina), pelvic congestion syndrome (veins in the pelvis become dilated), narrowing of the cervix after surgery, adhesions and tumours, polyps or cancers of the uterus or surrounding organs.

CURIOSITY

Extract from an 1831 medical text:

'If menstruation is suppressed, leeches should be applied to the vaginal lips, pubis or inguinal regions, and the frequent use of hot pediluvia recommended'.

PILES

The best way to look after yourself and prevent this miserably uncomfortable problem is to avoid both constipation and heavy weight-lifting when squatting.

ANATOMY

Haemorrhoids (also known as piles) are caused by dilation, damage to, bleeding from and blood clot formation in veins around the anus. Internal and external versions, depending on whether veins inside or outside the anus are damaged.

A vein circles around the anus close to the skin surface. When a motion is passed, the anal canal dilates, but if this dilation is excessive, these fine veins can be stretched, then rupture and form piles. They may be intermittent, painless swellings, or they can be excruciatingly tender and painful, and bleed profusely. Excessive bleeding from the pile may cause anaemia.

Once formed, a weak area will always be present, and even though one pile may settle, the same one may flare up again and again.

There is an inherited predisposition to develop piles.

CAUSES

Constipation is by far the most common cause of a pile. Passing a large, hard faecal motion over-stretches the anal canal to cause bleeding from the surrounding vein.

Straining to lift a heavy weight while **squatting** is another common cause, as excessive pressure builds up inside the anal veins. Advanced pregnancy has a similar effect.

Obesity may also place excessive pressure on the veins around the anus.

DIAGRAMATIC REPRESENTATION OF ANAL CANAL AND THE FORMATION OF A PILE

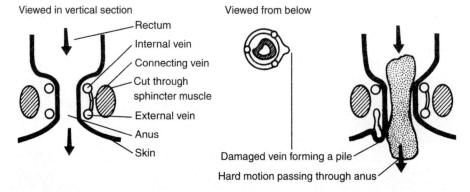

Viewed in vertical section

- Rectum
- Internal vein
- Connecting vein
- Cut through sphincter muscle
- External vein
- Anus
- Skin

Viewed from below

Damaged vein forming a pile

Hard motion passing through anus

Portal hypertension is an increase in the blood pressure in the veins of the abdomen that take nutrition from the intestine to the liver. Many different liver diseases may be responsible, and piles are a common effect.

*Patients with anal cancer often delay presenting
to a doctor because they think they have piles.*

INVESTIGATION

Looking and feeling are embarrassingly necessary for the problem to be appropriately diagnosed. This means that your doctor will examine the anus, and then feel inside with a gloved and lubricated finger to check not only for internal piles, but more serious causes of anal bleeding such as cancer.

Proctoscopy (passing an examination tube through the anus into the rectum) can be performed to examine the piles in greater detail, and see internal piles.

TREATMENT

Keeping the bowels regular and soft prevents piles. Initially, ice packs and simple soothing creams can be used in treatment, but if relief is not obtained, steroid and antiseptic creams or soothing suppositories are prescribed.

If there is a clot of blood in the haemorrhoid, it is cut open to allow the clot to escape.

If it persists, further treatment may involve clipping a rubber band around the base of the pile, injected or electrically coagulating the pile, or an operation to cut away part of the anal canal. The operation is normally successful in permanently removing the problem.

*Dark coloured blood on or in the faeces is a more
sinister sign, and probably not due to piles.*

ANAL BLEEDING

Bleeding from the anus at times when the patient is not passing a motion may be associated with piles or a fissure.

With a **pile** (haemorrhoid), the bleeding tends to occur after passing a motion, and blood is present on the toilet paper, but it may occur at any time, particularly if straining with heavy lifting. Piles can be painless, or very painful, depending on the degree of inflammation and the presence of a blood clot within the pile.

A **fissure** in the anus (fissure in ano), where the anus has over-stretched and torn during an episode of constipation, can also cause intermittent bleeding similar to that of a pile. Keeping the motions soft and using a medicated ointment usually settles the problem. Rarely, scarring and narrowing of the anus may occur. Generally the prognosis is good if constipation is controlled.

The possibility of a **cancer** in the anus, or above the anus in the rectum, must always be considered.

CURIOSITY

Extract from an 1820 medical text:

'Those who are liable to bleeding piles should avoid heating themselves with strong drink, nor must they fall into violent passions, either of love or anger'.

POISONING

A person can be poisoned by taking an overdose of drugs, either accidentally or deliberately, or by swallowing or inhaling some substance that upsets the functioning of their body.

It is necessary to act quickly to minimise the effect of the poison.

In children, a common cause of poisoning is raiding the family medicine chest or the kitchen cabinet with its supply of cleaning fluids, solvents and detergents.

Look after your family by ensuring that children do not have access to any potential poison, and knowing what to do if poisoning does occur.

FIRST AID

If someone is poisoned, ring an ambulance or hospital and ask them what to do in the case of the specific substance involved.

IN GENERAL TERMS:

- if the victim is unconscious (see separate entry in this book), place them on their side in the coma position and check that the airway is clear

- monitor their breathing and pulse constantly. If breathing stops, give expired air respiration, and if the pulse stops, give cardiopulmonary resuscitation

- consider inducing vomiting – if possible ask a doctor first.

DO NOT INDUCE VOMITING IF:

- the poisonous substance is unknown

- a corrosive substance such as battery acid, oven cleaner, toilet cleaner, a strong disinfectant or any acid or alkaline substance has been swallowed

- a petroleum-based product (e.g. kerosene, petrol, diesel oil, turpentine) is swallowed. If these substances are vomited they will burn the throat a second time, or damage the lungs by inhalation

- the patient is drowsy and may become unconscious. Such patients risk choking if they vomit.

Someone who has swallowed a **corrosive** substance can be given small sips of water or milk, but otherwise simply wipe the substance away from the mouth and face, make the victim as comfortable as possible and get urgent medical advice.

DO INDUCE VOMITING IF:

- the substance is a medicine or similar substance

- the victim is not elderly and frail

- the substance was swallowed within the previous half hour

To induce **vomiting**, give syrup of ipecacuanha according to instructions on the bottle, or stimulate the back of the victim's throat with a finger. Do NOT give salt or soapy water to drink. Keep a sample of the vomit in a clean jar to send to the hospital.

If the poison has been **inhaled**, move the victim away from the fumes or turn the fumes (e.g. gas) off at the source. Once the victim is in the fresh air, loosen any tight clothing and check breathing and pulse constantly – if either ceases or becomes weak, administer artificial respiration.

Do not become a victim yourself when dealing with gases or contact poisons.

Sometimes poisons are **absorbed** through the skin (e.g. pesticides, weed killer). In this case, remove the victim's clothes and get them to wash or shower thoroughly. If they become dizzy or sick, or complain of blurred vision or show any other sign of distress, get medical help immediately. Wash the contaminated clothes separately from other clothes.

FIRST AID TREATMENT OF POISONING

CHEMICAL/DRUG	EFFECT OF POISON	FIRST AID TREATMENT
Alkalis (household bleaches)	Burning, vomiting, shock, difficult breathing.	Dilute with milk, allow vomiting, give vinegar.
Antidepressants (Tryptanol, Sinequan, Tofranil etc.)	Coma, muscle spasm, convulsions, death.	Give charcoal or induce vomiting, assist breathing.
Aspirin (Aspro, Disprin etc.)	Rapid breathing, brain disturbance, coma, kidney failure.	Give charcoal or induce vomiting.
Barbiturates	Drowsiness, confusion, coma, breathing difficulty.	Give charcoal or induce vomiting, black coffee, assist breathing.
Codeine (in pain killers, cough mixtures, antidiarrhoeals)	Constipation, reduced breathing, stupor, coma, heart attack.	Give charcoal or induce vomiting, assist breathing.
Digoxin (Lanoxin)	Vomiting, irregular pulse, heart failure.	Dilute with milk or water then give charcoal or induce vomiting.
Insecticides	Vomiting, diarrhoea, difficult breathing, convulsions.	Dilute with large amount of milk, give charcoal or induce vomiting, assist breathing.

CHEMICAL/DRUG	EFFECT OF POISON	FIRST AID TREATMENT
Lysol and creosote	Burning of throat, vomiting, shock, breathing difficulty.	Dilute with large amount of milk. Do NOT induce vomiting.
Mushrooms	Varies depending on type.	Dilute with water, give charcoal or induce vomiting, assist breathing.
Narcotics (morphine, heroin)	Headache, nausea, excitement, weak pulse, shock, coma.	Give charcoal or induce vomiting if narcotic swallowed, assist breathing.
Paracetamol (Panadol, Dymadon, Panamax etc.)	Vomiting, low blood pressure, liver damage, death [>40 tabs].	Give charcoal or induce vomiting.
Petroleum products (petrol, kerosene, etc.)	Liver damage, lung damage.	Do NOT induce vomiting, dilute with milk.
Tranquillisers (phenothiazines)	Drowsiness, low blood pressure, rapid pulse, convulsions, coma.	Give charcoal or induce vomiting.

POISONOUS PLANTS

It is possible for the plants found in many gardens to fatally poison a child or foolish adult.

One of the prettiest and deadliest trees is the **Oleander**. These are widely grown throughout Australia as an ornamental tree, but are extremely poisonous. A leaf, a flower or a fruit is sufficient to kill a child, and the sap can be equally dangerous. The early symptoms of poisoning are vomiting, diarrhoea, palpitations and dilated pupils, which can lead to coma and death.

The **Castor Oil Plant** grows wild as a weed in many scrub areas along Australia's eastern seaboard. It has seeds the size of golf balls, which children often play with, but if eaten, can cause severe diarrhoea, cramps, vomiting and, rarely, death. Most councils consider it a noxious weed.

Dieffenbachia (also known as Dumbcane) is a decorative shrub often found in indoor plantar boxes. Chewing or biting the large fleshy leaves of this attractive plant produces copious salivation and severe burning and irritation of the mouth that may last for many days.

Angel's Trumpet is a small tree that may be three metres or more high and has white trumpet-shaped flowers. Eating any part of the plant, particularly the flowers, can cause severe gastrointestinal symptoms, delirium and death.

Other common plants that may cause severe illness, if not death, include the broad-leafed rainforest plant Cunjevoi; the stunted Pineapple Zamia palm; the blue-black plum-like fruit of the Wintersweet; the prickly Duranta Golden Dewdrop; the attractive fruit of the pot or rock plant called Coral Bush or Physic Nut; and the seeds of the Moreton Bay Chestnut Tree.

Children in the house? Ensure there are no poisonous plants in your garden.

ARSENIC

Arsenic (As) is an element used in industry and mining. It may be encountered in smelting (e.g. gold, lead, zinc and nickel), wood preservatives, pesticides, herbicides and some folk remedies. It may be accumulated slowly by workers in such industries, or acute poisoning may occur if the mineral is swallowed.

Symptoms of acute poisoning include a difficulty in swallowing, vomiting, diarrhoea, thirst and poor urine output. Death may occur in two or three days. The lethal dose is about 150mg.

First aiders should induce vomiting if arsenic is recently swallowed, and the patient should go to hospital, where the stomach will be pumped out and activated charcoal given. Copious fluids are then given by a drip into a vein to flush out the poison, and medications are given to neutralise it.

Chronic poisoning is characterised by nerve damage affecting sensation and muscle control, kidney damage, skin changes and irritation of the nose and mouth lining.

The prognosis depends on age and weight of patient, and dose of arsenic.

Arsenic can be detected in hair samples indefinitely after death from the poison.

CYANIDE

Correctly called hydrocyanic acid, cyanide is a potent poison that can be inhaled or swallowed. It has rapid toxic effects on many tissues in the body, causing them to fail due to an inability to process essential oxygen.

Cyanide is used in fumigation, photography, electroplating, rubber processing, metal cleaning and some other industries. It is found naturally in numerous seeds including cherry, plum, peach, pear and apricot. Lethal dose depends on form, but is about 250mg of sodium cyanide.

The **symptoms** of poisoning include headache, fainting, dizziness, anxiety, rapid heart rate, burning in the mouth and throat, shortness of breath, high blood pressure, nausea, vomiting, bitter almond breath, coma, convulsions and finally death.

Some medications may be effective as an antidote. The emergency treatment is pure oxygen given by a close-fitting mask. The prognosis depends on age, weight and fitness of patient, and dose of cyanide.

STRYCHNINE

Strychnine is a poison obtained from the seeds of the plant species *Strychnos*. It is a bitter tasting white powder in pure form, and acts as a powerful stimulant of the nervous system.

If swallowed, the victim will experience the **symptoms** of muscle spasms, convulsions and vomiting before brain death occurs. Symptoms start within 15 to 30 minutes of swallowing the poison.

In the hospital intensive care unit, medications are given to paralyse the patient and prevent convulsions, while life is sustained by artificial ventilation. The prognosis depends on the dose. If a patient survives for 12 hours, recovery is likely, but permanent heart, nerve or muscle damage is possible.

CURIOSITY
Mercury was used as an antibiotic to treat syphilis until the beginning of the twentieth century, and although reasonably effective, it is now known to be a cumulative poison.

PREGNANCY

E ntire books, even encyclopaedias, have been written about pregnancy, its progress and complications, so this must be a general overview.

To look after herself, a woman must keep her own body in good order so that her child has the best possible environment to develop.

DIAGNOSIS

SYMPTOMS

The first sign that a woman may be pregnant is that she fails to have a **menstrual period** when one is normally due. At about the same time as the period is missed, the woman may feel unwell, unduly tired, and her breasts may become swollen and uncomfortable.

Early in the pregnancy the breasts start to prepare for the task of feeding the baby, and one of the first things the woman notices is enlarged **tender breasts** and a tingling in the nipples. With a first pregnancy, the skin around the nipple (the areola) will darken, and the small lubricating glands may become more prominent to create small bumps. This darkening may also occur with the oral contraceptive pill.

Hormonal changes cause the woman to **urinate** more frequently. This settles down after about three months, but later in pregnancy the size of the uterus puts pressure on the bladder, and frequent urination again occurs.

Some women develop dark patches on the forehead and cheeks called **chloasma**, which are caused by hormonal changes affecting the pigment cells in the skin. This can also be a side effect of the contraceptive pill. The navel and a line down the centre of the woman's belly may also darken. These pigment changes fade somewhat after the pregnancy but will always remain darker than before.

PREGNANCY TESTS

Pregnancy tests are based on the detection of a hormone called human chorionic gonadotrophin (HCG), which is produced in the first few months of pregnancy by the placenta and can be detected in **blood** or **urine** as early as 12 days after conception (i.e. before a period is even missed). At this early stage, a false negative result is possible, and the tests are more reliable if carried out a couple of days after the missed period. A negative test may mean that the pregnancy is not far enough advanced to be detected, rather than that the woman is not pregnant, while a positive test is almost invariably correct.

The pregnancy test consists of mixing a few drops of the woman's urine with specific chemicals. If HCG is present, a chemical reaction will take place. In a test carried out in a test tube, the mix of urine and chemicals will form a characteristic deposit; but more often the urine is added to one side of a small flat plastic container and, as the urine moves across this, it interacts with chemicals that will change colour if the test is positive. To ensure a reliable result, the test is generally carried out two to seven days after the first missed period (i.e. 16 to 21 days after conception).

A pregnancy test can be carried out at home with a kit purchased from the chemist, but more reliable tests are performed by doctors using a sample of blood.

Although pregnancy actually occurs about two weeks after a woman has her last period, for convenience doctors always date a pregnancy from the first day of that last menstrual period.

PREGNANCY DATES

The date a pregnant woman is due to deliver (estimated date of confinement – EDC) can be calculated in the following way:

Add seven days to the day the woman's last period started,

and nine months to the month of her last period.

For example, if the last period started on 5 February 2005,

she will be due to deliver on 12 November 2005.

A pregnancy lasts 40 weeks (280 days) from the beginning of the woman's last period, but only 38 weeks from conception, because she ovulates two weeks after her period starts. It is not unusual for the pregnancy to be one or two weeks shorter or longer than this.

PRECAUTIONS

A pregnant woman should not smoke, because smoking adversely affects the baby's growth, and smaller babies have more problems in the early months of life. The chemicals inhaled from cigarette smoke are absorbed into the bloodstream and pass through the placenta into the baby's bloodstream, so that when the mother has a smoke, so does the baby.

Alcohol should be avoided, especially during the first three months of pregnancy when the vital organs of the foetus are developing. Later in pregnancy it is advisable to have no more than one drink every day with a meal.

No pregnant woman should smoke under any circumstances!

PREGNANCY PROGRESS

ANTENATAL CARE

After the pregnancy has been diagnosed, the woman should see her doctor at about ten weeks of pregnancy for the first antenatal check-up and referral to an obstetrician. At this check-up she is given a thorough examination (including an internal one), and blood and urine tests will be ordered to exclude any medical problems and to give the doctor a baseline for later comparison.

Routine **antenatal checks** will then be performed by the general practitioner or obstetrician at monthly intervals until about 34 weeks pregnant, when the frequency will increase to fortnightly or weekly. Blood pressure and weight measurement and a quick physical check are normally performed. A small ultrasound instrument may be used to listen for the baby's heart from quite an early stage. Further blood tests will be performed once or twice during this period, and a simple test will be carried out on a urine sample at every visit.

An **ultrasound scan** is usually performed to check on the size and development of the foetus.

Most women are advised to take tablets containing **iron** and **folic acid** throughout pregnancy and breast feeding, in order to prevent both the mild anaemia that often accompanies pregnancy, and nerve developmental abnormalities in the foetus.

MIDDLE TRIMESTER

As the skin of the belly stretches to accommodate the growing baby, and in other areas where fat may be found in the skin (such as breasts and buttocks), **stretch marks** in the form of reddish/purple streaks may develop. These will fade to a white/silver colour after the baby is born, but unfortunately they will usually not disappear completely.

About the fourth or fifth month, the thickening waistline will turn into a bulge, and by the sixth month, the swollen belly is unmistakable. The increased bulk will change the woman's sense of balance, and this can cause muscles to become fatigued unless she can make a conscious effort to maintain a good upright posture.

The nine months of a pregnancy is broken into
three month periods known as trimesters.

Care of the back is vitally important in later pregnancy, as the ligaments become slightly softer and slacker with the hormonal changes, and movement between the vertebrae in the back can lead to severe and disabling pain if a nerve is pinched.

During pregnancy, the mother must supply all the food and oxygen for the developing baby and eliminate its waste materials. Because of these demands, the mother's metabolism changes, and increasing demands are made on several organs. In particular, the heart has to pump harder, and the lungs have more work to do supplying the needs of the enlarged uterus and the placenta. Circulation to the breasts, kidneys, skin and even gums also increases. Towards the end of the pregnancy, the mother's heart is working 40 per cent harder than normal. The lungs must keep the increased blood circulation adequately supplied with oxygen.

As the mother is the baby's sole source of nourishment during pregnancy, she should pay attention to her diet. A balanced and varied diet containing plenty of fresh fruit and vegetables, as well as dairy products (calcium is required for the bones of both mother and baby), meat and cereal foods, is appropriate.

LAST TRIMESTER

During the last three months of the pregnancy, **antenatal classes** are very beneficial. Women are taught exercises to strengthen the back and abdominal muscles, breathing exercises to help with the various stages of labour, and strategies to cope

PREGNANCY AT FULL TERM

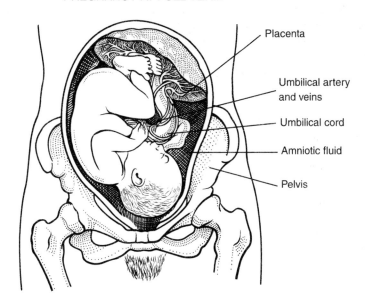

Placenta

Umbilical artery
and veins

Umbilical cord

Amniotic fluid

Pelvis

with them. Women who attend these classes generally do far better in labour than those who do not.

In the month or so before delivery, it will be difficult for the mother to get comfortable in any position, sleeplessness will be common, and the pressure of the baby's head will make passing urine a far too regular event. Aches and pains will develop in unusual areas as muscles that are not normally used are called into play to support the extra weight, normally between 7 and 12kg (baby + fluid + placenta + enlarged uterus + enlarged breasts), that the mother is carrying around.

Attending lectures run by the Nursing Mothers' Association (or similar organisations) to learn about **breast feeding**, how to prepare for it and how to avoid problems, is useful in the last few weeks of pregnancy and for a time after the baby is born.

Visiting the hospital or birthing centre that you have booked into for the confinement can be helpful, so that the facilities and the labour ward will not appear cold and impersonal when they are used.

*The number 40 is used as an abbreviation for the number of weeks
a pregnancy has progressed. The notation 15/40 in a doctor's notes
would indicate a pregnancy that has progressed to the 15 week stage.*

PREGNANCY PROBLEMS
BACKACHE
A pregnant woman's pelvis has to expand at the time of birth to allow the baby through. To facilitate this expansion, the **ligaments** that normally hold the joints of the pelvis (and other parts of the body) together become slightly softer and more

elastic, which makes them more susceptible to strain. The joints of the spine are particularly at risk because the expanding uterus shifts the centre of balance and changes posture. Standing for any length of time is likely to impose unusual stresses on the back, and this strains the supporting ligaments and results in backache.

Slight movements of the vertebrae, one on the other, can cause nerves to be pinched and result in pain such as **sciatica**. This nerve pinching is further aggravated by the retention of fluid in the whole body, which causes the nerves to be slightly swollen and therefore more easily pinched.

The best way to reduce the likelihood of backache is not to gain weight excessively and to avoid all heavy lifting. At antenatal classes, physiotherapists show the correct way to lift, and teach exercises to help relieve the backache.

BLEEDING

Extensive studies have not shown any increase in infant abnormalities after bleeding in early pregnancy. The bleeding may be due to a slight separation of the placenta from the wall of the womb as it grows, and it almost certainly does not involve the baby directly.

About 30 per cent of all pregnant women suffer from some degree of bleeding during pregnancy, and some have quite severe bleeds without losing the baby.

Vaginal bleeding in early pregnancy is common.

Bleeding in early pregnancy may also be a sign of an impending miscarriage. Unfortunately nothing except rest can help the mother in this situation. Doctors cannot usually prevent miscarriages once bleeding has started.

Other causes of bleeding in pregnancy include an ectopic pregnancy, vaginal ulcers or erosions, or hormonal imbalances.

CONSTIPATION IN PREGNANCY

Constipation is common in pregnancy and is thought to be due to a loosening of the muscles of the digestive tract caused by hormonal changes. In late pregnancy the enlarging womb presses on the intestines and aggravates the condition. It is not dangerous, but if worrying, a faecal softener can be used. No medications, including laxatives, should be used during pregnancy without discussing them with a doctor.

ECTOPIC PREGNANCY

A foetus normally grows within the womb (uterus). An ectopic pregnancy is one that starts and continues to develop **outside the uterus**. About one in every 200 pregnancies is ectopic. Conditions such as pelvic inflammatory disease and salpingitis increase the risk of ectopic pregnancies, as they cause damage to the Fallopian tubes. Other infections in the pelvis (e.g. severe appendicitis) may also be responsible for tube damage.

Symptoms of an ectopic pregnancy may be minimal until a sudden crisis from rupture of blood vessels occurs, but most women have abnormal vaginal bleeding

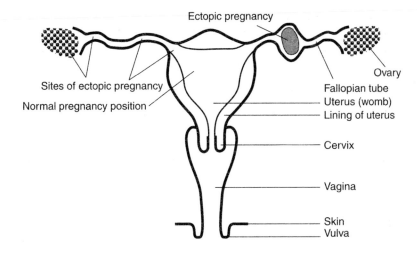

Ectopic pregnancy

Sites of ectopic pregnancy

Normal pregnancy position

Ovary

Fallopian tube

Uterus (womb)

Lining of uterus

Cervix

Vagina

Skin

Vulva

or pains low in the abdomen in the early part of the pregnancy. Many ectopic pregnancies fail to develop past an early stage, and appear to be a normal miscarriage. Serious problems can occur if the ectopic pregnancy does continue to grow.

The most common site for an ectopic pregnancy is the Fallopian tube, which leads from the ovary to the top corner of the womb. A pregnancy in the tube will slowly dilate the tube until it eventually bursts. This will cause severe bleeding into the abdomen and is an urgent, life-threatening situation for the mother. Other possible sites for an ectopic pregnancy include on or around the ovary, in the abdomen or pelvis, or in the narrow angle where the Fallopian tube enters the uterus.

If an ectopic pregnancy is suspected, an ultrasound scan can be performed to confirm the exact position of any pregnancy. If the pregnancy is found to be ectopic, the woman must be treated in a major hospital. Surgery to save the mother's life is essential, as a ruptured ectopic pregnancy can cause the woman very rapidly to bleed to death internally. If the ectopic site is the Fallopian tube, the tube on that side is usually removed during the operation. With early diagnosis and improved surgical techniques, the tube may not have to be removed. Even if it is lost, the woman can fall pregnant again from the tube and ovary on the other side.

It is rare for a foetus to survive an ectopic pregnancy.

DIABETES IN PREGNANCY

Pregnancy may trigger diabetes in a woman who was previously well but predisposed towards this disease. One of the reasons for regular antenatal visits to doctors and the urine tests taken at each visit is to detect diabetes at an early stage. If diabetes develops, the woman can be treated and controlled by regular injections of insulin. In some cases, the diabetes will disappear after the pregnancy, but it often recurs in later years.

If the diabetes is not adequately controlled, serious consequences can result. In mild cases, the child may be born grossly overweight but otherwise be healthy. In more severe cases, the diabetes can cause a miscarriage, eclampsia, malformations of the foetus, urinary and kidney infections, fungal infections (thrush) of the vagina, premature labour, difficult labour, breathing problems in the baby after birth, or death of the baby within the womb.

Diabetic women tend to have difficulty in falling pregnant, unless their diabetes is very well-controlled.

HEARTBURN IN PREGNANCY

Indigestion or heartburn affects about half of all pregnant women, because during pregnancy the muscle that closes off the upper part of the stomach from the oesophagus (gullet) loosens and allows digestive juices from the stomach to flow back up the oesophagus and irritate it. In late pregnancy the enlarging uterus presses on the stomach and aggravates the condition.

Heartburn can be very uncomfortable but is not harmful. Symptoms may be reduced by eating small, frequent meals, so that there is never too much food present but always enough to absorb the stomach acid. Antacids can usually be taken safely at most stages of pregnancy, and may be used to relieve more severe symptoms. The problem disappears when the baby is born.

MORNING SICKNESS

The nausea and vomiting that affects some pregnant women between the sixth and fourteenth weeks of pregnancy is called morning sickness, but it can occur at any time of the day. Its severity varies markedly, with about one-third of pregnant women having no morning sickness, one-half having it badly enough to vomit at least once, and in five per cent the condition is serious enough result in prolonged bed rest or even hospitalisation, when it is called hyperemesis gravidarum.

Half of all pregnant women have some degree of hyperemesis gravidarum (morning sickness) and one in twenty is severely affected.

Morning sickness is caused by the unusually high levels of oestrogen present in the mother's bloodstream during the first three months of pregnancy. Although it usually ceases after about three months, it may persist for far longer in some unlucky women. Severe cases may be associated with twins, and it is usually worse in the first pregnancy.

Because morning sickness is a self-limiting condition, **treatment** is usually given only when absolutely necessary. A light diet, with small, frequent meals of dry fat-free foods, is often helpful. A concentrated carbohydrate solution (Emetrol) may be taken to help relieve the nausea. Vitamin B6 and ginger (as pieces or extracts) may also be helpful. Only in severe cases, and with some reluctance, will doctors prescribe more potent medications. In rare cases, fluids given by a drip into a vein are necessary for a woman hospitalised because of continued vomiting.

Morning sickness has no effect upon the development of the baby.

OLIGOHYDRAMNIOS

In the womb, the baby is surrounded by, and floats in, a sac filled with amniotic fluid. This fluid acts to protect the foetus from bumps and jarring, recirculates waste, and acts as a fluid for the baby to drink. If **insufficient fluid** is present, the condition is called oligohydramnios.

Normally there is about a litre (1000mL) of amniotic fluid at birth. A volume less than 200mL is considered to be diagnostic of oligohydramnios. It may be caused by abnormal development of the foetus or abnormal function of the placenta, but in most cases there is no reason for the problem.

The condition is diagnosed by an ultrasound scan, and if proved, further investigations to determine the cause of the condition follow. Treatment will depend upon the result of these tests, but often none is necessary.

POLYHYDRAMNIOS

If an **excessive** amount of amniotic **fluid** is present, the condition is called polyhydramnios.

A volume greater than 1500mL is considered to be diagnostic of polyhydramnios, but it may not become apparent until 2500mL or more is present.

Polyhydramnios occurs in about one in every 100 pregnancies, and it may be a sign that the foetus has a significant abnormality that prevents it from drinking or causes the excess production of urine. Other causes include a twin pregnancy, and diabetes or heart disease in the mother. In over half the cases no specific cause for the excess fluid can ever be found.

The condition is diagnosed by an ultrasound scan, and if proved, further investigations to determine the cause of the condition must follow. The treatment will depend upon the result of these tests, but often none is necessary.

There is an increased risk to the mother of amniotic fluid **embolism**, a potentially fatal complication that occurs when some of the fluid enters the mother's bloodstream, but most pregnancies proceed relatively normally, although there is an increased risk of foetal abnormality.

PRE-ECLAMPSIA AND ECLAMPSIA

Eclampsia is a rare but very serious disease that occurs only in pregnancy. In developed countries it is very uncommon, because most women undertake regular antenatal visits and checks. Pre-eclampsia is a condition that precedes eclampsia, and this is detected in about ten per cent of all pregnant women. The correct treatment of pre-eclampsia prevents eclampsia.

High blood pressure in pregnancy is serious,
which is why doctors check it at every opportunity.

The exact **cause** of pre-eclampsia is unknown, but it is thought to be due to the production of abnormal quantities of hormones by the placenta. It is more common in first pregnancies, twins and diabetes. Pre-eclampsia normally develops in the last three months of pregnancy, but may not develop until labour commences, when it may progress rapidly to eclampsia if not detected.

The early detection of pre-eclampsia is essential for the good health of both mother and baby. Doctors diagnose the condition by noting **high blood pressure**, swollen ankles, abnormalities (excess protein) in the urine and excessive weight gain (fluid retention).

Not until the condition is well established does the patient develop the **symptoms** of headache, nausea, vomiting, abdominal pain and disturbances of vision.

If no **treatment** is given, the mother may develop eclampsia. This causes convulsions, coma, strokes, heart attacks, death of the baby and possibly death of the mother.

Pre-eclampsia is treated by strict rest (which can be very effective), drugs to lower blood pressure and remove excess fluid, sedatives, and, in severe cases, early delivery of the baby. The correct treatment of pre-eclampsia prevents eclampsia, and the prognosis is very good if detected early and treated correctly.

SEX IN PREGNANCY

Unless a doctor has recommended otherwise (e.g. for a threatened miscarriage), it is perfectly safe to engage in sex during pregnancy if both partners desire it.

Pregnancy does not preclude intimacy.

Some women find that their sex drive decreases at certain stages of pregnancy, while other women are the opposite. A man may also be affected, being more attracted to his pregnant wife, or deterred by the new life within her.

As a general rule, the foetus will not be affected by intercourse. In the last couple of months, only certain positions will be comfortable for the woman (e.g. woman sits atop lying man).

STRETCH MARKS

Stretch marks (striae) are the curse of pregnant women, when they develop on their belly and breasts, and overweight people whose stretch marks persist after they have lost weight. The tendency to develop striae is one that may be inherited.

They are caused by a breakdown and stretching of the elastic fibres in the skin by changes in the body's hormone levels as well as direct stretching of the skin. Once they form they usually remain permanently unless removed by plastic surgery or reduced by creams containing retinoic acids.

CURIOSITY

The labour of childbirth may be induced by the continued stimulation of the nipples of a woman in the last week or two of pregnancy.

A fear of pregnancy is called maieusiophobia.

PROSTATE GLAND

The prostate gland is a bit hard for its owner to look after, as its function is outside any voluntary control, and nothing a man does to look after himself (other than avoid venereal diseases) will affect any of the problems that may occur. On the other hand, if symptoms of difficulty in urination occur later in life, it may be due to the prostate, and proper assessment is essential.

ANATOMY

The prostate gland is situated behind the base of the penis. The bladder is above and behind the gland, and the tube which carries urine from the bladder to the outside (the urethra) passes through the centre of the prostate. It is found only in men and there is no female equivalent.

The prostate is about the **size** of a golf ball and consists of glands, fibrous tissue and muscle. Its primary purpose is to produce a substance that makes up part of the semen a man ejaculates during sexual intercourse. This substance is essential for the nutrition of the sperm as they try to fertilise an egg in the woman.

MALE GENITAL ANATOMY

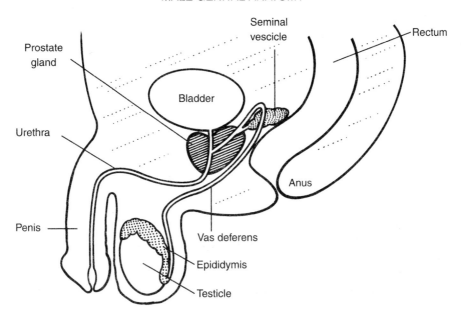

Most men are totally unaware of the presence of the prostate unless it causes trouble.

In younger men, the most common cause of disease is **infection**, when the gland may swell up and become very tender. In older men the disease process is quite different. Up to 20 per cent of all men over 60 may have an **enlargement** of the prostate which causes symptoms, and a small percentage of these may have **cancer** of the prostate.

> *Until the mid-twentieth century, doctors had*
> *no idea what the prostate gland was for.*

INVESTIGATION

Unless extraordinarily dextrous, no man can feel his own prostate, as this small organ which sits behind the base of the penis can only be felt by placing a finger through the anus, where the prostate can be felt as a firm lump on the front wall of the rectum (last part of the large bowel).

Doctors can often diagnose diseases of the prostate by **feeling** the gland. This involves putting a gloved finger in the back passage so as to gauge its size and hardness.

The most commonly used test on the prostate gland is the blood test to measure the prostate specific antigen (PSA). Ultrasound scans and biopsy of the gland may also be performed.

PROSTATE SPECIFIC ANTIGEN

A test for the prostate specific antigen (PSA) can be used to follow the success of treatment for prostate cancer and infection. If the levels drop, treatment is successful – if they rise, it is not.

There has been a lot of controversy about the use of this test as a **screening test** for prostate cancer. It has been argued that early detection leads to more effective treatment, and in younger men this is true, but it is an uncommon disease under 50 years of age. In older men, early detection does not necessarily mean a better outcome, as some cancers are dormant and do not need treatment, the treatment may have significant side effects, and some cancers are incurable even with radical treatment.

A level of PSA below 4 micrograms per litre is usually normal, while a level over 10 is probably due to cancer, but unfortunately many conditions other than cancer can cause the results to be high (e.g. infection or enlargement of the gland). On the other hand, a man with some types of prostate cancer can have a low level of PSA. As a result, it is not an absolute test for prostate cancer.

A combination of tests for different types of PSA (free and combined PSA) may be a better form of screening, but is still quite expensive.

To SUM UP, THE ADVANTAGES AND DISADVANTAGES OF PSA TESTING ARE:

ADVANTAGES

- side effects of treatment are fewer with early treatment of prostate cancer

- PSA increases the chance of detecting prostate cancer early

- modern treatment is often successful in curing early cancers

- most cancers detected with PSA are serious

- a low level of PSA is reassuring

DISADVANTAGES
- a raised PSA result may be due to other conditions other than cancer

- some prostate cancers are not serious and may be treated excessively

- a cure cannot be guaranteed with early detection

- there may be significant side effects from treatment

- the investigation of the raised PSA by biopsy can cause serious complications

- the treatment of prostate cancer is not straightforward and may lead to significant patient stress and confusion.

For men over 70 years, knowing they have prostate cancer can have more serious consequences than not knowing it is there, as the benefits of treatment may be very limited.

DISEASES
ENLARGED PROSTATE GLAND
If the prostate enlarges (**prostatomegaly**), the patient will have difficulty in starting the urinary stream, and when it does start, the urine will dribble out onto his shoes, rather than jet onto the porcelain. Up to 20 per cent of all men over 60 have benign enlargement of the prostate gland, which is usually associated with a drop in sexual activity. The absolute cause is unknown, but as the gland enlarges, it squeezes the urethra (urine-carrying tube) which passes through it, making it steadily harder to urinate.

With prostate enlargement the man develops increasing **difficulty in passing urine**, and eventually the urethra becomes completely blocked, causing extreme distress as the pressure of urine in the bladder increases. If back pressure of urine in the bladder becomes persistent, kidney damage can occur.

In the acute situation, a flexible tube is passed up the urethra through the penis into the bladder to release urine, but if this is unsuccessful a large needle must be pushed through the lower wall of the abdomen into the bladder.

In some cases drugs (e.g. finasteride, prazosin, terazosin) can be used to shrink the enlarged prostate slightly.

Most cases require surgery once symptoms develop. The operation can vary from simply dilating the urethra to scraping away the part of the prostate constricting the urethra by passing a specially shaped knife up it (transurethral resection of prostate – TURP), or completely removing the gland.

Treatment is almost invariably successful, with no subsequent effect on the general health of the patient, but there is sometimes subsequent sexual dysfunction.

PROSTATE CANCER

Prostate or **prostatic cancer** describes any one of several different types of cancer of the prostate gland, depending on which cells in the gland become cancerous. The cause is unknown, but those who have sex infrequently may be more susceptible. It is rare before 50 years of age, but up to 20 per cent of all men over 60 may have an enlargement of the prostate. The percentage of these men whose enlargement is due to cancer steadily increases with age, with virtually every male over 90 years of age having some degree of prostate cancer.

More men die with prostate cancer than from prostate cancer.

This is a very **slow-growing** cancer that may give no symptoms until many years after it has developed. Symptoms usually start with difficulty in passing urine and difficulty in starting the urinary stream. In advanced stages there may be spread of cancer to the bones of the pelvis and back.

It is treated with a combination of surgery, drugs and irradiation. Early stages may not be treated in the very elderly, because it is unlikely to cause trouble in their lifetime. **Brachytherapy** is a process in which tiny radioactive particles are injected into the prostate to create radiation which destroys the cancer. **Orchidectomy** (removal of the testes) is sometimes performed to remove all testosterone from the man's body, as this stimulates growth of the cancer.

If the cancer is localised to the gland itself, the five-year survival rate is over 90 per cent. With local spread, the survival rate drops to about 70 per cent, but with spread to the bone, only 30 per cent of patients survive five years.

PROSTATITIS

Prostatitis is an **infection** of the prostate gland by bacteria that may enter the prostate by moving up the urethra (urine tube) from the outside, from a sexually transmitted infection (e.g. gonorrhoea), or uncommonly from an infection spreading from other parts of the body.

Pain occurs behind the base of the penis, and there is a discharge from the penis, pain on passing urine and fever, and patients pass urine frequently. The infection may spread to the man's sexual partner, in whom it can cause pelvic inflammatory disease.

The **diagnosis** is confirmed by taking a swab from the urethra and identifying the bacteria present, and treatment requires taking a long course of antibiotics.

Acute cases usually settle with treatment, but recurrences are common and a low-grade persistent infection may develop, which is difficult to treat.

CURIOSITY

Use it or lose it – this old saying applies as much to the prostate as any other organ, as there is evidence that men who have frequent sex have fewer prostate problems than men who are celibate.

RASH

I is important to look after your skin by protecting it from sun and dryness, as the better you care for it, the better you will look, and the less likely you are to develop significant skin diseases.

THE SKIN

Skin is the outer covering of the body. It is much more complex than one might think, as it protects the body against infection and parasites and provides a tough resilient cushion to safeguard the tissues underneath from injury. It also helps to maintain body temperature and prevent the body from becoming dehydrated. The skin is also the main organ of the sensation of touch, which can perceive heat, cold, sharp, blunt, vibration and pain.

The skin consists of two main **layers** that are quite different from each other in the way they are made up and the way they function.

The top layer, the one we see, is the **epidermis**. This contains no blood vessels, nerves or connective tissue fibres and, in turn, is subdivided into two layers. The outer layer consists mainly of dead cells which are constantly being shed. The inner layer consists of cells with the capacity to multiply at a rapid rate, which they do continually, pushing up and replacing the discarded dead cells. The dying cells produce a protein called keratin which thickens and protects the skin. Keratin, developed in a particular way together with dead cells, also forms the hair and nails.

ENLARGED DIAGRAMATIC CROSS SECTION OF SKIN

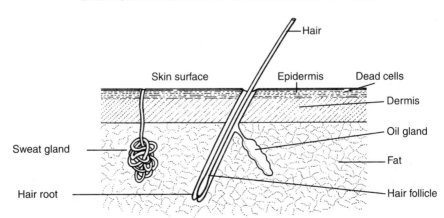

Under normal circumstances, from the time a skin cell is produced to the time it dies and flakes off takes about a month. However, if injury occurs, even just a minor scratch, the multiplication of cells speeds up to repair the damage. If the damage is repeated, deeper tissues may thicken to compensate and form a callus.

Every part of a person you are looking at or touching is made of dead skin cells.

The inner layer of the epidermis also produces the pigment **melanin**, which gives the skin its colour. Freckles are simply irregular patches of melanin. We all have the same number of melanin-producing cells, irrespective of our racial origin, but dark-skinned races produce more melanin than light-skinned races. Exposure to the sun encourages the production of melanin as a protection against the sun's rays, giving a suntan. Absence of the pigment melanin leads to the abnormally white skin and general appearance of people classified as albino.

Beneath the epidermis is the **dermis**, which is the so-called true skin. The dermis is well supplied with blood vessels and nerves and has a framework of elastic connective tissue, as well as the proteins collagen and elastin. The blood vessels provide the nourishment for the epidermis. The thickness of both the dermis and the epidermis varies so that some areas (e.g. the soles of the feet and the palms of the hands) are covered with thick layers, whereas other areas (e.g. the eyelids) are covered with thin and delicate layers.

The dermis rests on a layer of fatty tissue called the **subcutaneous** layer. The fat serves as both insulation and a reserve store of energy. Embedded in the dermis and extending into the subcutaneous layer are sweat and sebaceous glands, which are essential for the proper functioning of the body.

Most skin is covered by **hair**, with the exception of that on the soles of the feet and the palms of the hands. These areas are covered with alternately ridged and grooved patterns that increase the body's ability to grip at these points. These patterns are different in every single individual and remain the same throughout life, hence the use of fingerprints as a means of identification.

Disorders of the skin are not usually life-threatening but can be unsightly and psychologically damaging.

RASHES

Unfortunately, there are hundreds of things that can go wrong with our biggest organ, the skin. Some of the possible symptoms, and their explanations will be listed in order to allow you to make a more informed decision about your particular problem.

A rash is any visible abnormality of the skin.

BLISTERS

Blisters on the skin can vary in size from pin heads to several centimetres across. They may be full of clear fluid or creamy pus, and there may be one or hundreds of them.

A single blister full of clear fluid may be due to an insect or spider **bite** and can often appear as a clear blister in the centre of a small red patch of skin, or a significant burn will cause a clear blister to arise at the site of the burn.

Multiple blisters full of clear fluid may be due to **contact dermatitis** (a red rash that then develops multiple tiny blisters), **erythema multiforme**, and **herpes simplex** (type one causes cold sores on the face, while type two causes genital herpes).

Drug eruptions occur when a patient is sensitive or allergic to a medication and multiple large, clear fluid-filled blisters may erupt on many areas of the body.

Chickenpox is the most common infection to cause small scattered fluid-filled blisters. The rash usually starts on the head or chest as red pimples, then spreads onto the legs and arms, and develops into blisters before drying up and scabbing over.

Shingles is an infection of a spinal nerve caused by the same virus that causes chickenpox. At times of stress or reduced immunity, the virus may start to multiply again in one particular nerve, to cause sharp pain that gradually moves along the nerve on one side only from the back to the front of the abdomen. Shortly after the pain starts, a patchy blistering rash will appear in a line along the course of the nerve.

Shingles is a medical emergency, as the viral infection can be completely cured if treated within 72 hours of the rash starting.

Genital herpes and cold sores are caused by different forms of the *Herpes simplex* virus. **Genital herpes** causes a blister, which bursts to form a very painful, tender, shallow ulcer that persists for ten to twenty days.

Multiple blisters filled with creamy substance may be due to **molluscum contagiosum** (a common viral infection of the skin in children), **impetigo** (school sores – a bacterial infection), cellulitis (a skin infection that in severe cases may break down the overlying skin to form large, slack, pus-filled blisters) and **erysipelas** (a superficial infection of skin that causes blisters similar to cellulitis).

Virtually every child will eventually develop **hand foot mouth disease**, which is caused by a *Coxsackie* virus, and in severe cases, a child will develop blisters on the soles and palms, and mouth ulcers that persist for three to five days before settling.

LESS COMMON CAUSES OF SKIN BLISTERS INCLUDE:

- pemphigoid (a skin disease usually of elderly women)

- pemphigus (an autoimmune skin disease, large blisters develop)

- erythema multiforme (red blistering skin triggered by drugs or infections)

- epidermolysis-bullosa (inherited condition)

- toxic epidermal necrolysis (a severe but rare skin condition caused by exposure to a toxin or poison which causes large, clear fluid-filled blisters to form on extensive areas of the body).

BLUE SKIN

A blue tinge to the skin (**cyanosis**) is a serious symptom that can indicate significant disease, usually of the heart or lungs. Cyanosis is caused by the blood carrying too much waste carbon dioxide and not sufficient oxygen, and so remaining a dark blue colour rather than the bright red of well-oxygenated blood.

Cyanosis in an infant usually indicates a serious structural **defect of the heart** (e.g. ventricular septal defect) and/or lungs. These are usually congenital (present as a defect since the embryo stage).

In adults, cyanosis may be due to extensive involvement of both lungs with **pneumonia** (an infection of the small air bubbles – alveoli – in the lungs), **emphysema**, bronchiectasis, **heart failure**, pulmonary thrombosis (blood clot in lungs), severe **anaemia** and abnormal connections between major arteries and veins, or defects in the muscular wall between the right and left sides of the heart.

Blue fingers and toes are a common symptom of extreme **cold** in everyone. Initially they will go white, then if neglected will become blue and painful before the permanent damage of frostbite occurs. A specific form of this problem is **Raynaud phenomenon**, which is a spasm of arteries when tissue is exposed to only mild cold. It causes affected tissue to go white, then blue and red, before becoming swollen and painful. The hands and feet are usually affected, and it is far more common in women than men.

Many of the causes of blue skin may be
directly, or indirectly, caused by smoking.

Buerger's disease is damage to the small arteries in the feet and hands caused by smoking. Polycythaemia rubra vera is an uncommon condition in which there are an excessive number of red blood cells that can clog up the fine capillaries that supply blood to individual cells, leading to painful finger tips, itchy blue skin and a general tiredness.

In Pickwickian syndrome, grossly obese patients are unable to circulate sufficient blood due to heart failure.

DEPIGMENTED SKIN

A lack of skin pigment, even in northern Europeans, can be seen as a total lack of pigment everywhere on the skin, or patchy loss of pigment. The darker the natural skin colour, the more obvious the problem.

Severe burns and other skin injuries may heal with a **scar** that is dead white or significantly paler than the surrounding skin.

Pityriasis versicolor is a relatively common **fungal infection** of the outermost layers of the skin that occurs in warm climates. The fungus prevents the skin under it from tanning on exposure to the sun, so the patient appears to have white blotches of varying sizes scattered across their body. Pityriasis alba causes a similar effect.

Albinism is an inherited disorder in which the skin lacks pigment cells, and explains the occasional appearance of completely white Africans, or white animals that are normally dark-skinned. The iris (coloured part of the eye) also lacks pigment and appears pink because of the blood vessels in it.

Chediak-Higashi syndrome is an inherited condition that can pass to subsequent generations. It causes recurrent skin and lung infections, partial albinism (skin depigmentation) and sometimes liver, spleen and lung damage.

DRY AND SCALY SKIN

The skin is normally kept moist and supple by the production of oil from millions of tiny sebaceous glands that are distributed everywhere on the body surface. Dry skin (xeroderma) is often susceptible to infection, itchy, irritated and uncomfortable. There are many different causes for dry and scaly skin.

Seborrhoeic dermatitis is an inflammation of the skin oil glands in the affected area, which reduces oil production and causes a red, itchy, scaly rash.

High **fevers** from any cause can increase evaporation from the skin and make it feel both hot and dry.

The thyroid gland in the front of the neck produces the hormone thyroxine, which acts as an accelerator for every cell in the body. If there is a lack of thyroxine (**hypothyroidism**), all organs will function slowly, and symptoms will include intolerance of cold, constipation, weakness, hoarse voice, heavy periods, dry skin, hair loss, slow heart rate and anaemia.

Psoriasis is a skin disease characterised by plaques of red, dry, scaly skin, most commonly on the elbows, knees and scalp. Guttae psoriasis is a very active variant.

Some patients have an inherited tendency towards dry skin that can pass from one generation to the next. The extreme cases of this are known as **ichthyosis**.

Some **drugs**, such as cimetidine (Tagamet – for stomach ulcers), nicotinic acid (for high cholesterol) and retinoids (for acne) have dry skin as a side effect.

Uncommon causes of dry skin include a severe deficiency of vitamin A, sarcoidosis (widespread organ inflammation and damage), ichthyosis, leprosy and Refsum syndrome (loss of pain sensation in the arms and legs, deafness and dry skin due to an inherited biochemical abnormality).

The term ichthyosis, for scaly skin, comes from the Greek for 'fish-like'.

LIGHT-SENSITIVE SKIN

People with a pale complexion are obviously more sensitive to sunlight (photosensitive) than those with naturally darker skin tones, but there are a number of medical conditions that increase the sensitivity of any colour skin to sunlight.

Photodermatitis is a congenital (present since birth) allergy-type reaction to sunlight that results in a red, raised, itchy rash on sunlight-exposed skin.

Systemic lupus erythematosus (**SLE**) is an autoimmune disease (inappropriate rejection of the body's own tissue) that can affect tissues throughout the body, causing arthritis, mouth ulcers and discolouration, abnormal muscle movements, high blood pressure and a characteristic red rash across the sun-exposed areas of the cheeks and bridge of the nose in a butterfly pattern.

Other causes of photosensitivity include photosensitive eczema, porphyria, pellagra (lack of vitamin B3) and phenylketonuria (inability of the body to process proteins containing phenylalanine).

A wide range of **medications** may cause the skin to become more sensitive to the sun. Examples include tetracyclines (antibiotic often used for acne), phenothiazines (used in psychiatry), sulphonamides (broad spectrum antibiotic), thiazide and frusemide diuretics (fluid removers), malaria medications (e.g. quinine), griseofulvin (for fungal infections) and nalidixic acid (for urine infections).

LUMPS IN SKIN

Papules are small, discrete, firm, solid, raised lumps on or in the skin. They may be skin colour, red, brown or black. The lump created by acne, before it becomes filled with pus and blisters (becomes a pustule), is a typical papule.

Naevi are dark brown or black raised moles. More develop on the skin with age, and most are benign (not cancer) but there is always a chance that they may be nasty.

Melanomas are the most serious form of skin cancer, and may be black, brown, pink or blue. The surface of a melanoma is often uneven and bumpy.

Cancers of the deeper layers of the skin (basal cell carcinomas) are not nearly as serious as melanomas and appear as shiny, pink, rounded lumps that often change in size and colour.

Neurodermatitis (**nerve rash**) causes multiple small, red, itchy lumps to develop in response to stress or anxiety. The wrists, ankles, inside the elbows and behind the knees are the most commonly affected areas.

Various types of **dermatitis** can appear in many forms, including solitary or multiple small lumps. Contact dermatitis, where the skin is reacting excessively to a substance, is particularly likely to form papules.

OTHER CAUSES OF A PAPULAR RASH MAY INCLUDE:

- dermatofibromas (yellow-brown nodules)

- folliculitis (infection of the oil gland at the base of a hair)

- molluscum contagiosum (viral infection of the skin in children)

- xanthoma (creamy, yellow, soft, smooth, fatty lumps that often appear around eyes)

- granulomas (single, soft lumps that develop in response to skin damage)

- granuloma annulare (ring-shaped lumps)

- lichen planus (small, shiny, flat-topped growths that may join to form a plaque)

- milia (keratin cysts)

- heat rash (miliaria)

- tularaemia (bacterial infection of rats and rabbits spreads to humans via tick bite).

Large lumps under the skin may be due to enlarged lymph nodes, fatty cysts (lipomas), a glomus tumour or Von Recklinghausen's disease of multiple neuro-fibromatosis.

NODULES IN SKIN

Nodules are discreet, separate, lumps in or on the skin. There may be one solitary nodule (e.g. a wart) or hundreds (e.g. molluscum contagiosum) present, and they can vary in size from a couple of millimetres to over a centimetre.

Warts cause a persistent, rough elevation of an area of skin, usually less than 5mm in diameter. They are caused by a very slow-growing virus, and are most common in children from eight to 16 years of age.

The tendency to develop skin warts runs in families from one generation to the next, but does not affect all descendants.

Genital warts are caused by the human papilloma virus, which is passed from one partner to another during sex. These warts are usually external on the male, but internal in the woman. They can become itchy, but more seriously, the virus can cause cancer of the cervix in women.

Blood vessels in the skin may sometimes dilate and over-develop dramatically to form a small red lump that blanches on pressure, and bleeds dramatically if injured. These **haemangiomas** are harmless, but annoying and sometimes cosmetically unacceptable.

Cancers of the deeper layers of the skin are called basal cell carcinomas (BCC). They may appear as shiny, pink, rounded lumps that often change in size and colour, or they may present as an ulcer that fails to heal.

Molluscum contagiosum is a viral infection of the skin in children that causes dozens or hundreds of tiny pus-filled blisters with dimpled tops to appear on the body over a few weeks. They remain for several weeks or months before disappearing spontaneously.

Lipomas are soft, poorly defined, round lumps under the skin that consist of fat. They may develop due to an injury to the fat layer under the skin.

OTHER CAUSES OF SKIN LUMPS MAY INCLUDE:

- seborrhoeic keratoses (age spots)

- xanthomata (creamy, yellow, smooth, fatty lumps that occur around the eyes)

- Heberden's nodes (bony lumps that develop beside finger joints in patients with severe osteoarthritis)

- glomus tumours (hard, round lumps at base of nails)

- gouty tophi (white, hard lumps that develop beside joints affected by gout)

- chilblains (develop as a result of exposure to extreme cold)

- melanomas (serious form of skin cancer)

- rheumatoid nodules (around joints affected by rheumatoid arthritis)

- erythema nodosum (very tender, painful, red lumps on the front of the leg)

- Von Recklinghausen's disease of multiple neurofibromatosis (inherited)

- granuloma inguinale (a sexually transmitted disease).

PAINFUL SKIN

The most common and obvious cause of skin pain is an **injury** such as a bruise, graze, scald or sunburn, but the most important causes are infections.

Shingles is an infection of a spinal nerve caused by the virus *Herpes zoster*. This is the same virus that causes chickenpox. At times of stress or reduced immunity, the virus may start to multiply in one particular nerve, to cause sharp pain that gradually moves along the nerve on one side only from the back to the front of the abdomen. A day or so after the pain starts, a patchy blistering rash will appear in a line along the course of the nerve. Immediate treatment is essential.

A hot, red, painful rash must be seen by a doctor immediately.

Cellulitis is an infection of the tissue immediately under the skin, and can occur anywhere on the body, but is more common at points where the skin is more easily injured, such as over joints. The skin is hot to touch as well as red and painful, and often swollen and tender.

PIGMENTED SKIN

Excessive skin pigmentation can be patchy, but still normal as in **freckles**, but there are a multiplicity of medical conditions that can cause excessive pigmentation that is obviously more noticeable in those whose natural colouring is fair.

The most common cause of excessive skin pigmentation in Caucasians is **tanning** from excessive exposure to the sun.

Bruising is an obvious but temporary cause of skin pigmentation. The initially black bruise will fade to dark blue, brown and finally yellow before disappearing.

Many people have **naevi** (pigmented spots) of varying shades on their skin that increase in number with age and skin exposure. These are completely harmless, but may be mistaken for melanoma.

Lentigo is the technical name for the flat brown 'age spots' that increase in size and number on the skin of many elderly people. They are harmless, but may be cosmetically undesirable. Sebaceous moles are fatty, soft, irregular, raised lumps that also occur with age.

Some people heal poorly and any wound leaves a dark-coloured, and often raised, scar, known as a **keloid**.

The **Mongoloid spot** is an area of mid-brown pigmentation seen at the base of the spine of many people of Chinese and other Asian ancestry. It is an inherited characteristic.

> *Inherited Mongoloid spots on the back can be found in*
> *some families as far west as eastern Europe, as it was*
> *introduced by Ghengis Khan's Mongol invasions.*

Chloasma is a mark of motherhood, as pregnancy results in pigment being deposited in the skin of the forehead, cheeks and nipples. Unfortunately, it is also an uncommon side effect of using the contraceptive pill.

Long-standing **varicose veins** often cause pigmentation of the overlying skin due to tiny amounts of blood leaking out of the veins and staining the skin.

OTHER CAUSES OF EXCESSIVE SKIN PIGMENTATION INCLUDE:

- melanomas (serious form of skin cancer)

- Hutchison melanotic freckle (mild form of melanoma)

- haemochromatosis (excess iron in the body)

- carotenaemia (excessive eating of yellow fruit and vegetables)

- xeroderma pigmentosa (disfiguring fatty brown lumps that occur in the skin folds of people with high cholesterol levels)

- Cushing syndrome (over-production of steroids in the body, or taking large doses of cortisone)

- Addison disease (under-active adrenal glands)

- Von Recklinghausen disease of multiple neurofibromatosis (inherited condition)

- scleroderma (thickened skin from autoimmune disease).

PUSTULES

Pustules are small elevated skin blisters filled with pus. They are only caused by a bacterial or viral infection, but a number of diseases may be responsible.

Pimples (**acne**) are due to a blockage in the outflow of oil from the oil glands in the skin due to dirt, flakes of dead skin, or, most commonly, a thickening and excess production of the oil. The gland becomes dilated with oil, then inflamed and eventually infected to cause acne spots. Stress, an infection or hormonal changes may see the number of spots increase dramatically.

School sores (**impetigo**) are a very common bacterial skin infection that virtually every child will catch at some stage. It is most commonly caused by the bacteria

Staphylococcus aureus. The infection spreads easily to cause one or more itchy, tender, red, raised, weeping or crusting sores on the skin.

> *School sores can be caught by adults and pre-schoolers too,*
> *but are more commonly spread when people are in*
> *close contact in an institution such as a school.*

A virus called *Herpes zoster* causes **chickenpox**. It can be found in the fluid-containing blisters, breath and saliva of patients. The rash usually starts on the head or chest as red pimples, then spreads onto the legs and arms, and develops into blisters before drying up and scabbing over.

Shingles is an infection that causes a patchy blistering rash along the course of the nerve (see painful skin entry above).

Genital herpes causes a pus-filled blister which bursts to form a very painful, tender, shallow ulcer that persists for ten to 20 days. The virus that causes the infection (*Herpes simplex*) is highly contagious.

Other causes include folliculitis (bacterial infection of a hair follicle), rosacea (skin disease of the face), melioidosis and chancroid (bacterial sexually transmitted infection).

RED SKIN

Any **infection** (e.g. cellulitis, joint infection, mastitis – breast infection), **inflammation** (e.g. eczema, gout, arthritis), **injury** (e.g. sunburn, scald, bruise), or dilation of **arteries** (e.g. flush, allergy, alcohol) can cause the skin to become redder than normal (erythema). There are therefore literally hundreds of different causes of red skin. A number of typical examples will be explained below.

There are many different types of **dermatitis** which can cause red skin. Some examples include those caused by contact of the skin with substances to which it is sensitive (contact dermatitis), sitting or lying for prolonged periods (stasis dermatitis), inflammation of the outer layers of the skin that cause excessive peeling (exfoliative dermatitis), excessive sensitivity to sunlight (photodermatitis) and inflammation of the oil glands in the skin (seborrhoeic dermatitis).

The term **eczema** describes a large range of skin diseases that cause itching and burning of the skin. It typically appears as red, swollen skin that is initially covered with small fluid-filled blisters that later break down to a scale or crust. The many different forms of eczema also have innumerable causes, both from within the body (e.g. stress) and outside (e.g. allergies, chemicals). The appearance of an eczema depends more on its position on the body, duration, severity and degree of scratching than the actual cause. The specific diagnosis of the type of eczema is therefore quite difficult.

Viral infections such as measles, rubella (German measles) and infectious mononucleosis (glandular fever), as well as many other unnamed viruses, may cause a widespread slightly itchy, red rash (viral exanthema).

Urticaria (**hives**) is an allergy reaction in skin that causes marked swelling in patches across the affected area, which is also red and itchy. Any one of several trillion substances, from plants, animals or chemicals, may be responsible.

Cellulitis is a bacterial infection of the skin that may cause very thin-walled soft blisters over the site of an intense infection. These blisters burst very easily, while the skin underneath is hot, red, tender, swollen and painful. The patient may have a fever, and nearby lymph nodes are often tender and enlarged.

A red, butterfly-shaped rash across the cheeks and nose may be a sign of systemic lupus erythematosus (SLE).

OTHER CAUSES OF RED SKIN MAY INCLUDE:

- acne

- tinea (a fungal infection of the skin)

- psoriasis (scaling over red skin)

- intertrigo (caused by heat sweat and friction in skin folds)

- erysipelas (bacterial infection of the layer of fat just under the skin)

- rosacea (skin disease of the face found most commonly in middle-aged women)

- scarlet fever (Streptococcal bacterial infection)

- systemic lupus erythematosus (SLE)

- lichen planus (small, shiny, flat-topped growths that may join together to form a plaque)

- erythema multiforme (may be triggered by drugs, bacterial or viral infections)

- erythema nodosum (tender, painful red lumps that develop on the front of the leg)

- pellagra (a lack of vitamin B3)

- Lyme disease (an infection passed from mice and deer to man by tics).

RED PATCHES ON SKIN

Tinea is a fungal infection of the skin that may occur almost anywhere on the body, but most commonly on the scalp and in the groin. It starts as a red spot that slowly expands in size to form a red ring (ringworm) with a paler centre that may return to skin colour if the ring becomes very large.

Mycosis fungoides is a severe form of tinea that causes disfiguring raised plaques of red scaling skin.

Psoriasis is a skin disease characterised by plaques of red, scaly skin, most commonly on the elbows, knees and scalp. Guttae psoriasis is a very active form that tends to occur in young people.

Discoid lupus erythematosus is an autoimmune disease (inappropriate rejection of normal body tissue) that varies from the more common systemic lupus erythematosus (SLE) in that there are multiple red patches on the skin that occur most commonly on the face. The rash is not itchy or sore, but may have a fine scale and there may be permanent scar damage to the affected skin.

Many forms of dermatitis can cause red skin, but the redness is usually diffuse rather than occurring in distinct patches.

RED SPOTS ON SKIN

Petechiae and **purpura** are tiny and small red dots respectively (there is no defined cut-off size when one becomes the other) that appear in the skin when the smallest blood vessels (capillaries and arterioles) leak or burst. Leakage may be associated with a lack of platelets (blood cells that are required for the formation of clots), or one of the other factors that are essential for the formation of a blood clot.

Senile purpura occurs in the elderly, as their blood vessels weaken and break easily with advancing age.

An **injury** to the skin may cause a bruise which is surrounded by purpura.

Several severe **viral infections** may cause bleeding into the skin, including measles, cytomegalovirus (CMV), aseptic meningitis (infection of the membranes around the brain) and yellow fever.

Bacterial infections may also be responsible for purpura, the most serious being *Meningococcal* meningitis, which may cause death within hours. Other examples include endocarditis (heart infection), tuberculosis and septicaemia (blood infection).

> *The sudden appearance of widespread red spots in the skin that go white with pressure is a serious sign of a blood clotting defect.*

Thrombocytopenia is a lack of platelets in the blood, and without adequate numbers, abnormal bleeding and bruising occurs. Thrombocytopenia often occurs for no apparent reason, or it may be triggered by diseases of the bone marrow or liver, autoimmune diseases (inappropriate rejection of the body's own tissue), severe infections, alcoholism, many types of cancer, or a reaction to some medications (e.g. those used to treat cancer).

Many different **medications** may have bleeding into the skin as an unwanted or overdose effect. Examples include aspirin, warfarin and heparin (used to prevent blood clots), quinine (for malaria and rheumatoid arthritis), thiazide diuretics (remove excess fluid), and sulpha antibiotics.

OTHER CASES OF PETECHIAE AND PURPURA MAY INCLUDE:

- Cushing syndrome (over-production of steroids such as cortisone in the body, or taking large doses of cortisone)

- polyarteritis nodosa (inflammation of arteries)

- vasculitis (inflammation of blood vessels that occurs because of an allergy or reaction or an autoimmune reaction)

- uraemia (kidney failure)

- Henoch-Schoenlein purpura (self-limiting disorder of the immune system that causes bleeding into the skin)

- severe lack of vitamin K (which is normally produced by bacteria in the gut)

- scurvy (lack of vitamin C)

- aplastic anaemia (severe lack of red blood cells)

- inborn defects in the chemical pathways necessary to form a blood clot (e.g. haemophilia, Christmas disease).

THICK SKIN
Prolonged exposure to the **sun** over many years will lead to thickening of the skin, particularly on the forearms, back of the neck and face.

Skin that is constantly subjected to hard work, scratched or **irritated** for any reason will slowly thicken and harden.

OTHER CAUSES INCLUDE:
- scleroderma (an autoimmune disease in which the skin and gut are most commonly affected)

- porphyria (inherited condition that causes abdominal pains, nausea, vomiting and abnormal sensation)

- leprosy

- ichthyosis (congenital condition which causes widespread scaling and thickening of the skin)

- lichen sclerosis (scarring of the skin on one side of the penis).

THIN SKIN
The most common cause of skin thinning is without doubt **ageing**. Old people have far thinner and more fragile skin than the young due to the loss of connective tissue from the skin structure. The skin replaces itself every three weeks, but this process slowly falters with age. The average 80-year-old has skin only half as thick as when they were 20.

Cushing syndrome is caused by an over-production of steroids such as cortisone in the body, or taking large doses of cortisone to control a wide range of diseases, and causes headache, obesity, thirst, easy bruising, thin skin, impotence, menstrual period irregularities, red face, acne, high blood pressure, bone pain and muscle weakness.

In the same way, the excessive use of **steroid creams** on the skin for the treatment of eczema and dermatitis may cause thinning of the skin, particularly on the face.

Other causes include Ehlers-Danlos syndrome (joints that are excessively loose), Fröhlich syndrome (late onset of puberty) and the very rare Goltz syndrome (causes abnormally-formed nails and scar-like areas of thin skin on the scalp, thighs and sides of the belly).

Any skin break that fails to heal rapidly without
good reason must be seen by a doctor.

ULCER

A skin ulcer is a break in the skin that penetrates to the tissue layers beneath the skin and fails to heal in a reasonable time. There are a huge number of conditions that may be responsible.

Any cut, deep graze or other skin injury that becomes infected may become an ulcer, and a persisting **infection** usually prevents the ulcer from healing.

Constant **pressure** on an area of skin, from lying or sitting in the one position without moving for many hours, will prevent the normal circulation of blood to and from that area of skin, which will die and break down into an ulcer that may be very difficult to heal. This is a common problem in the elderly and those with some form of paralysis.

Sitting still for long periods may cause a **stasis** ulcer because blood pools in the feet and ankles to put pressure on the skin, which again may break down into an ulcer. Elevation of the feet, pressure stockings and regular movement of the legs of people who are unable to move their own legs will prevent this problem.

The **veins** in the legs contain one-way valves that allow blood to only travel up towards the heart when they are squeezed by muscle action. If these valves are damaged by increased pressure (e.g. during pregnancy, prolonged standing), obesity or direct injury, the blood is unable to move out of the leg as quickly, and the veins dilate with blood to form varicose veins. These may ache, put pressure on skin which may discolour and break down into an ulcer, as well as being unsightly.

Diabetes may be responsible for a wide variety of
skin problems, from fungal infections to ulcers.

Diabetes results in a higher than normal amount of sugar (glucose) circulating in the blood. The symptoms of untreated diabetes are unusual tiredness, increased thirst and hunger, excess passing of urine, weight loss despite a large food intake, itchy rashes, recurrent vaginal thrush infections, pins and needles, nerve damage, foot ulcers, dizziness, light headedness and blurred vision. Effective treatment is essential to prevent serious complications.

OTHER CAUSES OF ULCERATION MAY INCLUDE:

- skin cancers (basal cell carcinomas, squamous cell carcinomas and melanomas)

- chilblains (a result of exposure to extreme cold)

- blood clot in a vein or artery near the skin

- damage to the sensory nerves will reduce pain sensation and allow the patient to injure themselves without being aware of the injury

- cancer of an internal organ or tissue that is close to the skin surface (e.g. breast cancer)

- syphilis

- Buerger's disease (caused by smoking)

- polyarteritis nodosa (inflammation of arteries)

- bacterial sexually transmitted infections (e.g. chancroid, granuloma inguinale, lymphogranuloma venereum, leprosy)

Sometimes a biopsy of the edge of an ulcer is necessary to exclude skin cancer as a cause.

TREATMENT
The treatment of a rash will depend on its cause and the specific diagnosis. Creams, ointments, lotions and gels containing various medications are most commonly used.

ANTIBIOTIC CREAMS
Antibiotic creams may be used alone or in combination with antibiotic tablets to treat a bacterial infection of the skin (e.g. impetigo, infected ulcers). Examples include:

- **Bacitracin** (Cicatrin), which is now becoming old fashioned, as many bacteria are resistant to it and skin sensitivity is possible.

- **Framycetin** (Soframycin), which is often used in eye and ear infections.

- **Metronidazole** (Rozex), the use of which is restricted to to the unusual skin infection rosacea.

- **Mupirocen** (Bactroban), which is one of the more commonly-used creams for impetigo (school sores).

- **Silver sulfadiazine** (Silvazine), which is used mainly for burns.

- **Sodium fusidate** (Fucidin), which is another commonly-used and effective cream.

Most are very safe to use appropriately, but must not be used excessively or on rashes not due to bacteria.

ANTIFUNGAL CREAMS

Fungi are members of the plant kingdom and are one of the types of microscopic life that can infect the skin of human beings. Antifungals used on the skin include:

- **Amorolfine** (Loceryl paint), which is used for severe fungal nail infections

- **Amphotericin** (Fungilin, Fungizone), which is used for severe internal fungal infections, fungal mouth and gut infections

- **Griseofulvin** (Griseostatin, Grisovin), which is an oldie but a goodie that is used for fungal infections of skin, hair and nails, but may cause headache, nausea and sun sensitivity

- **Imidazoles** – some of the most effective antifungals come from this class of antifungals, including clotrimazole (Canesten), econazole (Pevaryl), miconazole (Daktarin) and itraconazole. They can be used for fungal infections of skin, mouth, vagina and scalp, and are safe in pregnancy and children.

- **Ketoconazole** (Nizoral), which is used for significant fungal infections of skin and internal organs, and dandruff. Nausea may be a side effect.

- **Nystatin** (Mycostatin, Nilstat) is a long established and widely-used antifungal that is safe in pregnancy and may be used for infections of skin, mouth, vagina and gut.

- **Terbinafine** (Lamisil) is a very effective medication for skin and nail fungal infections. It is available as a cream and tablet, but nausea, diarrhoea, rash and dizziness may be side effects of the tablets.

Never use a cream prescribed for someone else,
as some rashes are made worse by steroid creams
or masked by antifungal creams if used inappropriately.

STEROID CREAMS

Steroid-based creams act as powerful reducers of inflammation in damaged tissue. Artificial steroids have been synthesised to control a wide range of diseases, including dermatitis, eczema, and severe allergy reactions. They are an extremely useful group of drugs in a wide variety of conditions. Commonly-used creams include hydrocortisone, betamethasone, halcinonide, mometasone and triamcinolone. The actions of steroids include shrinking down inflamed tissue (e.g. in allergies, injuries, piles) to normal and reducing itching (e.g. in eczema and bites).

When used on the skin, side effects are uncommon. Creams and ointments that contain strong steroids should not be over-used, particularly in children and on the face, as they can cause skin thinning and damage. If used judiciously, steroids can dramatically improve a patient's quality of life, but doctors must always be aware of the pros and cons of their use in every individual.

ULCER

The treatment of an ulcer will depend on its cause, and may include covering the ulcer with a dressing that prevents irritation, removing excessive pressure on the area by regularly changing position or special mattresses or cushions, and special healing gels, plasters and dressings. Surgically excising a persistent ulcer and closing the defect by suturing or with a skin graft can be used in some cases.

CURIOSITY

The skin is the largest organ of the body, and about 2kg of it is made up of dead skin cells.

Every square centimetre of skin is covered with over 100,000 bacteria, even when clean.

RESUSCITATION

L ook after your family, friends and colleagues, by knowing how to perform emergency resuscitation. Your ability to act immediately and appropriately may save a life.

If someone has stopped breathing, it is necessary for someone else to breathe for them.
  When breathing stops, there will be no rise and fall movement of the chest, the face may be a bluish grey colour, and it will not be possible to feel any exhaled breath.

MOUTH-TO-MOUTH RESUSCITATION
The simplest and most effective form of expired air resuscitation is to exhale breath directly into the victim's lungs, usually by placing the first-aider's mouth over the mouth of the victim and performing mouth-to-mouth resuscitation. For obvious reasons this is also called the **kiss of life**.

MOUTH-TO-MOUTH RESUSCITATION:

To perform mouth-to-mouth resuscitation, the victim should be lying on their back. Then:

- check the victim's airway for any obstructions

- **tilt the head backwards** by placing one hand beneath the base of the head and lifting upwards

- put your face at right angles to the victim's face so that you have easy access to the mouth and **take a deep breath**

- **pinch the victim's nose** shut so that it does not provide an escape route for the air

- seal your lips around the lips of the victim and **blow firmly** so that your exhaled breath is pushed into the victim's lungs

- look to **see if the chest rises** – if it does not, check the airway again for any obstructions

- if the chest rises, remove your lips and look to **see if the chest falls**. At the same time, place your ear close to the mouth and listen for air leaving the lungs

- **repeat** the procedure again for four or five quick breaths

- feel the victim's neck **pulse**. If it is present, continue at the rate of one breath approximately every four seconds. If you cannot feel the neck pulse, start external cardiac compression (see below).

Recovery after up to an hour or more of
mouth-to-mouth resuscitation is possible.

Mouth-to-mouth resuscitation may be inappropriate if the person has facial injuries or their face is covered with poison, or if you are trying to operate in deep water. In this case **mouth-to-nose resuscitation** can be carried out following the same technique except that air is blown into the nose while the mouth is held shut.

The method of resuscitating a **baby** or young child is the same as for an adult, except it may be easier to seal your mouth over both the mouth and nose of the child. Do not tip the child's head back very far, because a child's neck and airway are more vulnerable to injury than an adult's. Blow gentle breaths of air into the lungs, one breath every two or three seconds (20–30 breaths a minute). Stop each breath when the child's chest starts to rise.

EXTERNAL CARDIAC COMPRESSION
External cardiac (heart) compression is a technique used to restart a heart that has stopped beating, and to maintain circulation so that damage caused by lack of oxygen to the brain and other vital organs is avoided. Basically it is intended to reproduce artificially the normal beating of the heart by rhythmically compressing the heart between the breastbone and the spine.

Before administering external cardiac compression it is important to **ensure that the heart has stopped beating**. If it is still beating, the procedure can be dangerous, even to the point of causing death. External cardiac compression can also damage vital organs as well as the ribcage if done incorrectly, so it should usually not be attempted unless you have learned how at an approved first aid course.

The need for external cardiac compression is indicated if the victim is unconscious, not breathing, and has no discernible pulse. Generally mouth-to-mouth resuscitation will be tried first. If the victim still shows no sign of life when the neck pulse is checked after the first five breaths, you should apply external cardiac compression together with the resuscitation. External cardiac compression must always be combined with mouth-to-mouth resuscitation as cardiopulmonary resuscitation.

CARDIOPULMONARY RESUSCITATION
Cardiopulmonary resuscitation (CPR) is a combination of **expired air resuscitation** and **external cardiac compression**. Essentially, it takes over both breathing and circulation in a person whose body has stopped carrying out these functions itself. It keeps vital organs supplied with oxygen and thus prevents death or brain damage. Although brain damage and death usually occur within three to six minutes, there are cases where breathing and circulation have stopped for longer than this and the person has survived (usually young people and in very low temperatures), so CPR should always be administered.

It is possible for CPR to be undertaken by one person alone who alternates the two forms of resuscitation, carrying out expired air respiration for a period and then external cardiac compression before returning again to expired air respiration, and so on. However, it is difficult and tiring, and it is far better if two people can work together, one on the airway and one on the heart.

If in doubt, perform CPR rather than wait
too long to see if a patient recovers.

Anyone proposing to give CPR should first check the victim's neck pulse. This is located between the Adam's apple and the large muscle running up the side of the neck. If there is no sign of a heartbeat, CPR is indicated.

CARDIOPULMONARY RESUSCITATION

To perform cardiopulmonary resuscitation, the victim should be lying on their back. Then:

- check that the airway is clear, and **tilt the head** back so that the passage to the lungs is unrestricted
- place the heel of one hand on the middle of the lower half of the breastbone, keeping the palm and fingers raised clear of the chest. Place the heel of the second hand on top. With the arms straight, **press down firmly** so that the **breastbone** is depressed 4–5cm. Keeping the hands in position, release the pressure
- **repeat** 15 times, about one compression per second or slightly faster (about five compressions in four seconds)
- give two **mouth-to-mouth** breaths (see above)
- give another **15 chest compressions**
- **continue** with a pattern of **15** compressions to **two** mouth-to-mouth breaths
- after one minute, **check** the neck pulse. If it has returned, stop the compression immediately
- if the neck **pulse** cannot be felt, continue with the compression and check the pulse every two or three minutes. Stop as soon as the heart starts beating again
- continue mouth-to-mouth resuscitation until the victim can breathe alone.

The same techniques of CPR can be used on babies and young children, but the breastbone should be depressed only 1cm in the case of a baby and 2cm in the case of a child. It is only necessary to use one hand to press down on the chest of a child, and two fingers are sufficient for a baby.

CURIOSITY

Due to the infrequent and scattered nature of CPR events, statistics on the success of CPR are hard to find, but in one American study, CPR was successful in 22 per cent of patients.

SEX

Sex is as natural an activity as eating, drinking, peeing and pooing, and is essential for the survival of the human race, if not for the survival of the individual.

The taboos that surround sex are primarily based on the possible significant consequence for a woman of having sex – pregnancy – and its associated risks and long-term responsibilities.

Having a healthy, mutually enjoyable and responsible sex life is an important factor in looking after yourself.

SEXUAL INTERCOURSE

The purpose of sexual intercourse is to produce a baby and perpetuate one's genes. However, humans also have sex because it feels good. In the Western world, people reproduce on average no more than two or three times in their lives, but they will probably engage in sexual intercourse one or two thousand times.

Statistically, 85 per cent of menstruating women will fall pregnant within one year if undertaking sexual intercourse at least once a week.

SEXUAL INTERCOURSE

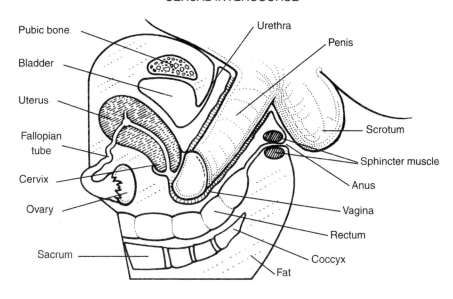

Sex is actually good for you. Having sex once or twice a week increases the level of immunoglobulin A in the blood, which protects against many infections, but daily sex reduces the level of immunoglobulin A to levels below those in people who totally abstain.

Intercourse consists of the man inserting his penis into the woman's vagina. Before he does this, ideally, each partner will become sexually aroused. In the man this means that the penis will become engorged with blood so that it becomes larger, stiff and erect. In the woman, the vagina lengthens, and glands in the vagina produce a lubricating fluid, which enables the man's penis to slide in easily. Thrusting movements by both partners stimulate the penis and vagina and produce pleasurable sensations that increase in intensity until a climax or orgasm is reached. In a woman an orgasm consists of contractions of the vagina, and the man will have an ejaculation of semen, which is a mix of seminal fluid and sperm.

Positions for intercourse vary. The most common is the so-called missionary position in which the woman lies on her back with her legs bent up and the man lies on top of her. Penetration is generally deepest in this position. Other common ones include the reverse of the missionary position, with the woman sitting on top of the man, the 'doggy' position with the woman kneeling on all fours and the man entering her from behind, and the spoon position with the man curled around the woman as she lies on her side. The choice of position is a matter of mutual preference, and no one position is necessarily better than another.

The **frequency** of sexual intercourse varies significantly between couples and with age. The frequency of sex in no way determines the affection a couple have for each other. In Australia, the average married couple of 30 to 35 years of age will have sex 106 times a year, while the average for couples between 50 and 55 years drops to 41 times a year. Social circumstances, pregnancy, children and individual preferences will result in couples varying significantly from these averages.

EJACULATION

In a man, **orgasm** and ejaculation go together. One usually does not occur without the other. Consequently, a man has to have an orgasm before he can father a child. The situation is different in women.

The ejaculation of semen from the penis is the culmination of sexual intercourse in men, and makes it possible for his female partner to fall pregnant. Ejaculation may also be stimulated by masturbation.

Orgasm in a woman is the equivalent of ejaculation in a man.

The man feels a build-up of pressure in the base of the penis and testicles, and then, with a release of pressure and pleasure, the semen is forced down the urethra by contraction of the seminal vesicles in the groin and the muscles at the base of the penis. Ejaculation may last in an intense phase for ten to thirty seconds, but semen may leak from the penis for some minutes afterwards. The penis usually becomes flaccid and soft shortly after ejaculation.

ORGASM

The female orgasm is a **reflex**, in the same way as a tap on the knee causes a reflex. Some people have a vigorous response to a knee tap, others have little. Thus it is difficult to determine what is a normal and abnormal reflex or orgasm.

An orgasm is the female equivalent of the male ejaculation.

The woman feels an intense sensation of **pleasure** sweeping over her, associated with contractions of the muscles in the vagina and uterus and tingling of the nipples. This may last for a few seconds or half a minute.

Different women require different degrees and types of **stimulation** to have an orgasm. Some can only orgasm by stimulation of the clitoris, others require prolonged intercourse, while others may orgasm frequently and easily with merely breast stimulation or thinking about sex. A woman may find that one particular sex position causes orgasm more easily than other positions.

A woman does not need to have an orgasm to conceive and some women who have active sex lives rarely or never achieve orgasm.

Sex is normally safe in pregnancy and, in very
late pregnancy, may stimulate labour.

SEX DURING PREGNANCY

Unless a doctor has recommended otherwise (e.g. for a threatened miscarriage), it is perfectly safe to engage in sex during pregnancy if both partners desire it. Some women find that their sex drive decreases at certain stages of pregnancy, while other women are the opposite.

A man may also be affected, being more attracted to his pregnant wife, or deterred by the new life within her. As a general rule, the foetus will not be affected by intercourse.

In the last couple of months, only certain positions will be comfortable for the woman (e.g. woman sits atop the lying man).

SEX FOR THE ELDERLY

There is no reason why elderly people should not maintain an active sex life until well into their seventies, but there are a number of factors which will make the task more difficult.

The main factor that can affect the elderly is the **menopause** in both men and women. Both sexes are affected, but the male menopause (andropause) is often forgotten, although there is no doubt that it does occur. From the mid-fifties onwards, the amount of male hormone in the system slowly decreases. Unlike the female menopause, where there is a relatively sudden drop in hormone levels, the drop in men is so gradual that it may not be noticed until the early seventies when sexual responsiveness and libido (desire for sex) starts to decrease. This will obviously vary from one man to another. The drop in libido in a woman may be more sudden, but a woman can still appreciate and enjoy the closeness and intimacy that sexual intercourse gives until an advanced age.

Some people think that their parents had sex only
often enough to conceive their children, but many
couples are sexually active into their eighties.

Other factors affecting the elderly can include **medical problems** as diverse as heart failure and arthritis, which may make sex physically more difficult, and medications (particularly those for blood pressure) that may affect a man's erection. Diseases such as diabetes and atherosclerosis cause the partial blockage of small arteries, and may also affect the ability to have an erection.

As other activities are undertaken at a slower pace in old age, so should sexual activity. Most problems can be overcome by patience, mutual understanding and sometimes the assistance of a doctor in modifying medication.

SEX PROBLEMS

Many problems encountered during intercourse are due to a lack of understanding of anatomy or physiology (how your partner works), or a lack of practice. Here you can read about common problems and be helped with the first two, but the last one is up to you.

LACK OF EJACULATION

The male ejaculation or discharge of semen at the time of sexual intercourse sometimes goes awry, and instead of travelling from the sperm storage sac (seminal vesicle) in the groin, into the penis and out through the urethra, the ejaculate goes backwards into the urinary bladder.

Causes include prostate surgery or disease, injury to the pelvis or the spinal cord, diabetes, or a tumour of the spinal cord. It may also be due to psychological stress, a stroke, tumour or cancer in the brain, compression to or damage of the nerves in the pelvis, Parkinson's disease, or an abnormality the individual was born with (when it will usually become evident soon after puberty).

Sometimes it may be a side effect of **medications** such as those used to treat high blood pressure, psychiatric conditions, and diuretics (which remove excess fluid from the body). Often no cause can be found.

FAILURE OF EJACULATION

An inability to ejaculate (ejaculatory failure or retarded ejaculation) during sexual intercourse is the male equivalent of a failed orgasm in the female. Some men can ejaculate when masturbating, or with oral sex, but not with vaginal sex.

This problem may be a drug side effect, or due to psychological problems, an inhibited personality, subconscious or conscious anxiety, or fear of losing self-control. Any significant underlying disease should be excluded.

Treatment involves progressive desensitisation with the assistance of a cooperative sex partner, who initially masturbates their partner to ejaculation, and, over a series of weeks, learns to bring him almost to the point of ejaculation by hand stimulation before allowing vaginal sex. Another technique involves additional stimulation of the penis during intercourse by the woman massaging the penis with her fingers while the man thrusts in and out of the vagina. Distracting the man from consciously holding back the ejaculation by passionate kissing or other stimulation of the face or back during intercourse may also help. Reasonable results can be achieved with commitment to the treatment program.

It takes two to tango, and to control premature ejaculation.
The co-operation of a man's partner is essential for successful treatment.

PREMATURE EJACULATION

Premature ejaculation can be very embarrassing for a man. He is just about to have sex, or has just started, when he finds he is no longer able to control himself and he ejaculates his sperm. The penis then becomes soft and flaccid. This leaves his partner sexually frustrated, may damage a relationship, and makes pregnancy impossible.

The most common **cause** is psychological stress, emotional upsets and performance anxiety. The more the man tries to please his partner, the more trouble he may have with the problem. The man may also be over-stimulated, excited and foreplay may have been too intense.

There are virtually no diseases or physical conditions which cause this problem.

Therapists can teach appropriate techniques, that involve the co-operation of the partner, to overcome premature ejaculation.

One simple technique is the **penis squeeze**. If a man feels that ejaculation is imminent, he indicates this to his partner, and all sexual activity ceases. The man, or his partner, uses the thumb and forefinger to squeeze the penis firmly from above and below, about one third of the way down the shaft from the head of the penis. This will cause the sensation of imminent ejaculation to cease, and the penis may start to become less rigid. Sexual activity can then recommence.

RETROGRADE EJACULATION

Retrograde ejaculation occurs if semen is ejaculated from the sac at the base of the penis (seminal vesicle), but instead of passing along the urethra in the penis to the outside, it travels in the other direction and enters the bladder. It is usually a complication of surgery in the area (e.g. to the prostate), due to advanced diabetes or a side effect of some uncommon drugs. The man has the sensation of orgasm during sex, but no ejaculation occurs.

Unfortunately, no treatment is available, but the resultant infertility may be overcome by microsurgical techniques to remove sperm from the man and artificially inseminate a woman.

FRIGIDITY

Frigid is a term, now outdated, usually intended to describe a woman who is unable to experience any pleasure or arousal from sexual stimulation. **Anorgasmia** is a term used to indicate an inability to have an orgasm.

Frigidity is usually a **psychological** problem and not a physical one, and may be the result of a woman's strict upbringing, or a loathing for sex that has been conditioned by a traumatic experience. Other causes include pain with intercourse, postnatal depression after birth, life stress (e.g. moving house or changing jobs), and the hormone drop associated with menopause. Certain prescribed drugs and hormones may also be responsible.

Frigidity is often a fear of the unknown and
can be helped by a caring gentle partner.

With sexual stimulation there is no lubrication of the vagina, enlargement of the nipples or clitoral tenseness. In extreme cases it may be responsible for infertility.

Treatment requires a very understanding partner and a very slow teaching process, usually with the help of a psychiatrist or psychologist. Stimulation of non-erotic parts of the body to relax the woman over a period of weeks, followed by stimulation of more erotically sensitive areas, slowly breaks down the barriers. Most women respond to appropriate treatment after many sessions over several months.

HOMOSEXUALITY

Homosexuality or homoeroticism is having intimate sexual contact with, or feelings for, a person of the same sex. The term may be applied to both men and women, and it is no longer considered to be a medical abnormality, but a variation of normal behaviour. There are many theories as to why some people are homosexual, but no absolute reason is known.

Six per cent of adult men and three per cent of adult women have partaken in some form of homosexual activity, but only about three per cent of men and half that number of women are exclusively homosexual. Homosexual women may be referred to as lesbians.

Virtually all boys and girls have some homosexual experimentation in their teenage years.

There is a higher incidence of sexually transmitted disease in homosexuals than in heterosexuals, mainly because of promiscuity. AIDS is the most common of these, although in undeveloped countries this is a condition that is spread by heterosexual sex (between men and women) more than anal intercourse. Gay bowel syndrome is an inflammation of the lower bowel caused by anal intercourse, which results in a constant urge to pass faeces (tenesmus), rectal discomfort and diarrhoea.

Individuals who have trouble accepting their sexual orientation because of peer or society pressures may require psychiatric assistance.

IMPOTENCE

See separate entry in this book.

REDUCED LIBIDO

Libido is the emotional **desire** for sexual intercourse and the natural instinct for sexual satisfaction. It is controlled by the brain and not the testes or ovaries, although diseases of these glands can certainly have an adverse effect on libido, as they do not respond to stimuli from the brain.

To enjoy, and be successful in achieving, sexual intercourse, both partners must be relaxed, secure and comfortable. Psychological stress of any sort will reduce sexual desire. Examples can be as wide-ranging as worries about work, money, pregnancy, discovery (will the children come in?), the relationship itself or disease.

Many psychiatric conditions, but particularly **depression**, will remove any desire for sex. Difficulty in sleeping, loss of interest in other activities and poor self esteem are other signs of depression.

Failure of any major organ of the body (e.g. heart, liver, kidney) or any other serious disease will affect the normal hormonal and chemical balances, as well as causing stress and anxiety, and sex becomes something to be remembered rather than sought.

Disease, infection, tumour (e.g. Fröhlich syndrome), injury or cancer of the pituitary gland under the centre of the brain will affect libido. This tiny gland is the conductor of the gland orchestra in the body, and is itself directly controlled by the brain. If for one of these reasons it does not produce the necessary hormones to stimulate the testes or ovaries, they will not release the appropriate sex hormones (testosterone and oestrogen) to allow appropriate sexual responses. Rarely, the pituitary gland may become over-active, and over-stimulate the sex glands to drain them of their hormones.

The part of the brain controlling the pituitary gland can itself be affected by a stroke, bleeding, injury, tumour, cancer or abscess. Parkinson's disease and other degenerative conditions of the brain will both reduce desire and ability.

Remember that the most erotic organ in the body is the brain, so talking and reading can be a bigger turn on than doing.

In **men**, any disease that reduces the production of testosterone (male hormone) in the testes will reduce libido. Examples include infections (orchitis), tumours (e.g. cancer), cysts and torsion (twisting to cut off the blood supply). Other causes of low libido in men include enlargement of the prostate gland and poorly controlled diabetes mellitus.

Women find that their libido varies during the month, usually being highest at the time of ovulation (when they are most likely to get pregnant) half-way between the start of one period and the next, and lowest during a menstrual period. Pregnancy also lowers libido for its duration, and breast feeding has a similar effect on the hormones. Other causes of low libido in women include tumours or cysts of the ovary, and during the menopause, when there is a lack of oestrogen, sex may be uncomfortable as well as undesirable.

Numerous **drugs**, legal, illegal and prescribed, can reduce libido. Examples include alcohol, heroin, marijuana, steroids, antihistamines (e.g. cold preparations), benzodiazepines (e.g. diazepam, oxazepam), fluid pills and some of those used to treat depression (tricyclics) and decrease high blood pressure (beta-blockers).

LACK OF ORGASM

The muscles in the wall of the vagina contract in pleasurable spasms when a woman has an orgasm during intercourse. This rhythmic contraction aids the movement of the ejaculated sperm towards the cervix and uterus. Some women rarely, or never, experience orgasm. A woman may be sexually responsive, enjoy sex and have the physical signs of erotic arousal, but she may still fail to have an orgasm.

Common causes of occasional or regular lack of orgasm (anorgasmia) include **psychological** or physical stress, anxiety, fatigue, over-indulgence in alcohol and poor sexual technique by her partner. Pain during sex is obviously not going to help the situation.

If a woman is relaxed about her sexuality,
she is far more likely to have an orgasm.

Infections (e.g. thrush, *Trichomonas*) or ulceration (e.g. *Herpes*) of the vagina or vulva will cause discomfort and reduce sensation.

Injuries to the spine (e.g. paraplegia) or nerves (e.g. pelvic fracture or surgery) that supply the vagina will affect the sensation of orgasm.

Under-activity of numerous **hormone**-producing glands in the body, including the ovaries (oestrogen), thyroid (thyroxine) and adrenal glands (adrenaline), because of infection, inflammation, tumours, cysts or cancer, will reduce all bodily responses and functions. The pituitary gland under the centre of the brain controls all other glands, and diseases affecting this gland can affect any other gland in the body.

If the woman is suffering some significant generalised **disease** (e.g. infection, cancer), or is in any pain, her responses will be reduced.

Some **medications**, including antidepressants, narcotics, sedatives and blood pressure drugs may reduce the ability to experience an orgasm.

Treatment is difficult. Obviously, any underlying cause should be treated, but if all these are excluded the following procedure may be adopted.

The woman should be taught relaxation techniques which are accompanied by masturbation by hand or mechanical devices in order to bring herself to orgasm. Once she has experienced orgasm in this manner, she can move to the next stage of treatment with a male partner. This may involve the man using his hand to stimulate her to orgasm, or by using different sex positions (e.g. man behind woman) during which the woman can stimulate her own clitoris. The supervision of a sex therapist (psychiatrist or psychologist) in this process is invaluable. Treatment is often successful if a woman and her partner are both well-motivated.

PAEDOPHILIA

Paedophilia is a psychiatric disturbance that results in the sexual abuse of a child by adult men (most commonly) or women. It may develop from childhood abuse of the paedophile by his or her parents, or other psychological traumas as a child. Paedophilia is NOT more common in homosexuals, but **pederasty** is by definition a homosexual act between a man and a boy.

The condition involves mentally disturbed adults who use children to become sexually aroused to the point of orgasm. Sexual contact varies from feeling, to oral sex, or sexual penetration that may progress to serious injury or, rarely, murder. Paedophiles have difficulty in establishing normal intimate relationships with adults of the opposite sex, have inadequate personalities, low self esteem, and male paedophiles are often impotent.

Treatment involves prolonged counselling by a psychiatrist and sometimes medications to reduce sexual desire and increase control. If discovered, paedophiles are invariably charged in the courts, but courts are more likely to treat leniently a person who comes forward voluntarily and seeks help. Unfortunately the long-term success of treatment is poor.

SMALL PENIS

A lot of rubbish is spoken of about penis size in locker rooms and other areas where men congregate, but medical texts indicate that the **average** male erect penis measured along the top is 12.9cm in length, and 90 per cent of men have an erect penis that is between 9cm and 17cm in length. The other ten per cent are evenly divided between longer and shorter. The longest medically-recorded erect penis was 32cm, but this is as much of a freak as the man who is 240cm (eight feet) tall.

There is no direct correlation between height, or any other obvious physical attribute, and penis size.

To a woman, sexual technique, affection and
attention are more important than size.

Usually no treatment is necessary, as a small penis has no effect upon a man's fertility, and does not determine whether a man is a good lover. During intercourse, the most sensitive part of a woman's sexual organs are the clitoris, which is at the outside entrance to the vagina, and the 'G spot', which is just inside on the front wall of the vagina, at a point where even the shortest penis can give stimulation. If desired, there are plastic surgery procedures available that will both lengthen and thicken the penis, but these may have significant complications.

No man with a relatively small penis should underestimate his sexual prowess, as he will be able to satisfy the sexual appetite of any woman if he approaches her in the right way. It is not the size of the equipment that counts, but how it is used.

PEYRONIE DISEASE

Peyronie disease is an uncommon problem that causes deformity of the erect penis. The cause may be **injury** to the penis, narrowing of the artery to one side of the penis (common with poorly-controlled diabetes or high cholesterol), abnormal nerve supply to the penis or, most frequently, have no known cause. The incidence increases with age.

These men have significant side-to-side (not vertical) **curvature** of the erect penis and a less firm than normal erection, as the normal tissue of the penis is replaced by fibrous tissue on one side only. A small degree of side-to-side curvature (up to 15°) is quite normal. A hard piece of tissue can often be felt at the base of the penis on the affected side. Ultrasound scans can show the abnormal fibrous tissue in the penis.

Most forms of **treatment** are not very successful. Surgery, steroid injections and radiotherapy may be tried, but the most radical, and most successful treatment, is surgical replacement of the contents of the penis with an inflatable bladder that can be pumped up when an erection is desired. This is up to 80 per cent effective.

PRIAPISM

Priapism is an abnormality in which the penis remains persistently, inappropriately and painfully erect for a long period of time. There are multiple possible **causes** including spinal cord injury, bladder stones, blood diseases (e.g. leukaemia in children), stroke, uncontrolled diabetes, some forms of widespread cancer, injury to the penis, excess dose of alprostadil (Caverject, Muse), illegal drugs (e.g. cocaine, marijuana) and prescription drugs (e.g. prazosin, heparin). It rarely occurs as a result of excessive sexual stimulation.

*An erection that just won't go away is very distressing
to a man, particularly if he needs to pass urine.*

Treatment involves warm packs, pseudoephedrine (Sudafed) tablets, and syringes to draw excess blood from the penis. Any underlying cause needs to be excluded by appropriate tests. Permanent damage to the penis may occur due to the constant pressure on the tissue if it is not treated within four hours.

SEXUAL SADISM

Sexual sadism is a **psychiatric aberration** that usually starts in males in their late teens and twenties, and sometimes persists long-term. The cause is unknown, but sometimes it is blamed on sexual assaults in childhood. Rarely, a brain tumour or disease may be found to be responsible for a personality change, and is detected by a CT scan.

The man has prolonged, recurrent and intense sexual urges and fantasies involving real or imagined acts in which physical or psychological suffering occurs in a victim. Humiliation is one of the more common psychological fantasies or acts. Most patients are unable to achieve sexual satisfaction in other ways. The victim may be consenting or non-consenting, and may be raped.

Psychotherapy and medications may be tried as treatments, but are often ineffective. Castration has historically been used as a last resort. Because of their interaction with the criminal justice system, many patients end up as long-term prisoners.

Sex is a two way process, and should be equally satisfying to both participants.

SEXUAL INTERCOURSE PAIN

Pain experienced by a woman during sexual intercourse is called **dyspareunia** by doctors. It may occur superficially near the outside as the penis initially enters the vagina, during deep penetration of the penis, or may be a mixture of both.

Infections of the vagina caused by a fungus (e.g. thrush) or a bacteria may inflame both the vagina and the vulval tissue around the outside. These infections are usually accompanied by a discharge. Irritation of the inflamed tissue during sex will cause pain.

Deeper infections in the lower part of the belly involving the bladder (cystitis), urethra (tube that drains urine from the bladder), bowel (e.g. diverticulitis), lining of the belly (peritonitis) or an abscess in the pelvis will be aggravated by intercourse.

A lack of the female hormone oestrogen after menopause may lead to a **dryness** of the vagina which makes sex difficult and painful. The natural lubrication of the vagina is maintained by glands that are stimulated by oestrogen. Some women may notice that their vagina is drier at some stages of their menstrual cycle than at others due to variations in the level of oestrogen. Under-active thyroid, pituitary or adrenal glands, which affect the functioning of all cells in the body, may also cause vaginal dryness.

A **prolapse** (dropping) of the uterus, usually as a result of childbirth, age or obesity, may cause a back ache that is aggravated by sex.

Causes of **superficial pain** during sex include vulvodynia (see below), Bartholin's gland infection (glands near the opening of the vagina that produce its natural lubricating fluid), genital herpes infection (painful ulcers around the vulva and the lips of the vagina), an episiotomy scar (cut in the back wall of the vagina performed to allow the baby's head to emerge more easily during birth), vaginismus (strong spasm of the muscles in the vagina that prevents the penis from entering), an allergy to soaps, perfumes, detergents in underwear or other substances may cause a swelling and inflammation of the delicate tissues of the vulva.

Causes of **deep pain** during sex include salpingitis and pelvic inflammatory disease (infections of the Fallopian tubes and other organs in the pelvis), endometriosis, fibroids (hard balls of fibrous tissue that form in the muscular wall of the uterus), an ectopic pregnancy (a foetus in the Fallopian tubes instead of the uterus) and tumours or cancer of the cervix, uterus or ovaries.

SEXUALLY TRANSMITTED DISEASES
See separate entry in this book.

VAGINISMUS
Vaginismus is a strong **spasm** of the muscles around the vagina. It is an unconscious reaction, normally triggered by anxiety related to sex. The initial trigger may be fear (of pregnancy, pain, etc.), guilt, lack of privacy, anxiety about expectations, lack of self confidence, previous rape or sexual assault, and other psychological factors. Sexual intercourse is impossible as the man is unable to penetrate the woman.

> *To a woman with vaginismus, a dildo can be the*
> *answer to both her prayers and those of her partner.*

Treatment consists of psychological counselling, medication to reduce anxiety and vaginal dilators (dildo – artificial penises) of gradually increasing width. Confidence must be gained in using one size of dildo before the next size is attempted. Treatment gives reasonable results if the woman is well motivated and has an understanding partner.

VULVODYNIA
Vulvodynia (burning vulva syndrome or vulvar vestibulitis) is a **painful** condition affecting the external genitals (**vulva**) of sexually active women due to inflammation of the tiny lubricating glands in the skin of the vulva. The cause is unknown, but attacks sometimes follow a vaginal thrush infection.

The vulva appears normal, but there is intermittent tenderness and pain of the vulva and opening into the vagina that is worse with pressure or friction (e.g. during sex, inserting a tampon, bike riding or tight clothing) and persists for an hour or more once triggered. Muscle spasms in the vagina triggered by fear of pain occurring may cause vaginismus and make sexual intercourse impossible.

Patients should apply heat to the area (hot bath, warm water bottle) when pain occurs. Steroid creams may reduce inflammation and amitriptyline tablets may relax the woman and help her cope, and patients should avoid using soap in the area. Sex can be assisted by an understanding partner, applying local anaesthetic ointment, adequate foreplay and the use of lubricants. The condition often persists for months or years before settling spontaneously.

CURIOSITY

The drug name 'belladonna' is Spanish for 'beautiful lady'. It was named thus because the drug was used in a very dilute form to dilate the pupils of Spanish women in the seventeenth and eighteenth century, in order to enhance their beauty. Large pupils are recognised by psychologists as a sign of sexual attraction.

The more a man thinks about sex, the faster his beard grows. Thinking about sex increases testosterone production which increases beard growth.

SEXUALLY TRANSMITTED DISEASES

Venereal (sexually transmitted) diseases are passed from one person to another by sexual contact. This includes homosexual, lesbian, oral and anal sex, as well as heterosexual intercourse.

Look after yourself by practising safe sex – always use a condom unless you are in a long-term, stable relationship.

Condoms have the advantage that they not only protect the woman against becoming pregnant, but they may also protect both partners against some sexually transmitted diseases. They are not infallible though, and may fall off or break, and contact between the pubic areas of both partners may spread diseases.

The common cold may be a sexually transmitted disease, as the responsible virus can pass from one person to another by sexual contact.

DISEASES

There are many different sexually transmitted diseases, and only the more common and serious ones will be discussed here.

AIDS

The **acquired immune deficiency syndrome** (AIDS) is an infection caused by a retrovirus known as the human immunodeficiency virus (HIV), which destroys the body's defence mechanisms and allows severe infections and cancers to develop. In the very early days of research into the virus responsible for AIDS, it was described as human T-cell lymphocytotrophic virus 3 (HTLV3).

The **history** of AIDS begins in central Africa, where it is now believed a form of AIDS has existed in apes for thousands of years. These animals come into close contact with humans in this area, and are butchered and eaten by the local population. At some stage in the early part of the 1900s, the virus spread from apes to humans. In apes, due to natural selection over many generations, the virus causes few or no symptoms, and is harmless.

The AIDS virus has been isolated from old stored tissue samples dated in the 1950s, found in Kinshasa Hospital, Zaire.

From Africa, AIDS spread to Haiti in the Caribbean. Haiti was ruled by a dictator (Papa Doc Duvalier), and many Haitian Africans fled to Africa to avoid persecution.

Once 'Papa Doc' and his son 'Baby Doc' were removed from power, these exiles returned, bringing AIDS with them. The virus mutated in humans and became more virulent, causing a faster and more severe onset of symptoms. Viruses mutate routinely (e.g. different strains of influenza virus appear every year).

American homosexuals frequented Haiti because it was very poor, and sexual favours could be bought cheaply. They returned home from their holiday with the AIDS virus, and it has spread around the world from there. The first cases were diagnosed in California in 1981, although cases occurred in Sweden in 1978 in the family of a sailor who had visited Haiti, but the disease was not identified as AIDS until years later. There may also have been some movement of the disease directly through Africa to Algeria and France.

Fortunately for most of us, it is a relatively hard disease to catch. AIDS is **spread** by the transfer of blood and semen from one person to another. It was initially only a disease of homosexuals and drug addicts, but although these remain the most affected groups in developed countries, it is promiscuous heterosexual contact that is the most common method of transmission in poorer countries. In the early days of the disease, some unfortunate recipients of blood transfusions and other blood-derived medications were inadvertently given the AIDS virus. Tests are now available to allow blood banks to screen for AIDS.

AIDS CANNOT be caught from any casual contact, or from spa baths, kissing, mosquitoes, tears, towels or clothing. Only by homosexual or heterosexual inter-course with a carrier of the disease, by using contaminated needles, or blood from a carrier, can the disease be caught. If someone does come into sexual or blood contact with an AIDS carrier, it is possible for the virus to cross into their body. The body's defence mechanisms may then fight off the virus and leave the person with no illness whatsoever, or the AIDS virus may spread throughout the body to cause an HIV infection.

Circumcised men are six to eight times less likely
to be infected with the HIV virus that causes AIDS
because of biological reasons, and not less risky behaviour.

The world-wide **statistics** for AIDS are horrendous. In 2001 there were 35 million people in the world with an HIV infection, 23 million of them in Africa and 95 per cent of them in developing countries. There are 7 million deaths world-wide every year from AIDS, and every day 20,000 people are infected with HIV. The incidence of HIV infection varies from two in every 100,000 people in China, to 115 in Australia, 2100 in Thailand, 20,000 in Uganda and over 50,000 in every 100,000 people in Botswana (the world's highest rate). The rate of infection is increasing in under-developed countries in Africa and Asia, but dropping in developed Western countries.

Those who are infected with the **human immunodeficiency virus** are said to be HIV positive. Once the HIV virus enters the body, it may lie dormant for months or years. During this time there may be no or minimal symptoms, but it may be possible to pass the infection on to another sex partner, and babies may become infected in the uterus of an infected mother.

The disease has been classified into several categories. A patient can progress to a more severe category but cannot revert to less severe one. The categories are:

- **HIV category 1** – a glandular fever-like disease that lasts a few days to weeks with inflamed lymph nodes, fever, rash and tiredness.

- **HIV category 2** – no symptoms.

- **HIV category 3** – persistent generalised enlargement of lymph nodes.

- **HIV category 4** (AIDS) – varied symptoms and signs depending on the areas of the body affected. May include fever, weight loss, diarrhoea, nerve and brain disorders, severe infections, lymph node cancer, sarcomas, and other cancers. Patients are very susceptible to any type of infection or cancer, from the common cold to pneumonia, septicaemia and multiple rare cancers (e.g. Kaposi sarcoma), because the body's immune system is destroyed by the virus.

Blood **tests** are positive at all stages of HIV infection, but there may be a lag period of up to three months or more from when the disease is caught until it can be detected.

It is frightening to think that almost one per cent of the entire adult population of the world is infected by HIV.

Treatments that slow the progression of the disease are available, but there is no cure or vaccine available for AIDS or HIV infection at present. Prevention is the only practical way to deal with AIDS. Condoms give good, but not total, protection from sexually catching the virus, and drug addicts may be educated not to share needles.

Once diagnosed as HIV positive, patients should not give up hope, because they may remain in the second stage for many years. Prolonging this stage can be achieved by the regular long-term use of potent antiviral and immunosupportive medications, stopping smoking, exercising regularly, eating a well-balanced diet, resting adequately and avoiding illegal drugs.

Patients may remain at the category 2 level for many years, possibly even decades. Up to half of those who are HIV positive do not develop category 4 disease for more than ten years. On the other hand, no one with category 4 HIV (AIDS) has lived more than a few months, and sufferers develop severe infections and cancers that eventually kill them.

CHANCROID

Chancroid is a sexually transmitted infection caused by the **bacteria** *Haemophilus ducreyi*, that is rare in developed countries, and more common in the tropics and Asia.

Three to five days after sexual contact with a carrier, a sore develops on the penis or vulva which rapidly breaks down to form a painful ulcer. Several sores and ulcers may be present at the same time. Lymph nodes in the groin then swell up into hard, painful lumps that may degenerate into an abscess and discharge pus. The patient is feverish and feels ill. Some patients develop a mild form with minimal symptoms, but they can transmit the disease. This is particularly common in women, where the sores may be hidden internally in the vagina. The condition is diagnosed by taking swabs from the sores and identifying the bacteria present in the pus, or skin tests that often remain positive for life.

Antibiotics (e.g. azithromycin, ciprofloxacin) cure the infection, but balanitis (infection of penis head) and phimosis (contracture of foreskin) are possible complications.

CRABS

Crabs (pubic pediculosis) is an infestation of the pubic hair with the **lice** (parasitic insect) *Phthirus pubis*, which lives by sucking blood from the soft pubic skin. It is caught by being in close bodily contact with someone who already has an infestation (e.g. during sex), but as the lice can survive away from humans for a time, they can also be caught from borrowed clothing, towels or bedding.

> *Technically, sexual intercourse is not necessary*
> *to catch crabs, just very close contact.*

Often there are no **symptoms** and many people are unaware of the presence of lice. In others the lice cause an itchy rash in the pubic area, which may be raw and bleeding from constant scratching. Secondary skin infections may develop in these sores, and this infection can cause further symptoms, including a fever and enlarged glands in the groin. Lice may be seen by examining the pubic hair through a magnifying glass.

A number of **lotions** are available to kill the crabs. The affected individual, and all sex partners, must be treated simultaneously to prevent reinfestations occurring. All clothing and bedding must be thoroughly washed in hot water. A repeat treatment after 24 hours and again after seven days is advisable in order to kill any lice that have hatched in the interim. Antibiotics may be required to treat secondary infections.

Correct treatment should result in a complete cure.

CYTOMEGALOVIRUS INFECTION

A cytomegalovirus (CMV) infection is an extremely common **viral** infection affecting between ten per cent and 25 per cent of the entire population at any one time. Infection rate may be in excess of 80 per cent in homosexual men. It may be a serious illness in patients who have reduced immunity due to treatment with cytotoxic drugs for cancer, have suffered other serious illnesses, are anaemic, suffering from AIDS or other immune affecting diseases, or who are extremely run-down from stress or overwork.

The virus passes from one person to another in saliva or as droplets in the breath, but may also spread through blood transfusions or sexual contact. In all but a tiny percentage of infected people, there are absolutely no symptoms, and they appear and feel totally well. Adults with reduced immunity develop a fever, headaches, overwhelming tiredness, muscle and joint pains, enlarged lymph nodes and a tender liver. In patients with severely reduced immunity, pneumonia and hepatitis may develop.

Normally a benign infection, in pregnant women CMV may be devastating.

If a **pregnant woman** with reduced immunity acquires a significant CMV infection, her baby may be affected in the womb and be born with liver damage (jaundice), enlarged liver and spleen, poor ability to clot blood, bruises and mental retardation, and one in six are deaf.

The infection can be detected by specific blood tests, and the virus may be found in sputum, saliva, urine and other body fluids.

There is no specific treatment. Aspirin and/or paracetamol are used to control fever and pain, and prolonged rest is required for recovery.

An uneventful recovery is expected in normal patients. In immune compromised patients, pneumonia and hepatitis may be fatal.

GENITAL HERPES

Genital herpes is a contagious **viral** infection of the genitals caused by the *Herpes simplex* type 2 virus, which is caught by sexual contact with someone who already has the disease. It is possible, but unlikely, for the virus to be caught in hot spa baths and from a shared wet towel.

If sores are present, there is a good chance of passing the disease on, but a patient is also **infectious** for several days before a new crop of sores develop. Condoms can give limited protection against spreading the disease.

Once a person is infected with the virus, it settles in the nerve endings around the vulva or penis, and remains there for the rest of that person's life. With stress, illness or reduced resistance, the virus starts reproducing and causes the **symptoms** of painful blisters and ulcers on the penis or scrotum (sac) in the male; and on the vulva (vaginal lips), and in the vagina and cervix (opening into the womb) of the female. The first attack may occur only a week, or up to some years, after the initial infection. An attack will last for two to four weeks and then subside, but after weeks, months or years, a further attack may occur. Women are affected more severely and frequently than men. The incidence of gynaecological cancer is increased in women with the infection and in rare cases it can cause encephalitis (brain infection).

Herpes simplex type one normally causes cold sores,
but with oral sex may cause genital sores too.

If a baby catches the infection from the mother during delivery, it can cause severe brain damage in the child. For this reason, if a woman has a history of repeated herpes infections, she may be delivered by caesarean section.

The infection is diagnosed by taking a swab from the ulcer or a blood test.

Rapid appropriate **treatment** is essential. Antiviral tablets and ointments will control an attack, but must be started within 72 hours of its onset, or they can be taken for months or years to prevent further attacks. Good control is possible with modern medications.

GENITAL WARTS

Genital or venereal warts (condylomata accuminata) are a sexually transmitted **viral** infection caused by the human papilloma virus (HPV), which is transmitted from one person to another only by sexual intercourse or other intimate contact, but condoms can give some protection against the infection. It is not possible to catch it from toilet seats or spa baths. The incubation period varies from one to six months.

Warts, sometimes of a large size, grow on the penis in men and in the genital area of women. They initially appear as flat, pale areas on the skin, or as dark-coloured, irregularly-shaped lumps. Both men and women can be carriers without being aware they are infected, and in women genital warts may develop internally where they are difficult to detect. A significant proportion of women with this infection will develop cancer of the cervix, which can only be detected at an early stage by regular Pap smears. Anyone with genital warts should also have tests performed to check for the presence of other venereal disease.

Genital warts can vary from barely visible
flat marks to growths the size of a golf ball.

Small warts can be more easily seen if a special stain is applied to the skin, then treatment can be given with antiviral imiquimod cream applied three times a week for up to four months, acid paints or ointments, freezing with liquid nitrogen, or burning with electric diathermy or laser. The treatment is often prolonged, and warts tend to recur, but with careful watching and rapid treatment of any recurrence, the infection will eventually settle.

GONORRHOEA

Gonorrhoea ('clap') is a common sexually transmitted **bacterial** infection caused by the bacterium *Neisseria gonorrhoeae*, which can only be caught by having sex with a person who already has the disease. It has an incubation period of three to seven days after contact. Some degree of protection can be obtained by using a condom.

The **symptoms** vary significantly between men and women.

In women there may be minimal symptoms with a mild attack, but when symptoms do occur they include a foul discharge from the vagina, pain on passing urine, pain in the lower abdomen, passing urine frequently, tender lymph nodes in the groin, and fever. If left untreated the infection can involve the uterus and Fallopian tubes to cause salpingitis and pelvic inflammatory disease, which can result in infertility and persistent pelvic pain. Babies born to mothers with the infection can develop a gonococcal conjunctivitis (eye infection).

In men symptoms are usually obvious with a yellow milky discharge from the penis, pain on passing urine and, in advanced cases, inflamed lymph nodes in the groin. If left untreated the prostate can become infected, which can cause scarring of the urine tube (urethra), permanent difficulty in passing urine and reduced fertility.

With the frequent use of antibiotics for throat and other respiratory infections, some forms of gonorrhoea are now antibiotic resistant.

With anal intercourse, a rectal infection with gonorrhoea can develop and cause an anal discharge, mild diarrhoea, rectal discomfort and pain on passing faeces.

Oral sex can lead to the development of a gonococcal throat infection.

Gonorrhoea may also enter the bloodstream and cause septicaemia. An unusual complication is gonococcal arthritis, which causes pain in the knees, ankles and wrists. Other rarer complications include infections of the heart, brain and tendons.

The **diagnosis** is confirmed by examining a swab from the urethra, vagina or anus under a microscope and culturing the bacteria on a nutrient substance. There are no blood tests available to diagnose gonorrhoea. Other sexually transmitted diseases should also be tested for when gonorrhoea is diagnosed, as they may be contracted at the same time. For this reason, blood tests are often ordered when treating anyone with any form of venereal disease.

Gonorrhoea has been readily **treated** with a course of penicillin until recently, but many strains are now resistant to penicillin and more potent antibiotics are required. All sexual contacts of the infected person need to be notified, as they may be carriers of the disease and unaware of the presence of the infection. After treatment, a follow-up swab is important to ensure that the infection has been adequately treated. More than 95 per cent of cases of gonorrhoea can be cured by the appropriate antibiotics.

GRANULOMA INGUINALE

Granuloma inguinale (donovanosis or granuloma venereum) is caused by the **bacteria** *Donovania* or *Calymmatobacterium granulomatis*, which pass from one person to another during sexual intercourse. The incubation period is one to 12 weeks and it causes painless nodules on or around the genitals that break down to shallow ulcers, and may join together into progressively larger ulcers that spread up onto the lower abdomen. Infection of the ulcers with other bacteria will cause them to fill with pus and become foul smelling. Microscopic examination of a biopsy or swab smear from the edge of an ulcer reveals the responsible bacteria and confirms the diagnosis.

Treatment is difficult, and it may be necessary to take antibiotics such as tetracycline for several months. Relapses are common unless a full antibiotic course completed.

HEPATITIS B

Hepatitis B (serum hepatitis – see Hepatitis entry in this book) is a **viral** infection of the liver that can only be caught by intimate contact with the blood or semen of a person who has the disease or is a carrier of the disease. Examples include receiving blood from a carrier, using a contaminated needle, rubbing a graze or cut on an infected person's graze or cut, being bitten by an infected person, or, most commonly, by having sex (homosexual or heterosexual) with them. Ninety per cent of babies born to mothers who are carriers catch the disease. The highest incidences are amongst homosexual men, drug addicts who share needles and Australian Aborigines, and the disease is widespread in South-East Asia. Blood banks screen all donations for hepatitis B. Splashes of blood into an eye or onto a cut or graze can spread the disease, and doctors, dentists, nurses and other health workers are therefore at risk.

There is a long **incubation period** of six weeks to six months, and the infection cannot be detected during this period. Once active, it causes the patient to be very ill with a liver infection, fever, jaundice (yellow skin), nausea and loss of appetite. Some patients develop only a very mild form of the disease but they are still contagious and may suffer the long-term effects.

In the 1960s, hepatitis B was described as Australia
antigen hepatitis because of its high incidence in Australian
Aborigines, in whom the disease was first identified.

Blood tests are available to detect antibodies against the various hepatitis viruses and diagnose the type of hepatitis and monitor its progress.

It has been possible to **vaccinate** against hepatitis B since the first vaccine was introduced in 1986. Three injections at intervals of one month and six months give at least five years protection. It should not be used during pregnancy unless essential, but accidental vaccination during pregnancy is unlikely to cause any significant problem. It may be used in children from birth onwards. Local soreness, swelling, redness and tissue hardness are the most common side effects. Unusually, a headache, dizziness, fever, muscle aches, tiredness, nausea, diarrhoea, joint pain and a rash may occur.

Treatment involves bed rest, and a diet that is low in protein and high in carbo-hydrate, and alcohol is forbidden. Sometimes it is necessary to give medication for nausea and vomiting and to feed severely affected patients by a drip into a vein for a short time. If it continues to worsen, drugs may be used to reduce the liver damage.

Patients must ensure that they are no longer infectious before having sex with anyone and have regular blood tests throughout their life to detect any liver damage. Nine out of ten patients recover completely after a few weeks, but one in ten become chronic carriers. Ten per cent of patients develop cirrhosis, failure of the liver or liver cancer, and about one per cent of patients develop a rapidly progressive liver disease that causes death.

HEPATITIS C

Hepatitis C is a **viral** infection of the liver transmitted from one person to another through blood contamination such as the sharing of needles by drug users. All blood donations are screened for this virus. Sexual transmission is possible but uncommon, and the incubation period is six to seven weeks.

The **symptoms** are usually mild, and the patient may only be vaguely unwell for a few days, but a minority progress to develop jaundice, liver enlargement and nausea. About a quarter of patients develop permanent liver damage, often after many years.

Blood tests are available to detect antibodies against the various hepatitis viruses and diagnose the type of hepatitis and monitor its progress.

Treatment involves bed rest and a diet that is low in protein and high in carbohydrate, and alcohol is forbidden. Sometimes it is necessary to give medication for nausea and vomiting and to feed severely affected patients by a drip into a vein for a short time. If it continues to worsen, drugs may be used to reduce the liver damage. Unfortunately it is not yet possible to vaccinate against hepatitis C.

No cure is available, but many patients lead normal long lives, although about half eventually develop cirrhosis and liver failure.

HEPATITIS D

Hepatitis D is a **viral** infection of the liver that can only be caught by patients who already have hepatitis B. The two diseases may be caught at the same time or separately. Hepatitis D is much more common in intravenous drug users with hepatitis B than in patients who have caught hepatitis B in other ways, and it is also more prevalent in countries around the Mediterranean.

Vaccination against hepatitis B also protects against hepatitis D.

If hepatitis D is caught at a later time than hepatitis B, there are usually no symptoms, but infection increases the risk of developing serious liver disease in those who already have hepatitis B. Blood tests are available to detect antibodies against the various hepatitis viruses and diagnose the type of hepatitis and monitor its progress.

Usually no **treatment** is necessary, but in severe cases, drugs may be used to reduce the liver damage. There is no specific vaccine against hepatitis D, but vaccination against hepatitis B will effectively prevent both diseases.

No cure is available, and most patients lead normal lives, but many eventually develop cirrhosis, liver failure or liver cancer.

LYMPHOGRANULOMA VENEREUM

Lymphogranuloma venereum is a sexually transmitted disease that is rare in developed countries but common in Africa and Asia. It is caused by the *Chlamydia* organism which is a **bacteria-like** germ that lives inside cells and destroys them. The incubation period after sexual contact is one to three weeks.

A **sore** develops on the penis or vulva, then the lymph nodes in the groin become infected, swollen, soften and suppurate (drain pus) onto the skin. The infection may spread to cause joint, skin, brain and eye infections. If anal intercourse has occurred, sores and pus-discharging lymph nodes may form in and around the anus. The initial sore and pus-discharging lymph nodes are not painful, and only if the disease spreads does a fever develop. It is diagnosed by special skin and blood tests.

Antibiotics such as tetracyclines are prescribed and surgical procedures to drain pus from lymph nodes may be necessary. If left untreated, disfiguring scarring will occur in the groin at the site of the infected lymph nodes, and the genitals may become permanently swollen, and if the infection spreads to other organs, they may be seriously damaged. The majority of cases are cured by appropriate treatment.

NON-SPECIFIC URETHRITIS

Non-specific urethritis (NSU) is also known as **Chlamydial urethritis** and non-Gonococcal urethritis, and is a sexually transmitted disease that is carried by women and infects men. Most (but not all) cases of NSU are caused by a Chlamydial infection, while unidentified bacteria are responsible for the other cases. *Chlamydiae* are a group of organisms that are not bacteria, but act as parasites inside human cells and eventually destroy the cell. They are spread by passing from the man to female sexual partners, where they remain in the vagina to infect the woman's next sex partner. In homosexuals, the infection may occur around the anus.

Men have a white discharge from the penis and painful passing of urine, but rarely other symptoms, although sometimes the infection may spread from the penis up into the testes or prostate gland.

In **women** there are usually no symptoms, but sometimes the infection may spread to cause salpingitis (infection of the Fallopian tubes).

Non-specific urethritis is the most common sexually transmitted disease.

Chlamydiae may be identified by specific blood and swab tests, but they are not always reliable, and a negative test does not mean that the infection is not present.

Antibiotics such as tetracyclines and erythromycins are used very successfully in treatment, and all sexual contacts should be treated when the infection is discovered.

PELVIC INFLAMMATORY DISEASE

Pelvic inflammatory disease (PID) is an **infection** of the uterus (womb), Fallopian tubes, ovaries and the tissues immediately around these organs. It is usually associated with the sexual transmission of bacteria from one person to another, although, less commonly, it may occur as a result of non-sexually transmitted infections. It is most common in young, sexually promiscuous women. The use of intrauterine devices (IUD) doubles the risk of developing PID, while condoms provide significant protection. A wide range of different bacteria may be responsible, and frequently two, three or more different types are present.

Symptoms may include pain low in the abdomen, fevers, a vaginal discharge, abnormal menstrual periods, pain with intercourse, and infertility. The pain may become very severe, and the patient appear extremely ill. One quarter of all women who develop PID will have long-term problems including repeat infections, infertility (ten per cent after one attack of PID, 55 per cent after three attacks of PID), persistent pain in the pelvis or with sex, and ectopic pregnancy (pregnancy that develops in the wrong position). There may be no symptoms in the male partner of the patient, although a discharge from the penis is sometimes present.

Swabs are usually taken from the vagina and cervix (opening into the womb) to determine the responsible bacteria and appropriate antibiotic.

Treatment involves antibiotics by mouth or injected in severe cases. Sex should be avoided until complete recovery, which may take several weeks or months. If an abscess develops in the pelvis, an operation will be necessary to drain it. Fortunately, many women are completely cured by early treatment.

SYPHILIS

Syphilis is an infection that is usually sexually transmitted, and which passes through three main stages over many months or years. It is relatively uncommon in developed countries, but still widespread in poorer societies. The cause is the spirochete **bacterium** *Treponema pallidum*, which is transmitted by heterosexual or homosexual contact, sharing injecting needles, blood transfusions, or from a mother to her child during pregnancy (congenital syphilis).

THE **SYMPTOMS** ARE TOTALLY DIFFERENT IN EACH OF THE
THREE STAGES:

- **First stage** syphilis causes a painless sore (chancre) on the penis, the female genitals, or around the anus of homosexuals, which heals after three to six weeks. There may be painless enlarged lymph nodes in the armpit and groin that also disappear.

- **Second stage** syphilis starts a few weeks or months later with a widespread rash, mouth and vaginal ulcers, and a slight fever. The patient is highly infectious but will usually recover and enter a latent period that may last many years.

- **Third** (tertiary) **stage** syphilis develops years later with tumours (gumma) in the liver, major arteries, bones, brain, spinal cord (tabes dorsalis), skin and other organs. Symptoms vary depending on organs involved but may include arthritis, bone weakness, severe bone pain, paralysis, strokes, heart attacks, internal bleeding from aneurysms, blindness, headaches, jaundice (liver failure), muscle spasms, skin ulcers, scars, nodules in the larynx and lungs, vomiting, confusion, mental illness and death.

Congenital syphilis occurs in newborn infants who have teeth abnormalities, deafness, misshapen bones, deformed nose, pneumonia, and mental retardation.

> *Yaws is a skin disease found in communities with*
> *very poor personal hygiene, which is identical in every way*
> *to syphilis except that it is spread by close non-sexual contact.*

It can be diagnosed at all stages by specific blood tests, or by finding the responsible bacteria on a swab taken from a genital sore in the first stage of the disease. All pregnant women should be routinely tested.

The first and second stages are **treated** by antibiotics such as penicillin (often as an injection), tetracycline or erythromycin. In the third (tertiary) stage antibiotics are also used, but can merely prevent further deterioration, as organ damage is irreversible. A child suffering from congenital syphilis is infectious when born and is treated with antibiotics.

There are many **complications** associated with a syphilis infection. In the first stage there are usually none, but in second stage syphilis there may be spread of the infection to involve the joints, brain, liver and kidney, which may be severely damaged. In the third (tertiary) stage almost any organ can be seriously damaged. Infants with congenital syphilis may develop more serious problems if the condition is not treated aggressively.

A course of antibiotics for a few weeks almost invariably cures the disease in its first two stages, but there is no cure for tertiary or congenital syphilis. Plastic surgery may correct the more obvious congenital deformities.

TRICHOMONIASIS

Trichomoniasis is an infection of a woman's vagina and the urethra (urine tube) of both men and women, caused by the **single-celled animal** *Trichomonas vaginalis*. It is transmitted from one victim to another by heterosexual or homosexual intercourse.

In women, vaginal infection **causes** a foul-smelling, yellow/green, frothy discharge, and there may be mild itching or soreness around the outside of the vagina. In men, there are often minimal symptoms, including discomfort on passing urine, often first thing in the morning.

The diagnosis can be confirmed by examining a swab taken from the vagina or urethra.

Antibiotic tablets (e.g. azithromycin) and/or vaginal cream are usually very effective, but all sexual contacts need to be treated at the same time.

VAGINITIS

Vaginitis is any form of inflammation of the vagina, or a vaginal infection by any of a number of different **bacteria**. Many bacteria may be responsible, including *Gardnerella vaginalis*, which is slightly unusual in that it requires an oxygen-free and alkaline environment. The upper end of the vagina can be oxygen-free, but is normally slightly acid. It may become alkaline with semen after sex, changing sexual partners, hormonal changes at different times of the month, and using antibiotics. Most other infections (e.g. gonorrhoea) are sexually transmitted venereal diseases. The infection may spread into the uterus and cause pelvic inflammatory disease, or to adjacent glands to cause a Bartholin cyst infection.

The woman develops a greyish fish-smelling **vaginal discharge**, with soreness and redness of the vagina. The diagnosis and type of bacteria present is determined by taking a swab from the vagina and having it examined and cultured.

Treatments include appropriate antibiotic tablets by mouth, antiseptic douches (e.g. iodine solution), and acidic gels or creams in the vagina. In recurrent cases the male sexual partner may need to be treated.

CURIOSITY

Syphilis was thought to have been introduced to Europe from America by the crew on Columbus' ships. This is now in doubt, as it is more likely that it was a modified form of the skin disease yaws that developed as hygiene improved.

Syphilis is called the French curse in England and the English disease in France.

SKIN CANCER

L ook after yourself and slip (on a shirt), slop (on sunscreen) and slap (on a hat) to prevent skin cancers.

Most skin cancers are caused by sun exposure, primarily in childhood, but some chemicals may also be responsible and there is sometimes a familial tendency. Tropical countries with a predominantly white-skinned population have a far higher incidence.

The various forms of skin cancer vary from the relatively innocuous to those which can spread rapidly enough to eventually kill.

Skin cancers fall into several different categories – squamous cell carcinomas (SCC), intraepithelial carcinoma (IEC), basal cell carcinomas (BCC), Bowen's disease and melanomas are the most common and are dealt with separately.

Signs to watch for in a spot or sore that may indicate that it is a skin cancer are any irregularity in colour, shape or outline; soreness or itchiness; bleeding or weeping.

A biopsy can give a definitive diagnosis, but it may be more practical to excise the whole growth.

They may be **treated** by freezing with liquid nitrogen, diathermy (burning), cutting out the growth, injecting anticancer drugs in and under it, or applying acid or anticancer ointments.

BASAL CELL CARCINOMA

Also known as a **rodent ulcer**, these shiny, rounded lumps are a cancer of the deeper (basal) layers of the skin. They are caused by prolonged exposure to sunlight, and occur most commonly on the face and back. They are not as serious as the more superficial squamous cell carcinomas (SCC), but occur at an earlier age than SCCs, although rarely before 25 years.

BCCs often change in size and colour, or they may present as an ulcer that fails to heal. The ulcer often has a pearly, rounded edge.

BCCs were originally called rodent ulcers because they formed an ulcer that failed to heal and gradually enlarged.

Whenever a BCC is suspected, it should be removed surgically. The specimen is then sent to a pathologist for examination to ensure that the diagnosis is correct, and that all the tumour has been removed. Alternate treatments in more difficult areas include anticancer creams, irradiation and diathermy.

If correctly treated, they can be completely healed, but if left until large, significant plastic surgery may be necessary, as they will slowly invade deeper tissues, and, after many years, may cause death.

BOWEN'S DISEASE

Bowen's disease is a precancerous skin condition that may be found anywhere on the body. It is caused by exposure to sunlight or arsenic compounds and appears as a sharply-edged red patch covered with a fine scale. Biopsy or excision is required to make a diagnosis.

Spots should be surgically removed or chemically destroyed, as they can progress to become a squamous cell carcinoma (SCC).

INTRAEPITHELIAL CARCINOMA

An intraepithelial carcinoma (IEC) is a common cancer in the outer layers of skin, similar to, but deeper in the skin than, a squamous cell carcinoma. They usually occur in patients who are over 50 years of age and are caused by prolonged exposure to sunlight. The rims of the ears, the face, scalp, arms and hands are commonly affected.

The cancer **appears** as an unsightly red spot covered in fine white scales that may be itchy or sore. Small IECs are easily removed by burning with a diathermy machine or freezing with liquid nitrogen. If larger, or if the diagnosis is not certain, it is necessary to excise the spot and surrounding tissue. Any IEC that recurs after freezing or burning must be surgically excised. Rarely, they may spread by blood or lymphatics to other parts of the body.

Treatment is very effective in early stages of the disease.

MELANOMA

A melanoma is the most **serious** form of skin cancer, and it starts in the skin cells that create pigment. In Europeans, these cells are relatively inactive, giving a pale colour to the skin, but in Asians they are moderately active, and in Africans they are very active, giving a darker skin colour.

The actual **cause** is unknown, but exposure to sunlight, particularly in childhood and teen years, dramatically increases the risk. Ultraviolet radiation, most of which is filtered out of sunlight by the ozone layer in the upper atmosphere, is the part of the spectrum that causes the damage. Fair-skinned people have a higher incidence than those with dark complexions, and it is rare in children, slightly more common in women than men, and most common between 30 and 50 years of age and on the legs and back. One in every 150 people in Australia will develop a melanoma at some time.

Although melanomas may be very serious, the majority
of people diagnosed with melanoma are cured.

It **appears** as a skin spot that may be black, brown, pink or blue, and the colours may be found individually or mixed. They usually have an irregularly edge, enlarge steadily, have an uneven and bumpy surface, and the pigment can be seen advancing into the surrounding skin. In advanced cases the spot will bleed, scab and ulcerate. They have a tendency to grow deep into the body and migrate to other organs, particularly the liver, lungs and lymph nodes in the armpit and groin. Melanomas can occur under the nail (where they may be mistaken for a bruise), in the mouth, under the eyelids, on the retina inside the eye, and in the anus, but the sun-exposed parts of the skin are the most commonly affected.

It is **diagnosed** by biopsy or excision of the suspected mole, then the melanoma and a large area of skin around and under it must be cut out. The lymph nodes around the melanoma may also need to be removed. If there is evidence that it has spread to other areas, the patient will also be treated with irradiation and injected medications to control its further growth.

In the very early stages there is a 97 per cent cure rate, but as the cancer enlarges, the cure rate drops dramatically. The thicker the melanoma the worse the prognosis, and ulceration of the melanoma at the time it is excised also worsens the long-term outcome. Unfortunately, sometimes the cancer may appear to be cured but can flare up decades later.

SQUAMOUS CELL CARCINOMA

A squamous cell carcinoma (SCC) is a cancer of the outermost layer of skin that occurs on sun-exposed parts of the body, usually in patients who are over 50 years of age. It is caused by prolonged exposure to sunlight or irritant chemicals. The rims of the ears, the face, scalp, arms and hands are commonly affected, but the cancer may also occur on the penis.

SCCs look like a red spot covered in fine white scales. They may be itchy or sore but often attract attention because they are unsightly. In severe cases they can spread by blood or lymphatics to distant parts of the body.

If suspected, excision or biopsy is necessary to make the diagnosis. Small SCCs are easily removed by burning with a diathermy machine or freezing with liquid nitrogen. If it is larger, or if the diagnosis is not certain, it is necessary to excise the spot and surrounding tissue. Any SCC that recurs after freezing or burning must be surgically excised.

Treatment is very effective in early stages of the disease.

CURIOSITY

The Gorlin-Goltz syndrome (or basal cell carcinoma naevus syndrome) is a rare inherited condition of children, characterised by the development of multiple basal cell carcinoma (BCC), skin cancers and other abnormalities, including calcification of areas of the brain, abnormal vertebrae and ribs, multiple cysts in the jaw and pitting of the palm. Excision of jaw cysts and basal cell carcinomas is the only treatment, but recurrence of skin cancers and jaw cysts after excision is common.

SMOKING

To look after yourself, never ever smoke, and don't live or work with people who smoke, because passive smoking is also dangerous.

If rhubarb, just for instance, was found not only to cause cancer in ten per cent of its heavy consumers, but eventually to bring 25 per cent to an early death, no one would consume it, and the government would long ago have legislated against growing it. Sadly, this is just what cigarette smoking does, but the sale of cigarettes is permitted, cigarettes are heavily promoted by advertising, and large profits are made from their sale.

HISTORY

Over the centuries, since the introduction of tobacco to Europe in the 1590s, more and more people have become addicted to nicotine. Women started smoking in public only during the First World War, and the habit reached a peak during the Second World War when 75 per cent of the adult population of most Western countries were smokers.

When today's grandparents were children, they were warned against smoking because 'it stunts the growth' (something it only does to the babies of smoking mothers), but generally it was not regarded as harmful, at least for adults. Cigarettes, cigars, lighters, pipes, ash trays, etc., were standard gifts at Christmas and birthdays for a generation. Vast factories poured out billions of cigarettes that were made, packed, wrapped and boxed untouched by human hand. Multi-national tobacco corporations gained enormous profits, and became powerful friends of government as tax payers and revenue earners. Governments even subsidised the growth of tobacco in some areas.

Then came the crunch. It was found that smoking tobacco killed people. There was a long delay, and more than half the smokers escaped, but there was little doubt about it – for many people smoking was lethal.

Nicotine is as addictive as heroin in some people.

NICOTINE

Nicotine is a highly **addictive** toxic alkaloid (chemical) found in tobacco, and one of the main reasons that smokers find it so hard to stop their health-damaging habit. Nicotine **stimulates** the pleasure centres in the brain, but tolerance develops, so that a greater dosage (i.e. more smoking) is necessary to obtain the same effect. Withdrawal causes anxiety, cravings, anger, frustration, inability to concentrate, increased appetite and irritability.

Nicotine also causes effects on the heart (increased blood pressure and pulse rate), increases blood sugar and has numerous other biological and physiological effects on almost every organ.

In addition to nicotine, tobacco smoke contains many other harmful chemicals, including tar and carbon monoxide. Tar released in the form of particles in the smoke is the main cause of lung and throat cancer in smokers and also aggravates bronchial and respiratory disease.

EFFECTS

We now know that 11 per cent of smokers will get lung cancer, and 90 per cent of these patients will die. Coronary heart disease will kill many prematurely. Chronic lung disease will cripple a large proportion of the remainder. Women smokers have an increased risk of cancer of the cervix.

SMOKING IS KNOWN TO INCREASE THE INCIDENCE OF A WIDE RANGE OF MEDICAL PROBLEMS INCLUDING:

- amblyopia (vision problem)

- aneurysm (dilation of arteries)

- angina

- asbestosis

- asthma

- bladder cancer

- bronchiectasis (chronic lung condition)

- Buerger's disease (poor circulation to feet and hands)

- cancer of the cervix

- cattarh (phlegm in throat)

- chronic bronchitis

- common cold

- cor pulmonale (disease of heart and lungs)

- depression

- emphysema (over-dilation of air spaces in lung)

- heart attacks

- high blood pressure

- histiocytosis X (replacement of lung tissue with fibrous tissue)

- hypercholesterolaemia (high cholesterol)

- kidney cancer

- laryngitis
- Legionnaire's disease (lung infection)
- lung cancer
- mesothelioma (form of lung cancer)
- mouth cancer
- mouth ulcers
- oesophageal cancer
- osteoporosis
- pancreatic cancer
- peptic ulcers
- pneumoconiosis (lung disease)
- pneumonia
- pneumothorax (air in sac around lung)
- reflux oesophagitis (heartburn)
- sinusitis
- sleep apnoea (breathing stops during sleep with snoring)
- small and sicker babies of pregnant women
- snoring
- strokes
- suicide
- tachycardia (rapid heart rate)
- talcosis (lungs affected by powder)
- throat cancer
- thrombosis (blood clots)
- tongue cancer
- viral and bacterial infections of the throat and lungs (e.g. influenza, tonsillitis).

It also alters the actions of many **medications** from betablockers to asthma inhalers.

Many of the effects above may affect not only the smoker, but those who live and work with smokers (passive smokers).

CONTENTS

Cigarette smoke contains hundreds of chemicals. Amongst the worst are:

CHEMICAL	MAY CAUSE
Tar	Cancer
Carbon monoxide	Suffocates and blocks oxygen uptake
Nicotine	Stimulation and addiction
Aromatic hydrocarbons	Cancer
Phenol	Tissue irritant
Arsenic	Poison
Carbazole	Accelerates cancer growth
Hydrocyanic acid	Cancer
Acetaldehyde	Slows function of cilia (fine hairs) in airways
Ammonia	Tissue irritant
Nitrosamine	Cancer
Formaldehyde	Stops phlegm clearance from airways
Indole dyes	Accelerates cancer growth
Vinyl chloride	Cancer

If governments actually recorded these substances officially, they would have to ban the sale of cigarettes, as no other product that contained these substances would be allowed on the market.

STATISTICS

At present, 26 per cent of the adult population in Western Europe smokes, but this figure is decreasing every year. The lowest rate of smoking in the world is in Australia where only 19 per cent of adults indulge. It will soon become so antisocial that it will only be permitted by consenting adults in private!

On the other hand, the highest rate of smoking amongst developed countries is in Japan, while in developing countries smoking is seen as a status symbol – the smoker can afford to burn money – and smoking rates of over 70 per cent are found in countries like Indonesia.

The medical facts are conclusive – smoking is the biggest health problem in the Western world. It contributes to more deaths than alcohol and illicit drugs together, and costs the economies of these countries millions of dollars a year. If nobody smoked, there would be 30 per cent less cancer.

SMOKING BEHAVIOUR	YEARS LIFESPAN GAIN MEN	YEARS LIFESPAN GAIN WOMEN
Never smoked	10.5	8.9
Quit aged 35	8.5	7.7
Quit aged 45	7.1	7.2
Quit aged 55	4.8	5.6
Quit aged 65	2.0	3.7
(Compared with lifelong smokers)		

SMOKING IN PREGNANCY

There is no doubt that the babies of mothers who smoke are **smaller** (by 200g on average) than those of non-smoking mothers. There is also an increased rate of **premature** labour (delivering the baby too early), **miscarriage** and stillbirth in these women.

After birth, babies of smoking mothers continue to suffer both directly and indirectly from their mother's smoking. The smoking by the mother appears to reduce their resistance to disease, in particular to **infection**, so that babies born to smoking mothers die in infancy more often than average. By inhaling the smoke from either of their parents, these infants have more colds, bronchitis and other respiratory problems than babies in non-smoking homes.

The most harmful legal thing a pregnant woman can do to her baby is smoke.

Any woman who smokes should ideally cease before she falls pregnant, but certainly should do so when the pregnancy is diagnosed. This is far easier said than done, but if her partner stops at the same time, support and encouragement is given by family and friends, and assistance is obtained from the family doctor, women who are motivated to give their baby the best possible chance in life will succeed in kicking this very addictive habit.

SMOKING CESSATION

Smoking dependence can be divided into two components – **addiction** to nicotine and **habit**. Those who are addicted will find it harder to stop than those who merely smoke out of habit. Usually it is not just addiction or habit, but a mixture of the two.

ADDICTION IS CHARACTERISED BY:

- desire to smoke immediately on waking

- difficulty in not smoking in places where it is forbidden

- smoking larger quantities of cigarettes

- smoking more often in the first two hours of each day

- smoking despite being ill

- becoming depressed if unable to smoke

Before anyone can stop smoking, they must really want to stop. No one who is half-hearted about wanting to stop will ever succeed.

ONCE YOU HAVE DECIDED TO STOP:

- set a time and date for the event

- tell everyone you know of your intentions

- take side-bets if you can, to reinforce your incentive

- make lists of reasons why you must stop, and leave them at home and work

- make sure that from the moment you stop, you have no cigarettes available to you

- resist the temptation to buy or beg for cigarettes

- start a savings account with the money you save by not smoking, and if you don't succeed, pay the balance to the Cancer Fund!

- nicotine-containing gum, inhalers or patches can be used to ease the craving for cigarettes

- see a doctor who can prescribe a medication (bupropion – Zyban) that can reduce the craving for nicotine

- consider group therapy sessions, hypnotherapy, psychological counselling, support groups, rewards at the end of each successful week and reinforcement visits to your doctor

- antidepressant medication may be useful in smokers who are very addicted.

PASSIVE SMOKING

Almost everyone is forced to inhale fumes containing toxins such as formaldehyde, acetone, arsenic, carbon monoxide, hydrogen cyanide and nicotine at some time. You have no choice in the matter and have to suffer the consequences, because these chemicals are just a few of the scores of irritants found in cigarette smoke.

Fortunately for most of us, the result of passive involuntary smoking is only a minor itch of the nose, a cough or a sneeze, but some people can develop life-threatening **asthma** attacks or have their **heart condition** aggravated by inhaling tobacco smoke. Being trapped in a vehicle or other enclosed space with a smoker can be a nightmare experience for such people.

Workers have successfully sued their employers for not
banning smoking because of the effects of passive smoking.

In some situations the non-smoker may be more affected than the smoker, because the smoke coming directly from a cigarette contains more toxins, nicotine and carbon monoxide than that inhaled by the smoker, which has been more completely burnt and passed through a filter.

The most unfortunate victims of passive smoking are the **children** of smokers. The incidence of pneumonia and bronchitis and the severity of asthma in children whose parents smoke are far higher than in the children of non-smokers. In babies of women who smoke, health problems caused by passive smoking begin before birth (see above).

In the **workplace**, more and more offices are becoming smoke-free zones. Unfortunately some people still smoke at work, and if their subordinates have adverse reactions to passive smoking, they may have to put up with it or change jobs. This situation may change in the future, as more and more workers are successfully claiming workers compensation payments for complications of passive smoking at work.

The non-smoking spouse or partner of a smoker is also at great risk. They have a significantly increased risk of lung cancer, reduced lung capacity, a higher incidence of asthma, and more respiratory infections than those whose spouses or partners do not smoke.

Smokers should now be aware of the health risks that they are taking every day, and they can no longer claim personal freedom to smoke where and when they like, as their habit is adversely affecting the health of those around them. All smokers should have the courtesy to only light up when there is no possibility of others inhaling the resultant toxic fumes. Legal suits by passive smokers against smokers for causing bodily harm have been successful in the United States.

CURIOSITY

Smokers just can't win in any way. In a Boston study smokers were found to have 50 per cent more traffic accidents and 46 per cent more traffic violation convictions than non-smokers.

SNORING

L ook after yourself by having your snoring treated, because it may cause sleep apnoea in you and significantly distress your significant other.

The noises, sounds, eruptions, gargles and other auditory traumas associated with snoring are impossible to express adequately in print. The effects upon a spouse or entire family may be sufficient to lead to arguments, fights or even divorce and mental illness. The greatest problem with snoring is that the snorer is often unaffected by the noise, but those around him (and most snorers are male) are the victims.

CAUSE

Snoring is the production of a harsh, rough sound caused by the passage of air through the mouth, throat and nose during sleep. It can occur intermittently during colds, flu or throat infections and with hay fever because of the excess production of **phlegm** and the swelling of tissues at these times, or it may occur almost every night.

In persistent cases, snoring is due to the vibration of the uvula or soft palate with the movement of air in and out of the mouth. The uvula is the piece of tissue that can be seen hanging down the back of the throat when the mouth is wide open, and the soft palate is the back part of the roof of the mouth, to which the uvula is attached. In some cases snoring is associated with periods when the breathing stops completely for up to a minute (**sleep apnoea**), which is due to the collapse of the soft tissues of the throat during sleep. It may cause significant health problems to the sufferer.

Snoring may be due to a floppy dingle dangle (uvula),
which is the flap of flesh hanging down from the roof of the mouth.

Other causes include enlargement of the tonsils or adenoids at the back of the throat, a broken nose that has an abnormal shape, polyps in the nose, or other distortions of the shape of the nose or throat.

The excessive use of alcohol, sleeping pills or sedatives will relax the tissues and muscles in the throat to make snoring more likely.

Smoking can increase the secretion of phlegm in the nose and sinuses, and cause persistent inflammation of the throat, which also increases the risk of snoring.

If severe, snoring may need to be investigated in a sleep laboratory, where the patient can be monitored through an entire night.

SLEEP APNOEA

A cessation of breathing (apnoea) during sleep most commonly occurs in over-weight middle-aged men due to a complete relaxation of the small muscles at the back of the throat. The throat tissue becomes very soft and flabby, and collapses as the patient breathes in, closing off the throat and preventing breathing. Snoring is caused in the same way. In elderly men with high blood pressure, there may be a suppression of the urge to breathe by the brain during very deep sleep.

In sufferers **breathing stops** for periods from ten to 60 seconds on many occasions during the night while asleep, resulting in tiredness during the day, morning headaches, personality changes, poor concentration, bed-wetting and impotence. The sleeping partner complains about the patient's loud snoring and thrashing restless sleep. Minor brain damage may occur with every episode of apnoea, and this eventually leads to a noticeable deficit in brain function.

The diagnosis is best made in a sleep laboratory, where the patient's sleep and breathing pattern can be monitored through an entire night.

A significant deterioration in the quality of life may occur unless successfully treated.

TREATMENT

Treatments that may be tried include changing the position during sleep from the back to the side, using pillows or straps if necessary. Patients should lose weight if obese, and stop sedatives, alcohol and smoking.

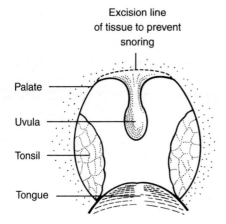

VIEW INTO MOUTH

Excision line
of tissue to prevent
snoring

Palate

Uvula

Tonsil

Tongue

Nose clips and dilating springs may prove successful. Sometimes medications (e.g. antidepressants, respiratory stimulants, anti-inflammatory drugs, steroids) may be beneficial.

In persistent cases a small mask is fitted to the patient's nose, and air is blown up the nose at a slightly increased pressure with a small electrically driven blower (continuous positive airway pressure – CPAP – see below).

In severe cases surgery to the back of the throat and nose to remove the uvula and part of the soft palate opens the airway.

CONTINUOUS POSITIVE AIRWAY PRESSURE MACHINE

Patients who snore excessively or develop sleep apnoea may be assisted by a continuous positive airway pressure (CPAP) machine that increases the air pressure in the mouth, throat and major airways of the lungs.

Untreated sleep apnoea can significantly affect the quality of life.

The machine is about the size of a shoe box, and from it runs a flexible hose that is attached to a mask. The mask is firmly applied to the face by means of elastic straps over the head, and the machine turned on. An electric motor pumps air into the mask at an adjustable pressure, and this higher pressure keeps the airway open while the patient sleeps to prevent the partial collapse of the airways, which is the cause of snoring and sleep apnoea.

Despite this description, many patients find that their sleep is less disturbed and more refreshing using this device, and their partners are certainly relieved by their quieter and more restful bed-mate.

These machines can sometimes be used in severely ill patients who would otherwise require a tracheotomy (hole cut through the front of the neck into the trachea – windpipe) in order for them to be able to breathe.

CURIOSITY

Snoring and sleep apnoea (brief stops in breathing during sleep) may be the cause of an early morning headache.

STRESS

L ook after yourself by learning how to handle stress, because no matter how hard you try, stress cannot be avoided.

CAUSE
Stress is **excessive anxiety** about problems of daily living. Mortgage repayments, marriage strife, young children, job security, family finances, separation and divorce, leaving home, poor health, work responsibilities, or a death in the family – all of these, and hundreds of other situations, are causes of stress.

EFFECTS
Stress may cause a very wide range of **symptoms** including a persistent headache, peptic ulcers, heart disease, migraines, diarrhoea, shortness of breath, sweating, passing excess urine, rashes and vomiting. Stress may worsen or trigger other physical illnesses, or progress to a neurosis, depression, or in severe cases, suicide is possible.

A hectic daily routine can be stressful. Whether at home, at work, bringing up children or studying, it's essential to take care of both your emotional and physical health. In a crisis – when a relationship breaks down or someone's been made redundant, for instance – it's even more important to be physically and mentally ready to deal with uncertainty and disruption. Unless you look after yourself, you may run into difficulty.

MANAGEMENT
Don't be afraid of stressful situations – overcoming them will help to increase your self-confidence. Stress management is not all about being passive, or lying down in a dark room with a wet washer on your head! Learn some active techniques to help you relax, rather than complaining, becoming depressed, introverted or drunk.

Write down the words that describe your daily routine (i.e. tiring, stimulating, stressful or reassuring). Put them in groups according to whether the adjectives are positive, neutral or negative. Work on solving the negative ones and look forward to the positive ones.

Talk to someone you trust about what makes you feel stressed. This is a useful way to let off steam and often helps to reduce stress. This can be as simple as a supportive chat over a cup of tea with a friend or colleague. There's a temptation to keep stressful feelings to ourselves for fear of what others might think of us, but, if you trust the other person, it may well be a chance to give and get mutual support.

When you are tired, everything becomes more difficult and even the simplest of decisions can seem impossible to make. Regular bedtimes, good diet, enough exercise, and less coffee and other caffeine drinks also help.

Alcohol is never the answer to stress.

SINGLE PARENTS

Although often considered stressful, single parenting can be satisfying and allow for extra closeness with your child. On the other hand, all the decisions and daily routines fall to you, which, if not handled properly, may lead to stress.

If you are a single parent it is wise to take extra care of yourself, by undertaking activities such as:

- Meet with other parents at least once a week. Friends and relatives with children may also enjoy meeting up.

- Participate in play groups and school parents and friends associations, which can bring parents together.

- Find time each day to for yourself without the children, even for just half an hour, and once a week for half a day. This can be done by arranging a child minding swap with another parent.

- Contact a parent support group, where volunteering can be a great way to get involved with others.

- Raise the issue of family-related stress at work. Many employers let staff vary their hours to cope with stress, and some offer stress counselling.

Laughter can relieve stress, and is recommended
for everyone on a daily basis.

TREATMENT

THERE ARE THREE POSSIBLE TREATMENT STRATEGIES FOR STRESS:

- Remove the **cause** of the stress, which is much easier said than done in most cases.

- **Rationalise** stress by talking over the problem with a spouse, relatives, friends, doctor or priest. Writing down details of the problem makes it appear more manageable, particularly when all possible options are diagrammatically attached to it to give a rational view of the situation. Professional assistance may be given by a general practitioner, psychiatrist, psychologist, marriage guidance counsellor, child guidance officer or social worker.

- **Medications** that alter mood, sedate or relieve anxiety are used in a crisis, intermittently or for short periods of time. Some antidepressant drugs and treatments for psychiatric conditions are designed for long-term use, but most of the anxiety-relieving drugs can cause dependency if used regularly.

The prognosis depends on the cause, but most people eventually cope with their problems.

POST-TRAUMATIC STRESS DISORDER

Post-traumatic stress disorder (PTSD) occurs after experiencing a situation that causes extreme stress and a feeling of horror and helplessness (e.g. armed hold-up, serious accident, war violence, being assaulted or raped, observing atrocities etc.).

Most symptoms start between two weeks and three months of the triggering catastrophe, but may start as late as six months.

There are no specific **diagnostic tests**, but patients must have at least one symptom from each of the following categories to be diagnosed:

GENERAL:

- symptom duration more than one month, with significant distress or inability to function normally in society

- re-experiencing phenomena

- experience intrusive recollections, nightmares, flashbacks as if the event was recurring, psychological distress on exposure to cues that may trigger memories, or physiological effects (e.g. rapid pulse, rapid breathing) on exposure to cues.

AVOIDANCE BEHAVIOUR:

- avoiding thoughts, feelings or conversations about the incident

- avoiding places, people or activities connected with the incident

- selective amnesia about the traumatic event

- reduced interest in everyday activities or detachment from others

- unable to look forward to future events with pleasure

- abnormal personality compared to before the incident.

Excessively Aroused:

- Insomnia, irritability, anger, poor concentration, increased vigilance or increased startle response to frights.

Treatment involves psychological counselling and debriefing immediately after the event, and a trained counsellor should follow up the victim for at least six months. Normal work and activities should be resumed as soon as possible. Referral to a psychiatrist is necessary if the patient does not appear to recover within six months, or deteriorates sooner, when medication may be necessary.

PTSD may become chronic and lead to recurrent minor illnesses, poor physical health, and, in extreme cases, suicide, but in most cases it usually settles within three to six months.

CURIOSITY

A century ago the post-traumatic stress disorder was known as shell shock.

STROKE

T o look after yourself and prevent a stroke, don't smoke, keep your blood pressure and weight under control, and choose the right parents.

EXPLANATION

A stroke is an accident involving the blood vessels in the brain, and is technically known as a cerebral infarct or cerebrovascular accident (CVA). If a **clot** or a piece of material from elsewhere in the body blocks an artery in the brain (cerebral thrombosis), or if an artery bursts in the brain, a stroke may occur.

The **risk** of stroke is higher in those who smoke, have high blood pressure, high cholesterol levels, are diabetic, and drink alcohol to excess.

Any blood vessel in the brain may be involved, so any part of the brain may be damaged, and the area damaged determines the effects on that person's body.

The **symptoms** can therefore be very varied. If a motor area of the brain that controls movement is affected, the patient becomes paralysed down the opposite side of the body, because the nerves supplying the body cross over to the opposite side at the base of the brain (the right side of the brain controls the left arm and leg). Other patients may lose their memory, power of speech, become uncoordinated, unbalanced, start fitting, have strange smells, hear abnormal noises or any of dozens of other possibilities.

The area of the brain affected may increase as a blood clot extends along an artery or bleeding into the brain continues.

Festination is walking with a quick shuffle and a
slightly bent back. It may be caused by a stroke.

INVESTIGATION

The **cause** of the stroke can be determined by using special X-rays, CT scans, MRI (magnetic resonance imaging), blood tests, tests on the fluid around the brain, and measuring the brain waves electrically (EEG).

TREATMENT

A wait-and-watch attitude is adopted in most cases, with medication given to prevent the stroke from worsening and to protect other organs.

Surgery to a bleeding or blocked artery in the brain may be appropriate in some cases. Physiotherapists, speech pathologists and occupational therapists will assist in recovery. Further strokes can often be prevented by the long-term use of low dose aspirin or warfarin, which prevent blood clots. Patients who are at a high risk can also use these medications.

It will be several days or even weeks before doctors can give an accurate prognosis. The brain does not repair itself, but it can often find different ways of doing a task and bypassing damaged areas.

Most improvement occurs in the first week, but full recovery may take months. Patients who become unconscious during a stroke generally have a poorer outcome than those who do not. Strokes are the third major cause of death in developed countries after heart disease and cancer.

*The primary benefit of moderate red or white wine consumption
is the reduction in the incidence of heart attacks and strokes.*

TRANSIENT ISCHAEMIC ATTACKS

A transient ischaemic attack (TIA) may be the cause for a type of **funny turn** in elderly people due to a temporary miniature stroke. The usual cause is hardening and narrowing of arteries (arteriosclerosis) in the neck and brain by excessive deposition of cholesterol that causes small blood clots to form. A clot may break off from the artery wall and travel through the arteries into the brain, where it may briefly obstruct an artery, causing temporary damage to the brain tissue beyond the blockage. Spasms of arteries caused by stress, toxins or allergies, and Fabry disease may also be responsible.

The patient feels strange and acts peculiarly. There may be weakness in one arm or leg, abnormal sensations (e.g. pins and needles, numbness), disturbances in vision, abnormally slurred speech, dizziness, confusion, tremor and blackouts. The symptoms may last for a few seconds or several hours. A TIA may be an early warning of narrowed arteries in the brain, and can forewarn of strokes.

All patients experiencing a TIA need to be fully **investigated** by blood tests, ultrasound examination of arteries in the neck, special X-rays of arteries in the brain, and CT scans of the brain to determine the cause.

There is no specific treatment, but aspirin or warfarin taken long-term in low doses prevent most TIAs, and often prevent strokes too, by preventing blood clots. The patient usually returns to normal within 24 hours.

CURIOSITY

The locked-in syndrome is an horrendous complication of certain types of brain damage caused by a stroke, to particular parts of the brain. The patient has total paralysis of limbs and facial nerves, but normal consciousness, and is able to communicate only by eye movements. No treatment is available, and death from pneumonia due to lack of movement and poor function of muscles of breathing is usually a blessed release.

THRUSH

N
o, we are not talking about a cute little bird found in English gardens, but a fungal infection that can affect any moist membrane in the body. Looking after yourself to prevent thrush involves good personal hygiene by yourself and those you are close to.

EXPLANATION

Thrush (**candidiasis** or **moniliasis**) is a fungal infection caused by the fungus *Candida albicans*, which occurs most commonly in the mouth and vagina.

Mushrooms, the green slime that forms on stagnant pools and tinea are all related. They are fungi. Fungi are members of the plant kingdom, and are one of the types of microscopic life that can infect human beings in many diverse ways. Fungal infections may be called mycotic infections or mycoses by doctors.

The most common site of infection is the skin, where they cause an infection that is commonly known as **tinea**. Fungi are also responsible for many gut infections, particularly in the mouth and around the anus. It is a rare infant that escapes without an attack of oral thrush. The white plaques that form on the tongue and insides of the cheeks are familiar to most mothers, and this is due to one of a number of fungi.

Around the anus, the fungus can cause an extremely itchy rash, but in women it may spread forward from the anus to the vagina to cause the white discharge and intense itch of vaginal thrush or candidiasis.

Fungi normally live in the gut, and are in balance with the bacteria that are meant to be there to help with the digestion of our food. Antibiotics may kill off the good bacteria, allowing the fungal numbers to increase dramatically, or they may migrate to unwanted areas. In these circumstances, they can cause trouble.

Every species of fungus (and bacteria, but not viruses) has two names – a family name (e.g. Candida) which uses a capital initial letter and comes first, and a specific species name (e.g. albicans) which uses a lower case initial letter and comes second. The fungus which causes thrush is thus called *Candida albicans* but may be abbreviated to *C. albicans*.

ORAL THRUSH

The **oral** form is quite common in infancy, particularly in bottle-fed babies, and may be triggered by a course of antibiotics that destroys the bacteria in the mouth that normally control the growth of excess fungi. Babies develop grey/white patches on the tongue, gums and inside of the cheeks that cannot be rubbed away with a finger tip or cotton bud. The infection may spread through the intestine and emerge to infect the skin around the anus, where it causes a bright red rash that is slightly paler towards the centre.

Milk curds may be confused with oral thrush in babies. Milk can be easily rubbed off the inside of the mouth, the white plaque of thrush cannot.

Antifungal drops or gels in the mouth, and antifungal creams around the anus rapidly settle the problem.

VAGINAL THRUSH

The **vaginal** form is very common in sexually active women. *Candida albicans* lives in the gut where it causes little or no trouble. When it comes out on to the skin around the anus, it usually dies off; but if that skin is warm, moist and irritated, it can grow and spread forward to the lips of the vagina (the vulva).

AGGRAVATING FACTORS FOR VAGINAL THRUSH INCLUDE:

- a warm climate

- tight jeans and pantyhose

- the contraceptive pill

- nylon bathers

- antibiotics

- sex.

These factors give the area between a woman's legs the right degree of warmth, moisture and irritation to make the spread of the fungus relatively easy. **Antibiotics** aggravate the problem, as they can kill off the bacteria that normally keep fungi under control. Entry of the fungus into the vagina is aided by the mechanical action of **sex** and the alteration in the acidity of the vagina caused by the contraceptive pill.

There are many causes of vaginal discharge other than thrush, so any persistent vaginal discharge must be checked by a doctor.

An unpleasant white vaginal **discharge** develops, along with intense itching of the vulva and surrounding skin, and often inflammation of the urine opening so that passing urine causes discomfort.

Swabs may be taken from the vagina to confirm the identity of the responsible fungus.

Antifungal vaginal pessaries (tablets), vaginal creams or antifungal tablets taken by mouth are the available **treatments**. The sex partner must also be treated, as he can give the infection back to the woman after she has been successfully treated. It is prevented by wearing loose cotton panties, drying the genital area carefully after swimming or showering, avoiding tight clothing, wiping from front to back after going to the toilet and not using tampons when an infection is likely.

Many women have repeated attacks, which may be due to inadequate treatment, contamination from the gut, or reinfection from their sex partner.

CURIOSITY

Yoghurt (unflavoured and without added fruit) may be used as a vaginal douche to both prevent and treat vaginal infections, including thrush.

TIREDNESS

Always ensure that you look after yourself by getting adequate rest, and assessing the cause of any tiredness so that action can be taken to investigate tiredness that cannot be reasonably explained.

DEFINITIONS

Fatigue is different to lethargy in that fatigue occurs with exercise, while **lethargy** is a tiredness that prevents any exercise in the first place. There is a great overlap in the causes of the two problems, so they will be dealt with together under this heading.

Fatigue is a very common problem, and trying to determine its cause can be extremely difficult, as often there are no other symptoms to give the examining doctor any clues.

CAUSES

There may be **lifestyle** factors that cause fatigue, such as excessive working hours, shift work, stress, long-term anxiety, grief, poor quality or inadequate diet, a sedentary lifestyle, obesity, and both a lack of sleep and over-sleeping. These may be overlooked by the patient, as they feel their way of life is relatively normal, but when a doctor analyses these factors, the problem may become obvious.

Any internal **infection** – bacterial (e.g. urinary infection, bronchitis, tuberculosis), viral (e.g. hepatitis, glandular fever, influenza) or fungal – will cause a person to tire excessively. In fact any long-term illness, persistent pain or even a recurrent allergy reaction can cause this effect.

Sleep apnoea from snoring is a very common,
but often overlooked, cause of persistent tiredness.

Snoring (see separate entry in this book) may be a sign of sleep apnoea (stopping breathing for half a minute or so while asleep), which results in a disturbed and unrefreshing sleep.

The chronic fatigue syndrome is a controversial diagnosis but may explain a persistent tiredness with numerous other symptoms that can vary from depression and irritability to arthritis and fevers.

OTHER CAUSES OF FATIGUE MAY INCLUDE:

- -

- cancer anywhere in the body

- anaemia (due to an excessive loss of blood, or a failure of the body to produce sufficient red blood cells)

- heart diseases of any sort (e.g. heart failure, angina, heart attack, damage to valves in the heart, myocarditis, endocarditis, subacute endocarditis)

- lung diseases (e.g. asthma, pneumonia, emphysema, pulmonary thrombosis)

- poorly controlled diabetes

- imbalances in any of the substances in the blood (e.g. sodium, potassium, calcium, magnesium, sugar and iron)

- failure or over-activity of the endocrine glands (e.g. thyroid, pituitary, adrenal) that secrete hormones

- depression (causes mood disorders, difficulty in sleeping, a loss of interest in life, early morning waking and both lethargy and fatigue)

- a mild stroke (cerebrovascular accident)

- autoimmune diseases (e.g. rheumatoid arthritis, systemic lupus erythematosus, scleroderma, multiple sclerosis)

- leukaemia (which may affect adults as well as children)

- agranulocytosis (a lack of white cells that leads to recurrent infections)

- thalassaemia (an inherited lack of vital blood ingredients)

- polycythaemia vera (an excessive number of red blood cells)

- kidney and liver disease

- AIDS.

Many **medications** can cause fatigue, and all medications being taken must be considered a potential cause of fatigue until specifically excluded. Antihistamines, sedatives, pain relievers, narcotics, betablockers (for heart disease, high blood pressure and migraines), and drugs used to control epilepsy and psychiatric conditions are particular suspects.

Recreational **drugs** (e.g. marijuana, ecstasy, heroin, cocaine, LSD) may initially cause a high, but this is often followed by a low and persistent fatigue, that is only relieved by another dose of the drug, rapidly leading to a vicious cycle of addiction.

EXCESS SLEEP

Excessive sleeping is usually due to exhaustion from extra physical exercise, mental activity, stress or anxiety, but may be due to some unusual medical conditions. It may be perceived as tiredness by the patient, but is actually a different problem.

Excessive sleeping from concussion after a **head injury** is relatively common, but if this becomes prolonged, or is associated with vomiting, confusion, changes in the size of the pupils in the eyes, bleeding from the nose or an ear, fits, spasms, severe headache or double vision, further medical assistance is essential.

Sleeping excessively and unnecessarily may actually be a cause of tiredness.

A number of **psychiatric** conditions may have excess sleeping as an effect, as the patient attempts to escape reality.

Epilepsy is a condition that causes recurrent seizures (fits). Fits can vary from very mild absences to the grand mal convulsion. After a major fit, it is very common for a patient to sleep, sometimes for some hours.

Narcolepsy is an unusual disorder of the brain's electrical activity that is characterised by sudden periods of sleeping for five to 30 minutes several times a day, hallucinations and sudden muscle weakness immediately before and during sleep. There is a wide range of severity, from those who merely appear to sleep excessively to those who are barely able to function or care for themselves. Patients may suddenly fall asleep in the middle of a sentence, or when halfway across a pedestrian crossing.

Other causes include a tumour, cancer, cyst, bleed or abscess in the brain or surrounding tissues that puts pressure on vital centres in the brain to affect sleeping patterns, and the Kleine-Levin syndrome (episodes every few months of severe excessive sleepiness, increased appetite, mood disturbances, increased sexual activity, disorientation, hallucinations and memory loss).

Excess sleeping may be the result of excess alcohol, or the effect of medications such as sedatives, antihistamines (used for allergy and colds) and tricyclic anti-depressants.

CURIOSITY

Extract from an 1891 Ladies' Guide:

'The baneful effects of tight-lacing corsets are now well understood and no medical person will venture to deny that the effects are harmful and although they attempt to shield themselves by denying that their figure is due to an excessively tightly laced corset, many young ladies may experience and complain of excessive fatigue as a result'.

TRAVEL

L ook after yourself and follow the **golden rule** when travelling in developing countries:

WASH IT, PEEL IT, OPEN IT, COOK IT OR TOSS IT

Getting sick on a holiday is always a major disappointment and in a strange environment can be very difficult to cope with. A few simple preparations can reduce the likelihood of disaster.

If you are going overseas, find out what the conditions are like in the country or countries you will be visiting. You should ask about the climate, the food, any local diseases against which you should be immunised, and the availability and cost of medical treatment.

REMEMBER, THE ONLY WAYS YOU CAN CATCH AN EXOTIC DISEASE IS TO:

- eat it

- drink it

- be bitten by it

- have sex with it!

Never travel overseas without health **insurance**. In developed countries you may be unlikely to be stricken with one of the more exotic Third World diseases, but medical treatment of any kind can be prohibitively expensive (e.g. in the United States) and you may find yourself unable to afford the care you need unless you are insured for the cost.

If you get ill in one of the less developed countries, you might need a hasty return home – even flying first class with special nursing care. Don't risk not being able to afford it.

The most important thing a Third World traveller can carry is a credit card that, in an emergency, can purchase an airline ticket home.

TRAVEL IMMUNISATION

The following countries require **no immunisations** or health protection for the benefit of the traveller, but may require proof of appropriate immunisation if coming from a country with serious health problems (e.g. yellow fever).

No immunisations are normally required for:

Australia, Austria, Bahamas, Belgium, Bermuda, Canada, Croatia, Czech Republic, Denmark, Estonia, Finland, France, Germany, Greece, Greenland, Grenada, Hong Kong, Hungary, Iceland, Ireland, Italy, Japan, Latvia, Lithuania, Luxembourg, Malta, Moldova, Nauru, Netherlands, New Zealand, Norway, Poland, Portugal, Slovakia, Spain, St. Vincent, Singapore, Slovenia, Swaziland, Sweden, Switzerland, Trinidad, United Kingdom, United States.

If you are visiting other countries, discuss your immunisation requirements with your doctor at least **six weeks before departure**.

TRAVEL **VACCINATIONS** AND **PRECAUTIONS** THAT MAY BE REQUIRED FOR OTHER COUNTRIES INCLUDE:

- **Cholera**. There are no vaccines that give really good protection. There is an oral vaccine available and injections are not normally given now. It is a very severe disease that causes incredibly profuse diarrhoea, and death can occur very rapidly from gross dehydration. Following the golden rule above is the best protection.

- **Typhoid** vaccine can be given as an injection which lasts for three years, or by three capsules taken by mouth over five days, which gives twelve months protection. Both typhoid and cholera are caught by eating contaminated food.

- **Yellow fever** is found in Central America, central Africa and around the Red Sea. The vaccine for this lasts for ten years. Yellow fever vaccinations are a condition of entry to some countries.

- **Malaria** occurs in practically every tropical country. Particularly vicious forms that are resistant to many medications occur in South-East Asia and some Pacific islands. To prevent malaria, it is necessary to take tablets regularly for up to a fortnight before departure and sometimes for a month after return. The malaria-carrying mosquito bites only between dusk and dawn, so travellers should take precautions against being bitten after dark – wear clothes that cover as much as possible, avoid perfumes, and use repellents and insecticides.

- **Hepatitis A** occurs worldwide, but is more prevalent in countries with poor hygiene, particularly those in South America, central Asia and Africa. One vaccination will give six to 12 months protection. A booster at this time will give long-term protection.

- **Hepatitis B**. Two vaccinations four to six weeks apart will give six months protection. Boosters at six months and five years will usually give long-term protection. South-East Asia is one of the areas with the highest incidence of hepatitis B, but it is not a routine travel vaccination, as it can only be caught by sex or contact with the blood of an infected person. A combined hepatitis A and B vaccination is available.

- **Immunoglobulin**. In situations where there has been exposure to hepatitis A or other serious illnesses, or there is insufficient time for a normal course of vaccinations, one immunoglobulin injection gives protection for six to 12 weeks against numerous viral infections, depending on dose.

- **Japanese encephalitis**. Two vaccinations, two weeks apart. It is required only for residence in rural areas of India, Nepal, China and South-East Asia.

- **Meningococcal meningitis**. One injection, five weeks before departure to live in areas of poor hygiene.

Always have a consultation with your doctor
at least six weeks before departing overseas.

TRAVELLER'S DIARRHOEA

Delhi belly, Montezuma's revenge, or Cairo cobbles, it doesn't matter what it is called, the most common ailment affecting overseas travellers is diarrhoea.

Most diarrhoea is caused by **contaminated water** resulting from inadequate water and sewerage systems. If you are travelling in any Third World or tropical country, you should avoid drinking the water unless it has been filtered and boiled. Bottled water is best (preferably fizzy water, so that you can ensure that it has not been replaced by tap water), and most reasonable hotels will provide bottled water in your room, but that still leaves the water you use to clean your teeth and ice blocks in all the long cool drinks you will undoubtedly consume. Don't have ice in your drinks, if necessary add mineral water from a bottle or can, and use bottled water to clean your teeth. If this is not possible, there are tiny purifying tablets you can pop into a glass, but these will give the water a taste (which you may be able to overcome with a small sachet of fruit-flavoured powder).

Food too can be a source of diarrhoea and food poisoning. Tempting as it is to try all those exotic dishes, steer clear of raw or underdone meat, uncooked seafood, unprocessed dairy products and uncooked fruits, vegetables and salad ingredients.

An attack of diarrhoea usually lasts only one to three days but, especially if you are travelling around, it can be very uncomfortable and embarrassing. Ask your doctor to prescribe antidiarrhoea tablets before you go, and keep them with you in your personal baggage.

Treatment involves giving a solution of water and electrolytes (vital elements) by mouth if possible, or intravenously. In an emergency, a mixture containing a level teaspoon of salt and eight level teaspoons of sugar or glucose into a litre of boiled water may be given by mouth. Plain water should not be given, as it will pass straight through the body. Because of their lower body weight, children will dehydrate far more rapidly than adults.

A decrease of five per cent in water volume can cause significant disease, and a ten per cent loss may be fatal in children. Fortunately there is a very good response to correct treatment.

CURIOSITY
A morbid fear of travel is called hodophobia.

UNCONSCIOUSNESS

L earn how to care for an unconscious person, so that you can look after others who may be close to you if they are affected.

COMA

If a person is unconscious (comatose), they cannot respond to their surroundings in a normal way and their usual reflexes may not operate. They cannot swallow or cough, and so clear the throat of any mucus or foreign objects. An unconscious person's muscles relax and may be so floppy that if they are lying on their back their tongue may fall backwards and block their airway.

THERE ARE THREE **LEVELS** OF UNCONSCIOUSNESS:

- the victim can be easily aroused but slips back into a sleepy state

- the victim can only be aroused with difficulty (semi-comatose)

- the victim cannot be aroused at all (comatose).

Any level of unconsciousness can lead to a difficulty in **breathing**, so it is essential to attend to the victim quickly and to get medical help. If a person does not respond to shaking or shouting they are unconscious.

CAUSES

Leaving aside a temporary faint from which the person usually recovers quite quickly, reasons for becoming unconscious include a stroke or heart attack, a blow to the head, an overdose of alcohol or drugs, and diseases such as epilepsy or diabetes.

Maintaining the airway without causing further harm is the prime imperative in the first aid of a comatose patient.

FIRST AID

Do not move an unconscious person unless they are in immediate danger, and do not leave them alone (send someone else for help). Carry out the ABC (airways, breathing, circulation) of first aid as soon as possible. If necessary, administer mouth-to-mouth resuscitation or cardiopulmonary resuscitation.

If the victim is breathing and has a pulse, put them in one of the positions described below and keep them there to ensure that the airway is kept clear. Monitor the airway and pulse continually until help arrives.

Do NOT give them anything to eat or drink – do not for example try to revive them with sips of water; they will be unable to swallow and may choke.

COMA POSITION

To put an unconscious person in the coma position:

- lie the victim on their back and kneel on one side

- place the near arm straight down beside the body, tucking the hand, palm up, under the buttocks

- cross the far arm over the chest

- cross the far leg over the near one

- protect and support the head with one hand, and with the other hand grasp the clothing at the hip furthest from you and pull the victim towards you so they roll onto the side

- readjust the head to make sure the airway is still open

- bend the upper arm into a convenient position to support the upper body. Bend the upper leg at the knee to bring the thigh well forward so that it supports the lower body

- carefully pull the other arm out from under the body and leave it lying parallel so the victim cannot roll back.

Do NOT use the coma position if you suspect the victim has an injured back or neck, unless breathing becomes noisy, laboured or irregular.

LATERAL POSITION

Provided there is adequate support for the head, an unconscious person may also be placed in the lateral position:

- place the victim on their back and kneel beside them

- extend the far arm out at right angles to the body

- place the near arm across the chest

- bend the near knee so the leg is at right angles to the body, keeping the far leg straight

- grasp the victim's near shoulder and hip and roll them on to their side so that they are facing away from you. Keep the back straight

- place the top arm so that it rests comfortably across the lower arm

- tilt the head backwards with the face slightly downwards to maintain a clear airway.

GLASGOW COMA SCALE

The depth of a patient's unconsciousness may be assessed by the Glasgow coma scale.

THE SCORE IS DERIVED FROM THE FOLLOWING
OBSERVATIONS AND POINTS:

EYE OPENING (E)	POINT SCORE
• Spontaneous opening	4
• Open to verbal command	3
• Open to pain	2
• No response	1

MOTOR RESPONSES (M)	
• Obeys verbal command	6
• Responds to painful stimuli by:	
– localising pain	5
– withdrawings from painful stimulus	4
– abnormal flexion	3
– extensor response	2
– no response	1

VERBAL RESPONSES (V)	
• Oriented and converses	5
• Disoriented and converses	4
• Inappropriate words	3
• Incomprehensible sounds	2
• No response	1

COMA SCORE = E + M + V
3 = very deeply comatose   15 = completely conscious and alert

FAINT

A faint (syncope) is a sudden, unexpected loss of consciousness that may be preceded for a few seconds by a feeling of light headedness. If a person has fainted, they should be made to lie flat with their legs raised to increase the flow of blood to the brain.

FIRST AID

Tilt the head backwards and make sure the **airways** are clear. Loosen any tight clothing. The person should regain consciousness within a few minutes. If the victim does not recover spontaneously within a short period, turn them on their side in the coma position and get medical help. Recovery usually occurs within a minute or two, and it is not associated with any convulsion or passing of urine or faeces.

A faint, by definition, is a brief, temporary form of unconsciousness.

CAUSES

Low blood pressure (**hypotension**) and poor blood supply to the brain are the absolute causes of a faint, and these in turn may be due to a number of conditions, including stress, anxiety, fright, over-exertion, lack of sleep, lack of food, heat, dehydration, lack of ventilation, prolonged standing and hormonal fluctuations.

A significant **infection** of any sort, from a bad dose of influenza to pneumonia or gastroenteritis, may lead to a faint, particularly if the patient is trying to push on and not rest.

Stokes-Adams attacks are caused by a sudden change in the **heart rate**, with the heart slowing down markedly for a few seconds or minutes, and then recovering. It is due to a problem with the conduction of electrical impulses through the heart muscle.

OTHER CAUSES OF A FAINT MAY INCLUDE:

- vasovagal syndrome (response to stress)

- heart attack (myocardial infarct)

- pulmonary thrombosis (blood clot in the lung)

- stroke (cerebrovascular accident)

- sudden changes in emotional state

- transient ischaemic attacks (temporary blocking of a small artery in the brain)

- low blood sugar (from starvation, or overuse of insulin or sugar lowering tablets)

- micturition syncope (faint that occurs when urine passed)

- pregnancy

- hardening of the arteries (arteriosclerosis)

- severe anaemia

- dehydration

- alcohol intoxication

- narrowing (stenosis) of the main artery from the heart to the body (the aorta)

- sudden episodes of irregular heart beat

- high blood pressure (may sometimes cause a faint as the increased pressure on the brain prevents it from working properly)

- migraines

- epilepsy (may be mistaken for a faint)

- severe allergy reaction (anaphylaxis)

- Wolf-Parkinson-White syndrome (peculiar abnormality of the electrical conduction system in the heart)

- drugs (e.g. those that lower blood pressure, narcotics, sleeping tablets, anxiety relieving medications).

Some psychiatric patients may fake a faint as an attention-seeking device.

No **investigations** are usually necessary, but if repeat attacks occur, the more serious diseases above that may cause this condition (e.g. low blood sugar, low blood pressure, irregular heart beat, infections, anaemia) must be excluded by blood tests and electrocardiographs.

The patient usually recovers quickly once lying down, but should only rise slowly and when completely well.

CURIOSITY
Always remember that illegal drugs may be used to spike a drink and render a person unconscious.

URINE

L ook at your urine and look after yourself. Always note any change in colour, frequency, odour or discomfort associated with passing it, and check with a doctor to find the cause if it persists or recurs.

EXPLANATION

The body produces three waste products – urine from the kidneys, faeces from the bowels, and bile, which passes from the liver via the gall bladder to the small intestine and mixes with the faeces.

After being produced by the nephrons in the kidney by filtration of blood, urine moves down the ureters to the bladder, where it is stored before being expelled when convenient through the urethra to the outside of the body.

Urine consists mainly of water, with a very large number of dissolved waste products (e.g. urea), salts (e.g. urate), ammonia, enzymes, vitamins (e.g. vitamins B and C), minerals, proteins (e.g. creatinine), fats and carbohydrates. Many toxic substances and medications are removed from the body in the urine.

The concentration of urine will depend on the amount of water in the body (hydration). If the person is well hydrated, dilute urine will be passed. If the person is dehydrated, the urine will be far more concentrated. The colour of the urine varies depending on its concentration from almost completely clear (dilute) to a dark yellow.

The yellow **colour** comes from the pigment that gives blood its red colour, and is removed from the body as red blood cells are broken down and recycled.

Good quality urine is essential for good health, as most waste products are removed from the body in it.

SYMPTOMS

BLOOD IN URINE

Blood may be seen in the urine as a red tinge, dark red colour or even blood clots, but often the amount present is so small that no difference in colour can be detected by the patient.

Doctors can **test** for extremely small amounts of blood in urine (haematuria) very simply by using a plastic strip with a spot of chemical on it that changes colour if blood is present. The greater the colour change, the greater the amount of blood present in the sample of urine. Examining the urine under a microscope will reveal red blood cells if blood is present.

Diseases of the kidney, ureter (tube from kidney to bladder), bladder, urethra (tube from bladder to outside) and prostate may cause bleeding into the urine. Blood may also find its way into the urine by contamination of a sample during a woman's menstrual period, bleeding piles or from a bleeding sore on the genitals. Red coloured foods (e.g. beetroot, some medications) may give a false impression of blood.

By far the most common cause of blood in a urine sample is a bacterial bladder **infection** (cystitis). The patient will experience a fever, feel pain low down in the front of the belly, will pass urine more frequently, and pain will be felt when passing urine. Virtually every woman will have cystitis at some time, but it is far less common (and usually indicates more serious disease) in men.

Pyelonephritis is a bacterial infection of a kidney. The symptoms include a fever, loin pain (usually only on one side), frequent passing of urine, general tiredness and sometimes blood in the urine.

Glomerulonephritis is a degeneration of the filtering mechanism (glomeruli) of the kidney that occurs in two forms – acute and chronic. Acute glomerulonephritis is often triggered by a bacterial infection (e.g. tonsillitis) but may start as a result of other diseases in the body. The patient feels tired, has no appetite, develops headaches and has a low-grade fever. Some patients do not recover from acute glomerulonephritis, and are considered to have chronic glomerulonephritis. There are usually no symptoms until the kidneys start to fail and excessive levels of waste products build up in the bloodstream.

Other causes of blood in the urine include **prostatitis** (bacterial infection of the prostate gland), a **stone** in the kidney, extremely vigorous exercise (e.g. running a marathon) and a tumour or cancer that develops anywhere in the urinary system.

An **injury** to the kidneys, bladder or genitals (e.g. car accident, fall, sport) may cause damage to these organs and bleeding. If the bleeding persists for more than a couple of days, investigations are necessary to find the exact site of bleeding so that it can be corrected.

Patients who are taking **warfarin** to thin their blood because of a risk of blood clots, and patients who have poor blood clotting due to other diseases (e.g. haemophilia), often have small amounts of blood found in their urine.

Some people with **haematuria** can have no cause found for the condition, and it is thought that they may have been born with kidneys that leak blood into the urine without any disease being present. This diagnosis is only made after all other possibilities are excluded.

Rare causes of haematuria include haemolytic anaemia (excessive breakdown of red blood cells), tuberculosis involving the kidneys, septicaemia (blood infection), autoimmune diseases (e.g. systemic lupus erythematosus, polyarteritis nodosa, rheumatoid arthritis, scleroderma), leukaemia and bilharzia (transmitted by a species of snail that is found in freshwater streams, rivers and lakes in Egypt, tropical Africa, the Caribbean and South America).

ABNORMAL URINE COLOUR

The urine normally varies in colour from a very pale clear straw colour to dark brownish yellow, depending on whether the body is trying to get rid of excess fluid, or preserve fluid when dehydrated. Any other colour may indicate a significant disease.

WHITE – Whitish urine may be due to the presence of white cells (pus), or excess protein or fat.

RED/BROWN – Urine containing blood may appear brown or red. Red urine may also be due to eating lots of red food (e.g. beetroot) and some medications (e.g. phenytoin, phenothiazines, phenindione, rifampicin).

PURPLE – In the disease porphyria, brown urine is passed, which turns purple on exposure to sunlight.

The unusual disease porphyria runs in the English royal family,
although none of the current generation are sufferers.

BROWN – Excess bilirubin from liver failure will make urine brown, as will eating lots of deeply coloured foods (e.g. rhubarb, fava beans, liquorice) or medications such as nitrofurantoin (for urine infections).

BLACK – Blackish or very dark urine may be caused by the medication methyldopa, cascara and old blood.

ORANGE – With dehydration and diseases of the liver that cause jaundice, the urine may become a dark orange colour. The medications primaquine, riboflavin and sulfasalazine may also give urine an orange colour.

BLUE/GREEN – A few medications and naturopathic remedies may cause the urine to take on a blue/green tinge. Examples include amitriptyline (used in psychiatry), triamterene (used to increase urine production), phenol and indigo.

DIFFICULT URINATION

Despite having a full bladder, it is sometimes difficult to pass urine because of anxiety, stress or the location in which it is being attempted. A number of diseases, almost invariably affecting men, may also be responsible.

The **prostate** gland at the base of the penis is responsible for producing some of the fluid (semen) which is ejaculated during sex. With increasing age this tends to enlarge, putting pressure on the urethra (urine tube from bladder to the outside), which passes through the middle of the gland, and making it more difficult to pass urine. In extreme cases, it may become impossible to pass any urine, and the bladder will increase to an enormous size causing considerable pain.

A difficulty in passing urine is very appropriately
described as stranguary.

Cancer of the prostate is a common condition of elderly men, but it progresses very slowly in most cases, and its presence may not be noticed until the enlarging cancer puts pressure on the urethra to make passing urine difficult. An aching pain at the front of the pelvis is the other possible symptom.

Other causes include prostatitis (a bacterial infection of the prostate gland), urethritis (infection of the urethra), an injury to the urethra, an inserted foreign body, and a stone, polyp, tumour, cancer or blood clot in the bladder that may block the opening of the bladder into the urethra.

Rarely, the nerve supply to the bladder may be damaged by an injury to the lower back or pelvis, making bladder emptying difficult or impossible.

FREQUENT URINATION

Passing more urine than normal (**polyuria**) may be due to drinking more fluid (particularly coffee, tea, cola or alcohol which stimulate urine production), cold weather, pregnancy (when pressure is put on the bladder by the growing baby), anxiety, fright or fear, but there are many different kidney, bladder and other organ diseases that may also be responsible.

Virtually every man over 60 and woman over
50 years has to get out of bed to pass urine,
so this is considered a normal phenomenon.

If the bladder becomes infected by bacteria (**cystitis**) the patient will have a fever, feel pain low down in the front of the belly, will pass urine more frequently, and pain will be felt when passing urine. In severe cases the urine will be cloudy and sometimes blood will be seen in the urine.

Diabetes mellitus results in a higher than normal amount of sugar (glucose) circulating in the blood. The symptoms of untreated diabetes are unusual tiredness, increased thirst and hunger, belly pains, excess passing of urine, weight loss despite a large food intake, itchy rashes, recurrent vaginal thrush infections, pins and needles, dizziness, light headedness and blurred vision.

A **prolapse** (bulging) of the bladder into the front wall of the vagina in a woman will make passing urine difficult and uncomfortable, and increases the risk of infection. The bladder cannot be completely emptied, so the woman will find that she has to pass small amounts of urine very frequently. Damage to the vagina during childbirth is the most common cause of a prolapse.

Other causes of frequent urination include **prostatitis** (bacterial infection of the prostate gland), kidney failure (from persistent infection or inflammation of the kidney, a poor blood supply to the kidneys, severe high blood pressure, or a number of rarer diseases) and systemic lupus erythematosus (autoimmune condition). A number of psychiatric conditions, particularly those associated with anxiety and depression, may increase bladder irritability.

Diuretics are medications designed to increase urine production in conditions such as high blood pressure, heart failure and kidney failure. Other medications may have increased urination as a side effect.

All forms of alcohol and caffeine increase urine production.

Rare causes of frequently passing urine include diabetes insipidus (failure of the pituitary gland in the centre of the head), Hand-Schueller-Christian syndrome, Cushing syndrome (over-production of steroids in the body, or taking large doses of cortisone), Addison disease (adrenal gland failure), and hyperparathyroidism (over-activity of the parathyroid glands in the neck).

REDUCED URINE PRODUCTION

A markedly reduced production of urine (oliguria) is a **serious** symptom, while a total absence of urine (anuria) is a medical emergency. Kidney diseases and severe dehydration are the usual causes.

Glomerulonephritis is a degeneration of the filtering mechanism (glomeruli) of the kidney that occurs in two forms – acute and chronic. Acute glomerulonephritis is often triggered by a bacterial infection (e.g. tonsillitis) but may start as a result of other diseases in the body. The patient feels tired, has no appetite, develops headaches and has a low-grade fever. Other symptoms can include a low urine output, loin (kidney) pain, swelling of the ankles and around the eyes, and cloudy urine. Some patients do not recover from acute glomerulonephritis, and are considered to have chronic glomerulonephritis. There are usually no symptoms until the kidneys start to fail and excessive levels of waste products build up in the bloodstream.

Other causes of **kidney failure** include infection of both kidneys, severe generalised infections (e.g. septicaemia, yellow fever), long-standing high blood pressure, blockages to the arteries supplying the kidneys or cysts replacing the kidney tissue. The main symptoms of kidney failure are slowly decreasing urine production, swelling of feet and hands (oedema), headaches, high blood pressure, and eventually lung and heart damage.

Severe **dehydration** will result in reduced urine production, particularly when associated with massive diarrhoea in diseases such as cholera.

Massive bleeding from an injury, or internally from disease, may result in a dramatically reduced blood volume in the body (shock), and a shutdown of kidney function that can lead rapidly to death if not treated as an emergency.

Some **poisons** and toxins can cause serious kidney damage that results in reduced urine production. Compounds that contain mercury are particularly insidious in their action as poisons, while carbon tetrachloride (used in dry cleaning) may cause quite a rapid deterioration in kidney function.

GASSY URINE

Very rarely a patient will notice that they are passing gassy urine (pneumaturia). This is a **serious** symptom that may be caused by a bladder or kidney infection with a gas-producing bacteria, or a connection between the bladder and a hollow organ such as the gut or vagina allows air into the bladder.

A number of serious bowel diseases, including Crohn disease (an inflammation and thickening of the bowel wall), bowel or bladder cancer, diverticulitis (outpocketing of the colon) and an abscess on the bowel may weaken tissue so that the walls of the bowel and bladder break down to form a connection (fistula) between them.

A difficult childbirth in Third World countries may result in
damage to the front wall of the vagina and a persistent
connection between the vagina and bladder.

In a complicated childbirth, the front wall of the vagina may be damaged and an opening into the bladder may be formed that will allow urine to leak constantly into the vagina and air into the bladder.

INVESTIGATIONS

After blood tests, urine tests (urinalysis) are the most frequently ordered diagnostic tests.

URINE TESTS

During the course of the day, all the blood is filtered through the kidneys, which means that not only are diseases of the urinary system and kidneys detectable in urine, but also a number of diseases that occur elsewhere in the body, the most common of which is diabetes. However, for something to show up in the urine, it must be a substance that is isolated by the kidneys or picked up as the urine flows from the kidneys to the bladder and out of the body. This does not include disease-fighting antibodies, some hormones, proteins and fats, and many other substances which are symptoms of disease – blood tests are necessary for these. Substances that are found in the urine include sugar, blood, pus, crystals, bile and some proteins.

Urine can be analysed by its appearance, by mixing it with various chemicals and noting the reaction, and by placing a specimen under a microscope to see if organisms are present.

A **midstream** urine sample is usually collected, so that the patient must pass a small amount of urine into the toilet, then about 10mLs into a sterile container, then the rest may be passed into the toilet. This reduces the risk of contamination from the skin around the urine opening. On occasions a urine sample is collected straight from the bladder by means of a catheter.

The act of passing urine is called micturition in medical terminology.

A routine **urinalysis** begins with an evaluation of the colour, clarity and odour of the sample. Normal urine is clear, pale yellow to dark amber, and has an easily recognisable odour. If the urine is cloudy or has a foul odour, it may indicate the presence of infection. If it has a pinkish tinge, blood may be present, and if it is brownish, there is too much bilirubin – a pigment produced by the liver which is present in excess if the person is suffering from liver disease such as hepatitis. Certain foods, food colourings and drugs turn urine orange.

Urine that **smells** of ammonia may be a sign of cystitis, whereas the urine of someone suffering from diabetes smells like new-mown hay. What is eaten may be reflected in the smell urine gives off – the pungent smell of garlic is evident in the urine as well as in the breath, spinach produces an acrid smell, mushrooms produce a fetid odour, and truffles a stagnant smell. Even certain deodorants and talcum powders can be detected in the urine.

The most common form of analysis is a **dipstick** – a plastic strip impregnated with bands of chemicals that change colour when exposed to certain substances. Diabetes, kidney disease, urine infection, liver disease and dehydration can all be diagnosed in this way.

Urine can also be examined under a **microscope** for the presence of bacteria and cells. Although blood may be visible to the naked eye, the presence of blood cells will normally be confirmed by a microscope analysis. Blood indicates kidney disease or a stone, an infection, ulcer or tumour in the urinary system. If pus is present, it generally shows that there is infection or ulceration somewhere in the urinary passages.

If bacteria are present, they can be cultured to confirm the type, and then tested against various antibiotics to see which one will work most effectively.

CURIOSITY

For thousands of years, doctors have been making remarkably accurate diagnoses by looking at, smelling, and even tasting urine. Today, an experienced doctor can still tell a lot about a patient before even testing a urine sample in much the same way, using many of the clues outlined above, but very few now taste urine for the sweetness of diabetes.

VISION

Most people consider vision to be the most important of their five senses. To look after your vision, make sure that your eyesight is checked as a child, teenager and regularly from mid-life onwards. Mid-life checks should cover increased pressure and cataracts as well as vision. Properly protect your eyes when playing sports such as squash, or using grinders, slashers, impact tools or similar.

VISION PROBLEMS
CHANGES IN SIGHT

Because of their complexity, the eyes sometimes function less than perfectly. There are four main types of vision problems:

- People who are short-sighted (**myopia**) have eyeballs that are too long. This means that the light cannot accurately be focussed by the lens and a blurred image results.

- The reverse problem occurs in long-sighted people (**hypermetropia**) where the eyeball is too short. These people can see objects at a distance but when close objects are seen, the muscles that change the shape of the lens to focus the light rays cannot cope with the shortened eyeball.

- Older people whose sight slowly deteriorates suffer from **presbyopia**, or the inability of the lens to change shape sufficiently to see objects that are close to

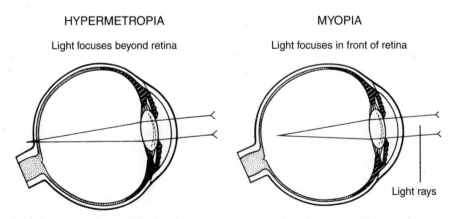

HYPERMETROPIA

Light focuses beyond retina

MYOPIA

Light focuses in front of retina

Light rays

them. This is caused by a weakening of the tiny muscles that pull on the lens to change its shape.

- The last group are those with **astigmatism**. These people have an uneven curve of the refractive surfaces at the front of the eye (i.e. the lens and cornea), so that some parts of the vision are clear while other parts are blurred at the same time.

All these problems can be corrected by placing a lens (spectacles or contact lenses) in front of the eye to help the natural lens of the eye focus the image. Reshaping the cornea with laser surgery can also be used to help people with myopia.

Patients often present to a doctor concerned about their
vision when they discover their blind spot.

BLIND SPOT

When we see something, light reaching the retina at the back of the eye stimulates nerve cells, which convert it into electrical impulses and send these along the optic nerve to the brain. The point where the optic nerve leaves the retina has no light-sensitive cells and so forms a blind spot. You can find your blind spot by the following simple test.

Hold this page at arms length and close your left eye. Look at the cross with the right eye, and move the page slowly towards you. When the dot disappears, its image has fallen on the blind spot of the right eye.

BLIND SPOT TEST

VISUAL ACUITY

Visual acuity tests are tests administered to determine if there are any defects in vision, what they are, and how severe they are.

The patient looks at a **chart** on a wall 6 metres away with letters on it and is asked to read it line by line. The letters vary in size from row to row. The top row has one large letter, the next row smaller letters, the next smaller letters still, and so on. A person with normal vision should be able to read letters 6mm high at a distance of six metres.

The doctor will generally guess at which line the patient will be able to see, and asks them to start there and read the letters out. If they cannot see them, the doctor will move up a line until the patient reaches a line they can read without difficulty.

The result is given as two figures (e.g. 6/12). The first figure refers to the distance at which the letters (6m) are read. The second figure describes the distance at which a person with normal vision can read the smallest letters that the patient was able to read correctly. For example, if the smallest letters read from a distance of 6m would be seen from 12m by a person with normal sight, the result is 6/12. The results may be different for each eye. 6/12 is the minimum visual acuity permissible for a normal driver's licence.

Since the adoption of the metric systems in every country except the USA, 20/20 vision is now 6/6 vision.

Poor reading of the chart usually means that the eyes have an impaired ability to refract light – the basis of sight – either near-sighted (myopic) or far-sighted (hypermetropic). Occasionally it indicates a serious eye disease, such as glaucoma.

If the vision is faulty, the doctor or optometrist will ask the patient to look through a selection of lenses of different magnifications and to read the chart again, covering up one eye at a time. The combination of lenses which enable the person to see best are then prescribed as glasses or contact lenses.

Even people with previously good sight usually find that they are having difficulty reading and seeing things up close as they get older, and most people need a visual acuity test by the time they are in their mid-forties.

MANAGEMENT
SPECTACLES
Spectacles (glasses) are lenses that are held in a frame in front of the eyes to aid vision. The lenses may be the same over their entire area, bifocal (divided into two halves with different degrees of magnification and focal lengths), trifocal (three divisions) or graduated (gradual change across the lens from one degree of magnification and focal length to another). Astigmatic lenses vary their focal length and magnification in varied patterns across the surface of the lens to match the variations in the patient's vision.

CONTACT LENSES
Contact lenses must be prescribed by an ophthalmologist or optometrist. This is the case even if you don't normally wear glasses and just want contacts to change your eye colour. Contact lenses are medical devices that need to be properly fitted.

Lenses can be used to correct myopia (short-sightedness) and hyperopia (long-sightedness) as well as some cases of amblyopia. They can have a fixed focal length (curvature), be bifocal or graduated in focus to allow both close and distant vision.

The selection of contact lenses available is vast. Contact lenses can be broken down into several main categories based on what they're made of, how often you need to replace them and whether you can sleep in them.

Contact lenses are made of many different **types** of plastic, but they are divided into two main groups – soft or rigid gas permeable. Soft contacts contain from 25–79 per cent water, are easy to adjust to and are quite comfortable. Rigid gas permeable (RGP) contact lenses take longer to adjust to, but are more durable and more resistant to deposit build-up. They tend to be less expensive over the life of the lens (but the upfront cost is higher) and can offer some people crisper vision than they would get with soft contacts.

The **replacement** schedule of a contact lens refers to how long you can safely wear it before you need to throw it away. With RGPs, you generally replace them every several years. Because they're so hardy, it is not necessary to replace them more often. Soft contact lenses come in a wide variety of replacement schedules that vary from daily to monthly.

Thirty-day continuous wear contact lenses are available. They are made out of a different type of material than other soft lenses, and allow a lot more oxygen to reach the eyes while wearing them, making them a much safer and more comfortable option.

REFRACTIVE SURGERY

Refractive surgery involves one of a number of procedures on the cornea (transparent front surface of the eye over the pupil) to alter its curvature and correct short- or long-sightedness. These procedures can revolutionise the vision of a person who is short-sighted, but the patient must be at least 18 years of age, and normally under 70.

Anyone considering refractive surgery should always seek a second opinion from another ophthalmologist before proceeding.

All procedures are expensive and only undertaken after very careful discussion, then mapping and measuring of the eye surface and the degree of vision correction required. The patient usually returns at a later time for the procedure. Both eyes may be done at once, but the eyes must remain bandaged for 12 to 24 hours after the procedure. There is often some pain for the first day after the operation, and the eyes must not be rubbed or knocked for a couple of weeks, but much clearer vision is usually obtained as soon as the eye patches are removed.

Originally radial keratotomy was performed using tiny radial knife cuts in Russia, but now lasers are used to reshape the cornea.

Laser photorefractive laser keratectomy (PRK) was the next procedure developed. The patient is placed on a table under a computer-driven laser machine, and is given a light anaesthetic in order to keep the head and eye totally still. The ophthalmic surgeon then removes the outer surface of the cornea with a fine scalpel, and the laser is applied for 30 to 60 seconds to reshape the deeper layers of the cornea. The cornea usually heals within 72 hours, but a haze may develop and persist for a few months. This does not affect vision but sometimes causes glare with lights at night. It may take six months for the eye surface shape to stabilise.

Laser in-situ keratomileusis (LASIK) is the latest and now most common procedure. Up to -16 myopia can be corrected by this technique, and it has less postoperative pain and more rapid stabilisation of vision than PRK. Under the same circumstances as PRK, the surgeon lifts a small flap on the surface of the cornea in front of the pupil. The tissue under this is then given a carefully programmed momentary burn with the laser to reshape it to focus the light appropriately. The flap is then replaced and the eye bandaged.

Vision symptoms
BLINDNESS
Loss of the sense of vision is one of the most devastating things that a person can experience. Fortunately sudden total blindness is rare, but a partial loss of sight is quite common.

Common causes include a serious **injury** to the eye or the part of the **brain** that is responsible for perceiving vision (e.g. by a stroke, tumour, cancer, abscess or direct injury), or an **ulcer** on the surface of the eye (cornea) from infection, injury or an object in the eye.

Other possible causes of blindness include:

- trachoma (a type of conjunctivitis)

- cataract (clouding of the lens in the eye that causes gradual loss of sight over many years, usually in the elderly)

- glaucoma (an increase in the pressure of the jelly-like fluid inside the eye)

- macular degeneration (due to a poor blood supply to the retina at the back of the eye in the elderly)

- retinal detachment (the light-sensitive retina at the back of the eye becomes detached from the globe of the eye)

- inflammation of the optic nerve (optic neuritis)

- malignant hypertension (extremely high blood pressure)

- poorly controlled diabetes

- bleeding into the fluid in the eye

- craniopharyngioma (form of brain tumour)

- retinitis pigmentosa (pigment deposition in the retina)

- certain poisons (e.g. methanol)

- medication overdoses (e.g. quinine) will damage or destroy the retina.

AMAUROSIS FUGAX
Amaurosis fugax is a sudden, painless, temporary loss of vision due to a disruption to the blood supply to the optic nerve or brain. It may be associated with narrowing of the carotid artery in the neck, or a tiny blood clot in the arteries supplying the retina at the back of the eye.

*The temporary blindness of amaurosis fugax is very
frightening, and as a result is usually adequately
investigated, which is essential to prevent recurrences.*

DOUBLE VISION

Everyone normally sees double, because we have two eyes, but the brain learns from infancy to merge the two images into one seamless image. Double vision (**diplopia**), is seeing two images instead of one, rather like a badly ghosting television set. It is a disorienting and confusing symptom that can be caused by eye or brain diseases, or conditions elsewhere in the body that have an effect on these organs.

A **squint** occurs if the eyes do not align properly, and look in slightly different directions. If a squint occurs from infancy, the image from one eye is suppressed by the brain, and the child effectively sees with only one eye. A squint developing later in life is usually due to damage to the nerves supplying the muscles that control eye movement, or damage to the muscles themselves. The damage is usually a result of a tumour, cancer, direct injury (e.g. fractured skull) or inflammation of the nerves or muscles.

An **injury** to an eye or surrounding bone or other tissue, which prevents it from moving normally, will also cause double vision.

Migraines are often associated with visual symptoms including flashing lights, double vision, shimmering, seeing zigzag lines and loss of part of the area of vision.

In a **stroke** (cerebrovascular accident), various parts of the brain may be affected by having their blood supply cut off by a blockage in an artery, or a blood vessel in the brain may burst, causing bleeding and damage to part of the brain. The onset is almost instantaneous and may be associated with a wide variety of symptoms, from paralysis and headache to weakness, loss of sensation, double vision, anaesthesia, confusion and coma.

A **head injury**, causing concussion, may affect the part of the brain responsible for receiving and interpreting sight, as may a tumour, cyst, cancer, abscess or infection affecting the relevant parts of the brain.

Less common causes of double vision include myasthenia gravis (a disease affecting muscle control), multiple sclerosis (a nerve disease), Wernicke-Korsakoff psychosis (associated with alcoholism), and hyperthyroidism (excess thyroxine production).

*Although double vision is a recognised symptom, triple or
quadruple vision is a figment of the patient's imagination.*

BLURRED VISION

Seeing things that can't be focussed and that remain blurred is very frustrating, and the most obvious causes are **long-sightedness** (inability to see close objects and read, usually associated with advancing age), **short-sightedness** (inability to see distant objects and often a problem from childhood), or **astigmatism** (uneven focus). These problems can be corrected by spectacles or contact lenses, but there are some eye and other diseases which may cause blurred vision.

A **cataract** is clouding of the lens in the eye that will cause gradual blurring and loss of sight over many years in the elderly. Rarely, babies are born with a cataract.

Glaucoma is due to an increase in the pressure of the jelly-like fluid inside the eye. This may come on gradually, or may be quite sudden. If inadequately treated, total blindness may result. Early symptoms include an eye ache or pain, blurred vision, seeing halos around objects, red eye, a gradual loss of peripheral vision, and there is an hereditary tendency.

The **retina** is the layer of light-sensitive cells at the back of the eye. If this is damaged by a poor blood supply from narrowed hardened arteries, a blood clot in a tiny artery, or separation of the retina from the back of the eyeball, the vision will be blurred or totally absent in the affected area.

OTHER CAUSES OF BLURRED VISION INCLUDE:

- iritis (inflammation of the coloured part of the eye)

- conjunctivitis (bacterial or viral infection on the surface of the eye)

- ulcer on the surface of the eye

- severe allergy reaction affecting the surface of the eye

- exposure of the eye to the brilliant white light of an arc welding torch

- prolonged exposure to ultraviolet light (e.g. in a disco)

- migraines

- amblyopia (a decrease in vision in one eye)

- poorly controlled diabetes

- stroke (cerebrovascular accident)

- uraemia (kidney failure)

- medications such as atropine (used in eye surgery)

- nicotine in tobacco (smoking over 40 cigarettes a day)

- illegal drugs (e.g. cocaine).

HALF LOST VISION
If you cover one eye, and, while looking with the other eye, find that you cannot see half of the objects in front of you, you are said to have hemianopia.

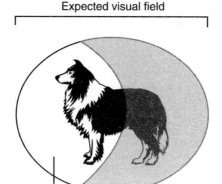

Expected visual field

Actual visual field

The most serious cause of this problem is damage to the **optic nerve**, which carries the sight nerve messages from the eye to the brain. This damage may be caused by a poor blood supply to the nerve, or a tumour, cancer (e.g. cranio-pharyngioma), abscess or infection in the nerve, brain or other surrounding tissues.

Far more commonly, a **migraine** may be responsible, and may not always be accompanied by a headache. Migraines are often associated with visual symptoms including flashing lights, shimmering, seeing zigzag lines and loss of part of the area of vision. Any headache usually occurs on only one side of the head, is described as throbbing, and causes intolerance of exercise, light and noise. Nausea and vomiting are common.

A temporary loss of half the area of vision
is most commonly due to a migraine.

In a **stroke** (cerebrovascular accident) part of the brain is affected by having its blood supply cut off by a blockage in an artery, or a blood vessel in the brain may burst, causing bleeding and damage to part of the brain. The onset is almost instantaneous, may be associated with paralysis in various parts of the body, headache, shortness of breath and other abnormalities that can vary from minor discomfort, confusion and visual disturbances to widespread paralysis and coma.

Temporal arteritis is an inflammation of the artery in the temple. There is severe tenderness over the artery, searing pain into the jaw and temples, and the eye may be affected in various ways.

BLACK SPOTS IN VISION

Seeing black spots floating across the vision, or fixed in one spot in the visual field (everything that can be seen), can be a frightening experience. Most causes are associated with diseases of the layer of light-sensitive cells at the back of the eyeball (the retina).

The most common cause is suddenly noticing the **blind spot** (see above) in the visual field of one eye. It is a phenomenon that only occurs when one eye is covered and you are looking with the other. When both eyes are used, the brain compensates for this defect in the visual field by using information from the other eye.

Migraines are often associated with visual symptoms including flashing lights, black spots, shimmering, seeing zigzag lines and loss of part of the area of vision. They usually occur on only one side of the head, are described as throbbing, and cause intolerance of exercise, light and noise. Nausea and vomiting are common.

Floaters appear as a spot in the vision that won't go away, and may continue to move across the vision after the moving eye comes to rest. A floater is a collection of cells in the half-set jelly-like substance that fills the eyeball that cast a shadow on the light-sensitive retina at the back of the eye, which the brain perceives as an object in front of the eye. They may be due to bleeding into the eye, a detached retina (which itself may cause a black spot or patch in the visual field) and infection, or no apparent cause may be found.

Other possible causes include some forms of epilepsy, a cataract (clouding of the lens in the eye), tumours of the optic nerve which takes nerve signals from the eye to the brain, and a poor blood supply to the eye because of hardening of the arteries (arteriosclerosis) or a blood clot (thrombosis).

PHOTOPHOBIA

If looking at bright light causes pain in the eyes (photophobia – fear of light), it can be a sign of anything causing **inflammation** of the eyes or eyelids. Foreign matter in the eye, an infection causing conjunctivitis or, more seriously, an inflamed iris (iritis) or acute glaucoma may be responsible. Migraine can also make it painful to look at bright light.

Less commonly, photophobia can be a symptom of viral infections such as measles and rare diseases caused by tiny parasitic organisms, usually passed on through animals or insects. Very rarely a disorder of the parathyroid gland (surrounding the thyroid in the neck) is involved.

VISUAL FLASHES

Seeing flashing lights, often at the edge of vision, when there are none actually present, can be both an annoying and a serious symptom. There are only two possible causes.

By far the most common cause is a **migraine**. These are often associated with varied visual symptoms including flashing lights, shimmering, seeing zigzag lines and loss of part of the area of vision. Pain usually occurs on only one side of the head, and is described as throbbing, and causes intolerance of exercise, light and noise. Nausea and vomiting are common.

Damage to the **retina** (the layer of light-sensitive cells at the back of the eye) is the other much more serious cause. If the retina starts to lift off the back of the eye (retinal detachment), or if there is bleeding into or under the retina, the light-sensitive cells will send inappropriate signals to the brain, which are interpreted as flashing lights. If treated early, this problem can often be cured, but if left for too long, permanent damage to the sight may occur.

VISUAL HALO

When looking at a street light on a misty night, everyone sees a faint halo of light around it, but if this phenomenon occurs all the time and in all degrees of light and dark, a person is considered to have abnormal visual halos.

A halo around objects is a serious symptom
and always requires medical assessment.

The most serious cause of this effect is **glaucoma**. This is caused by an increase in the pressure of the jelly-like fluid inside the eye.

Other causes include cataracts (clouding of the lens in the eye), allergic conjunctivitis (reaction to a pollen, dust, chemical or other substance that enter the eye) and any injury, ulceration or infection which causes swelling of the surface of the eye to cause distortion and blurring of vision.

Contact lenses may be responsible if they are poorly fitting, the wrong strength, contaminated, or left in place for too long.

SQUINT

A squint occurs when the eyes appear to look in slightly different directions away from each other. When the eyes are both turned inwards the condition is called esotropia. It is critical that this is detected and treated when it occurs in childhood, because if allowed to persist, the brain will permanently suppress the vision in one eye in order to overcome the double image it receives. Even if the good eye becomes blind later in life, the eye in which vision has been suppressed will not be able to see.

The medical term for a squint is strabismus.

In **children** a squint is usually due to an inherited tendency with weakness or abnormal development of the tiny muscles within the eye socket, which move and align the eyes, or abnormal vision in one eye due to a cataract (cloudy lens).

In older patients a squint may be caused by damage to the muscles that control eye movement from a direct blow to the eye or surrounding skull, a poor blood supply to the muscles of one eye, a stroke that affects the nervous control of the eye muscles, a tumour or cancer in the eye socket, an over-active thyroid gland (causes eyes to protrude slightly) or multiple sclerosis (affects nerves to eye muscles).

Special **spectacles** may be used long-term to correct the problem by reducing the angle of the squint. In more severe cases, an eye patch may cover the good eye to strengthen the poorer one and eye exercises may be added. In marked degrees of squint, it is necessary to operate to change the tightness of the tiny muscles that control eye movement, which is a technically a difficult operation for the surgeon, but relatively minor surgery for the patient. Provided medical advice is followed, the long-term cosmetic and vision results are excellent.

CURIOSITY

A patient who survives an electrocution may develop deteriorating vision several months later due to the formation of cataracts in the eye lens.

Wine in moderation may give older people better vision, as it helps to prevent the eye disease macular degeneration.

VITAMINS

It is important to look after yourself by having an adequate intake of vitamins in your diet, but it is an unusual person in modern society who does not obtain an adequate vitamin intake provided that they eat reasonable amounts of fruit and vegetables.

There is no evidence that vitamin **supplements** benefit anyone on a normal diet and in good health. The cheapest and most effective way to obtain adequate vitamins is to eat a well-balanced diet. Most vitamin supplements are expensive, pass rapidly through the body, and merely enrich the sewers.

Vitamins are a group of totally unrelated **chemicals** that have only one thing in common – they are essential (usually in tiny amounts) for the normal functioning of the body. All vitamins have been given letter codes, sometimes with an additional number to differentiate vitamins within a group. The missing letters and numbers in the series are due to substances initially having been identified as vitamins but later being found to lack the essentials for the classification.

Sugar contains no minerals, vitamins or fibre.

VITAMIN A
A fat-soluble vitamin, **retinol** (vitamin A) is found in milk, butter, eggs, liver and most fruit and vegetables. Very high levels are found in orange-coloured foods (e.g. pumpkin, carrots, pawpaw, etc.). It is essential for the normal function of the skin and eyes, but there is no evidence that extra amounts can improve vision in people with sight problems or can cure skin problems.

A vitamin A **deficiency** (hypovitaminosis A) may occur with starvation, tropical sprue, a poor or fad diet that lacks vitamin A, and alcoholism or narcotic addiction that may lead to the other causes. Symptoms include reduced night vision, dry eye surface, eye ulceration and dry skin. Permanent damage to the retina (light-sensitive area at the back of the eye) is possible. Blood test measurements of low vitamin A levels are inaccurate, and the diagnosis must be made by history and clinical signs.

An **excess** of vitamin A (hypervitaminosis A) causes carotenaemia, which is characterised by yellow skin, palms and soles, and may cause foetal abnormalities in pregnant women.

VITAMIN B
This vitamin is divided into several subgroups numbered 1, 2, 3, 5, 6 and 12. All are water-soluble and occur in dairy products, meats and leafy vegetables. Vitamin B1

has the chemical name of **thiamine**, B2 is **riboflavin** and B5 is **pantothenic acid**. Vitamin B6 (**pyridoxine**) may be useful in mouth inflammation, morning sickness and nervous tension. Vitamin B12 (**cyanocobalamin** or hydroxocobalamin) is used as an injection to treat pernicious anaemia. **Nicotinic acid** (vitamin B3) is specifically found in peanuts, meat, grain and liver. It is used in the treatment of certain types of headache, nervous disorders, poor circulation and blood diseases.

Most vitamin B supplements end up in the sewer, because once the body stores are full, the rest merely passes through the kidneys and out in the urine.

It is almost impossible to have a **lack** of only one in the group. If one is missing, several will usually be missing. A lack may cause anaemia and other blood diseases. Beriberi is caused by a lack of vitamin B1, and pellagra by a lack of vitamin B3, while pernicious anaemia is due to a lack of vitamin B12. A lack of vitamin B6 (pyridoxine) may be an uncommon side effect of some medications (e.g. isoniazid, penicillamine), genetic disorders and poor nutrition. It causes epileptic-like seizures, dermatitis, mouth sores and dryness, vomiting, weakness and dizziness. The blood levels of pyridoxine can be measured to confirm the diagnosis, which is easily corrected by vitamin B6 supplements.

Excessive blood levels of any of the B group vitamins may be due to taking too many vitamin B supplements. Usually there are no serious effects, as excess passes out in the urine. Very high doses of pyridoxine (vitamin B6) may cause nerve damage and poor coordination, numbness around the mouth, clumsiness, muscle weakness and loss of position sense. Very high doses of niacin (vitamin B3) may cause severe flushing, itchy skin, diarrhoea and liver damage. Long-term complications are uncommon.

VITAMIN B17

Laetrile (also known as amygdalin and vitamin B17) is purported to be a treatment against cancer, but there is no evidence to support this. It is mainly used by unethical fringe practitioners who prey on desperate patients who will try (and pay) anything for the faintest chance of a cure.

In orthodox medicine it is considered to be a poison, and is certainly not a vitamin, as it breaks down to cyanide in the body. As such, its use is restricted in many countries. Detailed research has shown no clinical benefit from the use of the drug in many clinical trials.

Laetrile is found in, and extracted from, the seeds of apricots.

VITAMIN C

Ascorbic acid (vitamin C) is water-soluble and found in citrus fruits, tomatoes and greens, but its level in food is reduced by cooking, mincing and contact with copper utensils. Vitamin C can also be synthesised from non-food sources, and the synthetic form cannot be differentiated from the natural in any way.

It is essential for the formation and maintenance of cartilage, bone and teeth, and is used in moderate amounts to promote the healing of wounds and during convalescence from prolonged illnesses. Unfortunately there is no evidence to support its use in preventing or treating the common cold.

Three thousand Californian users of Vitamin C supplements followed for ten years had the same incidence of common colds as a control group of nonusers.

A lack of vitamin C in the diet will result in the disease **scurvy**.

Excess vitamin C in the body from taking too many vitamin C (ascorbic acid) supplements may have several unusual effects including increased blood levels of oestrogens, which cause breast tenderness and menstrual period irregularities, increased risk of kidney stones, reduced absorption of vitamin B12 and the development of pernicious anaemia, and rebound scurvy in babies born to mothers who take too much vitamin C during pregnancy. The level of vitamin C can be measured in the blood. If the patient stops vitamin C supplements, long-term complications are uncommon.

VITAMIN D

This is a fat-soluble chemical found in egg yolks and butter, and it may be formed by a reaction of sunlight on skin. It is essential for the balance of calcium and phosphorus in the bones and bloodstream, but it is not used routinely in the treatment of disease. Vitamin D is actually composed of a number of chemicals, including **calcitriol** and **ergocalciferol**.

A **lack** of vitamin D causes rickets and osteomalacia, while an excess causes hypercalcaemia (high blood calcium levels), constipation and nausea.

Vitamin D **supplements** must be used with caution in pregnancy, breast feeding and children, kidney disease or kidney stones, and heart disease.

VITAMIN E

Readily available in most foods, vitamin E (**tocopherols**) is a fat-soluble vitamin that acts as an antioxidant.

High doses may cause serious diseases and abnormalities, including blood clots, high blood pressure, breast tumours, headaches, tiredness and diarrhoea. It may be harmful to the foetus in pregnancy, and prevent blood clotting in those who are taking warfarin. Vitamin E is quite a dangerous substance, and is only rarely used in medicine.

A **lack** of vitamin E from starvation, poor diet or malabsorption of fats may result in nerve damage. The patient has reduced reflexes, abnormal gait (way of walking), decreased senses of position and vibration, and eye movement abnormalities. Permanent degeneration of the spinal cord is a rare complication. The diagnosis is confirmed by measuring vitamin E levels in the blood. There is a good response to vitamin E supplements provided there has not been permanent nerve damage.

VITAMIN H

Biotin (vitamin H) has no specific medical use. A lack occurs only in severe starvation and in some rare diseases in which there is poor absorption.

VITAMIN K

Essential for the clotting of blood, vitamin K (**phytomenadione** or phylloquinone) is fat-soluble and is found in most vegetables, particularly those with green leaves.

It is also manufactured by bacteria living in the gut. It is not commonly used clinically.

A **lack** of vitamin K is relatively common in newborn infants, or may rarely be due to diseases that prevent fat absorption from the gut and long-term potent antibiotic use. Excessive bleeding and bruising are the symptoms, but it is easily and well-treated by vitamin K injections, which, rarely, may be given to infants. The excessive bleeding may lead to anaemia if left untreated.

Excess vitamin K may occur with taking too many vitamin K supplements. This stops anticoagulants (e.g. warfarin) from working and may lead to strokes or heart attacks. In pregnancy, the baby may be born jaundiced (yellow skin due to liver damage) due to anaemia in infants from the breakdown of red blood cells.

VITAMIN M

Folic acid is sometimes classed as vitamin M. It is essential for the basic functioning of the nucleus in cells, and extra amounts may be needed during pregnancy, breast feeding, and in the treatment of anaemia and alcoholism. It assists in the uptake and utilisation of iron. During pregnancy, supplements may prevent spinal cord defects in the baby. It is found naturally in liver, dark green leafy vegetables, peanuts, beans, whole grain wheat and yeast.

The level in blood can be measured and the normal range is 9.1 to 57nmol/L (4 to 25ng/mL). The amount in red blood cells can also be measured (normal range is a level greater than 318nmol/L or 140ng/mL), which gives a longer term picture than the normal folic acid level in blood that may be affected by recent changes in diet.

Low levels can be due to long-term alcoholism, oral contraceptive use, anti-convulsant medications, malnutrition, sprue (poor food absorption), sickle cell anaemia, cytotoxic drugs (used to treat cancer), pregnancy and food malabsorption syndromes.

On the other hand, a low intake in the diet can cause pernicious anaemia.

Vitamins C and E are antioxidants, and so foods high in
these vitamins have a significant antioxidant effect.

ANTIOXIDANTS

Antioxidants are **chemicals** that prevent the addition of an oxygen atom (oxygenation) to an existing molecule or element.

Adding oxygen to a fat molecule makes the fat rancid. The presence of natural antioxidants in wine and chocolate (the latter having a lot of fat) prevents them from going off, and, in particular, allows chocolate to remain fresh for years without refrigeration or special storage.

Antioxidants are **found naturally** in red wine, chocolate, tea (particularly green tea), fruit (e.g. apples, blackcurrants), vegetables (e.g. onions). Vitamins C and E are antioxidants, and so foods high in these vitamins have a significant antioxidant effect.

By interacting with, and neutralising, free radicals in the body, antioxidants are able to give some protection against heart disease and cancer, and may slow ageing to some extent.

The presence of antioxidants in red wine is said to explain the so called French paradox, in which the French have a low incidence of heart disease despite a high fat diet, because of their regular consumption of red wine with meals from an early age. Similarly, the Japanese have a low rate of heart disease and the longest average lifespan in the world with their consumption of green tea, but the Japanese also have a low fat diet, and consume more than an average amount of seafood.

CURIOSITY

Humans cannot exist without bacteria. They allow us to digest food, synthesise vitamins in the gut, break down carbohydrates, convert nitrogen into amino acids, and destroy unwanted microbes.

VOMITING

L ook after yourself by ensuring that any prolonged episode of nausea and
vomiting is attended to and not tolerated.
   Vomiting, and the nausea that usually precedes it, are some of the most
common symptoms experienced by humans, and are almost unavoidable at some
time in life. An enormous range of infections, gut diseases, liver disorders, brain
conditions, glandular disorders, and even urinary tract abnormalities, as well as
many other problems that cannot be easily categorised, can cause nausea and
vomiting.

CAUSES
There are a huge number of possible causes for nausea and vomiting.
   Gastroenteritis (see separate entry in this book) is the most common infective
cause of vomiting, and it is usually associated with diarrhoea. A viral infection is the
normal cause, but bacteria may sometimes be responsible. The infection is passed
from one person to another by close contact or on the breath, and usually occurs
in epidemics, often in springtime.
   The nausea and vomiting associated with **sea sickness**, car sickness and other
motion-induced forms of vomiting is due to an inability of the brain to coordinate
what it is sensing from the balance mechanisms in the inner ears with what is being
seen by the eyes. In a ship, the cabin appears to be perfectly still, while the balance
senses movement. For this reason, watching the horizon while on the ship deck
enables the brain to see the motion and reconcile the visual and balance senses.

Although distressing, the vomiting associated with migraines is not harmful.

   Migraines are often associated with nausea and vomiting, as well as head pain and
visual symptoms (e.g. flashing lights, shimmering, seeing zigzag lines and loss of
part of the area of vision). Pain usually occurs on only one side of the head, and is
described as throbbing, and causes intolerance of exercise, light and noise.
   Morning sickness usually occurs between the sixth and fourteenth weeks of pregnancy, but in some women may persist for much longer. It is caused by a hormonal
effect on the brain, probably arising from the developing placenta (afterbirth). See
page 455 for further information on this topic.
   Bulimia is a psychiatric condition in which anxious patients consume excessive
amounts of food (often sweets or fatty foods), and then vomit to get rid of the food
and so stay slim. The patient (almost invariably high achieving, middle to upper class

young females) may gorge and vomit or purge themselves for hours, days or weeks. The condition may be associated with anorexia nervosa. Complications can include menstrual period irregularities, sore throat, bowel problems, dehydration, lethargy, and dental problems due to the repeated exposure of the teeth to stomach acid.

Severe **pain** of any cause may result in nausea and vomiting as a reaction to the pain.

AN ENORMOUS NUMBER OF OTHER CONDITIONS MAY ALSO CAUSE NAUSEA AND VOMITING. THEY INCLUDE:

- meningitis (infection of the supporting membranes around the brain)

- many different bacterial and viral infections (e.g. cystitis, sinusitis)

- labyrinthitis (infection or inflammation of the balance mechanism in the inner ear)

- gastritis (inflammation of the stomach from acid irritation)

- appendicitis

- mesenteric adenitis (infected lymph nodes in the abdomen)

- cholecystitis (inflammation or infection of the gall bladder)

- gall stones

- hepatitis (several different types of liver infection)

- cirrhosis (damaged liver)

- stroke (cerebrovascular accident)

- Ménière's disease (dizziness, deafness and ringing in the ears)

- an increase in the pressure of the cerebrospinal fluid (CSF) which surrounds the brain and spinal cord due to a head injury, tumour, cancer, abscess or infection in the brain or surrounding tissues

- kidney stones

- uraemia (kidney failure)

- malaria

- stomach cancer

- Crohn disease (inflamed and thickened intestine)

- intussusception (infolding of the gut on itself, usually in children)

- blood clot in the main artery supplying the gut

- epilepsy

- a reduction in the blood supply to the brain (from suffocation, near drowning, inhalation of smoke or toxic gases, narrowing of the arteries to the brain, or any form of heart failure)

- abnormalities of most glands (may affect the body's chemical balances)

- premenstrual tension syndrome (hormonal changes that precede a menstrual period)

- poorly controlled diabetes

- hyperthyroidism (over-active thyroid gland)

- Addison's disease (adrenal gland failure)

- glaucoma (increased pressure in the eye)

- altitude sickness

- severe high blood pressure

- myocardial infarct (heart attack)

- congestive cardiac failure (damaged heart is unable to beat effectively)

- Chinese restaurant syndrome (reaction to preservatives and flavour-enhancers in food)

- anaphylactic reaction (immediate, severe, life-threatening reactions to an allergy-causing substance)

- polyarteritis nodosa (inflammation of arteries)

- AIDS.

In infants, particularly boys, severe projectile vomiting may be due to **pyloric stenosis** (narrowing of the drainage valve from the stomach).

Many illegal drugs, including ecstasy, ketamine, amphetamines
and heroin, may have nausea and vomiting as side effects.

Alcohol abuse, either a binge or long-term overuse, will lead to vomiting. Binge drinking and intoxication causes vomiting, headaches and hangovers because of the effect of alcohol on the brain and stomach.

Many **medications** may have nausea and vomiting as a side effect. Common examples include most medications used for the treatment of cancer, narcotics (e.g. morphine), digoxin (used in heart disease), theophylline (used in lung diseases) and overdoses of hormones (e.g. contraceptive pill, hormone replacement therapy).

Radiotherapy (powerful X-rays) and nuclear irradiation used for the treatment of cancer often cause nausea and vomiting as a side effect.

Vomiting may sometimes be caused by psychological disturbances and used as an attention-seeking device.

VOMITING BLOOD

Vomiting blood (**haematemesis**) can vary from a few specks of red in copious vomitus to vomiting large amounts of blood with no other substance being present. Vomiting a small amount of blood on one occasion is not normally a reason for any concern, but if even small amounts are vomited repeatedly, or a large amount only once, medical attention must be obtained.

Prolonged vomiting from any cause may result in vomiting of blood as the junction between the oesophagus (gullet) and stomach becomes torn. This is known as the Mallory-Weis syndrome.

A **peptic ulcer** in the stomach is caused by the concentrated hydrochloric acid in the stomach penetrating the protective mucus that normally lines the organ, and eating into the stomach wall to cause significant pain. If a vein or artery is penetrated by the ulcer, severe bleeding into the stomach may occur.

Varicose veins can occur not only in the legs, but also in the lower oesophagus (gullet), when liver disease (e.g. **cirrhosis** from alcohol, liver tumours or hepatitis) increases the pressure in the veins that drain from the gut into the liver. The dilated veins in the oesophagus (oesophageal varices) can be damaged and bleed torrentially because of vomiting, reflux of acid into the oesophagus (e.g. with a hiatus hernia), straining with heavy lifting, or swallowing hard or sharp objects.

Uncommon causes of haematemesis include swallowing a sharp foreign body (e.g. a pin, sharp bone), cancer of the stomach or oesophagus, abnormal arteries and veins that may be present in the stomach or oesophagus from birth, and yellow fever (a severe infection of the liver transmitted by mosquitoes).

Some medications, such as aspirin, anti-inflammatory medications (used for arthritis), and, more seriously, warfarin (used to thin blood), may cause bleeding into the stomach and vomiting blood.

TREATMENT

Obviously, the best way to stop vomiting is to treat the cause, but this may not always be practical as the cause may not be known, the cause may be impossible to remove (e.g, pregnancy), further investigations may be necessary to identify the cause, the treatment of the cause may take time or there may be no treatment for the cause.

Wine may be used in small quantities to ease
nausea if no medication is available.

Antiemetics are medicines that stop vomiting. They are often impossible to give in tablet or mixture form, so many of them are also available as an injection or suppository (for insertion into the back passage). There are many different drugs in this category, from the mild over-the-counter travel sickness pills such as dimenhydrinate (Andrumin, Travacalm) to the more effective and potent prescription drugs such as prochlorperazine (Stemetil), domperidone (Motilium) and metoclopramide (Maxolon). These are also available as injections. Prochlorperazine may also be used for Ménière's disease, and prochlorperazine for dizziness.

Side effects may include constipation, dry mouth, tremor, drowsiness and blurred vision.

MORNING SICKNESS

The nausea and vomiting that affects some pregnant women between the sixth and fourteenth weeks of pregnancy is called morning sickness, but it can occur at any time of the day. Its severity varies markedly, with about one third of pregnant women having no morning sickness, one half having it badly enough to vomit at least once, and in five per cent the condition is serious enough to result in prolonged bed rest or even hospitalisation.

Morning sickness is known technically as hyperemesis gravidarum.

Morning sickness is caused by the unusually high levels of **oestrogen** present in the mother's bloodstream during the first three months of pregnancy. Although it usually ceases after about three months, it may persist for far longer in some unlucky women. Severe cases may be associated with twins, and it is usually worse in the first pregnancy.

Because morning sickness is a self-limiting condition, treatment is usually given only when absolutely necessary. A light diet, with small, frequent meals of dry fat-free foods, is often helpful. A concentrated carbohydrate solution (Emetrol) may be taken to help relieve the nausea. Vitamin B supplements and ginger are also known to ease morning sickness. Only in severe cases, and with some reluctance, will doctors prescribe more potent medications. In rare cases, fluids given by a drip into a vein are necessary for a woman hospitalised because of continued vomiting.

Morning sickness has no effect upon the development of the baby.

CURIOSITY

Extract from an 1821 medical text:

'In some particular forms of disease in infants, champagne will prove itself to be of the greatest possible value. It is most efficacious when given ice cold in cases of obstinate vomiting'.

WARTS

L ook after yourself by treating warts earlier rather than later, as the smaller they are, the easier they are to destroy.

TYPES
SKIN WART
A wart is an unsightly, hard, rough, raised growth on the skin caused by a very slow-growing virus (papillomavirus), which takes months or years to cause a wart.

They are most common in children from 8 to 16 years of age, but people with warts should not be isolated for fear of spreading the disease, as the virus is widespread in the community. The most common sites affected are the knees, elbows, hands and feet.

Treatments that may be tried include acid paints (e.g. keratolytics) applied regularly to eat away the wart tissue, freezing (cryotherapy) with liquid nitrogen, which causes the wart to fall off after a few days, burning the wart tissue away with a high voltage electric current (diathermy) or laser, injecting a cell-destroying substance (bleomycin) under the wart, immunotherapy (inducing a skin reaction under and around the wart), or, rarely, cutting the wart out surgically. Warts may recur after all forms of treatment, and only warts that are causing disfigurement or discomfort should be treated, as a scar may remain after any form of surgery, diathermy or cryotherapy.

Warts usually go away by themselves without any treatment, but this may take many months or years. The average life span of a wart is about 18 months, but some may last several years.

Plantar warts are known as verruca in England.

PLANTAR WARTS
A plantar wart is a type of wart that grows on the soles of the feet, and they tend to grow inwards rather than out. The cause is the same human papillomavirus that causes normal warts.

A hard, slightly raised, scar-like growth forms on the sole of the foot, and becomes painful with walking. Plantar warts are like icebergs, with only a small part showing on the surface and a much larger area affected deeper in the sole. They may become large, widespread and painful, so that walking is very difficult.

456

There are numerous treatments available, including diathermy (burning), acid ointments, freezing, cutting out, or injecting under the wart. After surgery, a far larger hole than expected is usually left in the sole that may take some weeks to heal. Unfortunately, recurrence is common despite the best treatment.

GENITAL WARTS
See the entry in this book under sexually transmitted diseases.

TREATMENTS
KERATOLYTICS
Keratolytics are skin preparations that are designed to remove the outermost layer of the skin (the keratin layer) and therefore act as the ultimate skin cleanser. Most are available without prescription and are used to treat diseases such as warts as well as acne, psoriasis and some forms of dermatitis. Excessive or inappropriate use may cause reddening, burning and discolouration of the skin, particularly on the face. It is wise to make a test application on an area of skin that is not cosmetically important before applying a keratolytic to the face. They are available as creams, lotions, pastes, gels, ointments or soaps.

Examples include benzyl peroxide, salicylic acid, tretinoin, glutaraldehyde and triclosan.

Side effects may include stinging, redness, skin swelling and skin peeling. Patients should avoid eyes, mouth, nostrils and wounds. Care is necessary with sun exposure. Tretinoin must be used with caution in pregnancy.

DIATHERMY AND EXCISION PROCEDURE
A local anaesthetic injection is given into the sole of the foot, which can be painful for 20 to 30 seconds. After this, the wart area will be completely numb.

Although initially painful, and apparently radical, diathermy and excision is the best way to deal with all but the smallest plantar warts.

A diathermy machine is used to burn the wart and surrounding tissues, and then a scalpel or scissors are used to cut away the burnt tissue. Burning is necessary to prevent as much bleeding as possible. The resultant hole in the foot is not sutured, but filled with an antiseptic cream and covered with a dressing.

It will be sore for a couple of days, then uncomfortable for a week, but probably no more so than before the procedure. You should be able to walk on it normally after a week or ten days, but the hole may take up to three months to close and fill up with scar tissue. A permanent scar will be left on the sole.

CRYOTHERAPY
Cryotherapy (freezing) to remove warts, skin tumours or sunspots is usually carried out using a liquid nitrogen spray or probe cooled to -196°C, although carbon dioxide snow (dry ice) is sometimes used. Stinging is felt at the time of freezing, and often a slight ache later as the area thaws. Pain killers are not normally needed, but some patients may wish to use paracetamol tablets after the procedure.

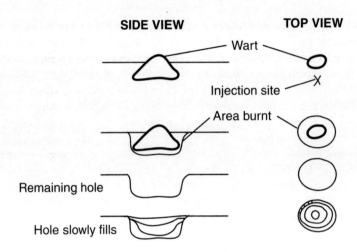

SIDE VIEW   **TOP VIEW**

Wart

Injection site

Area burnt

Remaining hole

Hole slowly fills

THE FROZEN SITES MAY GO THROUGH ANY OR ALL OF THE FOLLOWING STAGES DURING RECOVERY:

- Dry, swollen, mildly inflamed areas. These should be left uncovered, except when a dressing is necessary to prevent the area becoming dirty (e.g. if gardening with a freeze site on the hand). Avoid using make-up on the site until inflammation settles.

- Blistering. If the blister is intact and contains clear fluid, leave it alone. Bursting a blister makes it more likely to become infected. If the blister is very uncomfortable, it may be drained by pricking with a needle that has been soaked in disinfectant or methylated spirits.

- Blistering with weeping. Clean lesions as often as practical with saline (salty water). Continue until sore is dry, which usually takes several days, but occasionally two to three weeks.

- Dry crusts. Apply Vaseline or petroleum jelly three times a day.

- Infection. This is uncommon, but if the freeze site has a red border more than 2mm wide surrounding it, is painful, or a pus-filled blister is present, it is infected. Avoid prolonged wetting and dry well after a shower. Burst infected blisters with a disinfected needle, and apply an antiseptic ointment three times a day. If these measures don't lead to rapid improvement, return to see your doctor.

Cryotherapy is only successful on small, thin, superficial warts, and may need to be applied several times.

Almost every spot treated by cryotherapy will develop some **scar**. All scars are bright pink for one to four months, then usually fade. White scars may persist for many months after this, especially where a particularly thick wart has required a longer freeze spraying time.

Keloid scarring is a less common form of healing that appears as a pink smooth nodule (proud flesh) in the centre of the freeze site, or as a thin, straight ridge of thickened scar tissue. Keloid scars may last for several years, but eventually most fade and flatten. Scarring can be reduced by treatment with steroid creams that can be prescribed by a doctor.

Wart **recurrence** is most commonly seen as a faint pink or slightly scaling area 2–3mm wide arising adjacent to a freeze site. A recurrence is often larger than it looks, but is usually teated by excision rather than refreezing.

CURIOSITY

Only about a quarter of the population is susceptible to the wart virus – the rest have natural immunity.

WEIGHT LOSS

An unintended weight loss, or one that cannot be explained by a change in diet or activity, requires you to look after yourself by consulting a doctor to see if there is a medical cause for the problem.

CAUSES

There are many different causes for an unintended weight loss.

Diseases that increase **metabolic rate** (the rate at which the body's basic functions work), a lack of nutrition, an increase in exercise, excessive sweating, an inability to absorb food (malabsorption), diarrhoea or any disease or inflammation that puts stress on the body can cause weight loss.

Any condition that causes persistent **diarrhoea**, nausea or vomiting will lead to weight loss. Sometimes, the diarrhoea and vomiting may be self-induced in order to lose weight, or may be part of a number of different psychiatric conditions, including depression.

Weight loss that is not easily explained is a significant
symptom that needs to be investigated by a doctor.

Anorexia nervosa is a psychiatric condition that normally occurs in young women who have a distorted image of their own body. They believe that they are fat when they are not, and so starve themselves in order to lose excessive amounts of weight. The patient can become seriously undernourished and emaciated, to the point of death, if adequate treatment is not available. Other symptoms include a cessation of menstrual periods, diffuse hair loss, an intolerance of cold, a slow pulse, irregular heart beat and other complex hormonal disorders. Patients practise deceit to fool their family and doctors by appearing to eat normal meals but later vomit the food, use purgatives to clean out their bowel, or hide food during the meal.

OTHER POSSIBLE CAUSES OF WEIGHT LOSS INCLUDE:

- persistent infection (e.g. tuberculosis, hepatitis, AIDS, brucellosis)

- autoimmune disorders (e.g. rheumatoid arthritis, dermatomyositis, SLE)

- cancer of almost any organ

- cirrhosis (damage to the liver)

- cholecystitis (inflammation or infection of the gall bladder)

- peptic ulcer in the stomach

- ulcerative colitis (lining of the large intestine ulcerates and bleeds)

- over-active thyroid gland (hyperthyroidism)

- severe asthma

- uncontrolled diabetes

- parasites of the intestine

- kidney failure

- congestive heart failure

- emphysema (incurable lung disease caused by smoking)

- alcoholism

- addictive drug abuse.

There are many rare conditions which may cause loss of weight, including Crohn disease (inflammation of the small or large intestine), pancreatitis, tropical sprue (long-term intestinal infection) and Addison disease (underactive adrenal glands).

CHILDREN

Failure to thrive is a term use to describe babies and young children under two years of age who are lighter than 97 per cent of children their age, and who do not put on weight or develop at the expected rate.

Obviously the most common cause is **neglect** and starvation, and sometimes this can be difficult for doctors to detect, and it is only when the child is hospitalised, or information is given by friends or relatives that this problem becomes apparent.

Unfortunately, one of the most common, and hardest to detect, causes for a child not to gain weight is neglect, which may be unintended and due to poor education and a failure by the parents to cope.

Persistent **infection**, particularly of the urine, is another common cause. Infections may be low grade and not apparent, and urine infections may have no symptoms in young children, and collection of urine samples is difficult, making them hard to detect.

Infestations of the gut with various **worms** and **parasites** must be excluded by examination of a sample of faeces in a laboratory.

Genetic factors must also be considered. If both parents are very small, then the child may be also be small, but completely healthy.

A wide range of uncommon diseases can cause failure to thrive. If one of the common causes listed cannot be found, it may be necessary to undertake extensive investigations to find a long-term disease that is affecting the child's growth.

EXAMPLES OF DISEASES THAT MAY CAUSE WEIGHT LOSS OR FAILURE TO THRIVE IN CHILDREN INCLUDE:

- diabetes (rare under two years)

- pyloric stenosis (narrowing of the outlet of the stomach)

- Down syndrome (mongolism)

- Turner syndrome (girls born with only one X chromosome instead of two)

- Fanconi syndrome (failure of the kidneys)

- major heart valve and artery abnormalities (e.g. Fallot's tetralogy, patent ductus arteriosus)

- cystic fibrosis (failure of the glands throughout the body)

- coeliac disease (intolerance to gluten in flour)

- failure of any of the body's major hormone-producing glands (e.g. thyroid gland, pituitary gland, adrenal glands and parathyroid glands)

- diet deficient in iron or other essential nutrients.

Numerous other rare congenital and acquired conditions may also cause failure to thrive.

CURIOSITY
One of the most common symptoms to indicate that a person with an HIV infection is developing the final stage of AIDS is a sudden loss of weight.

WORMS

The very thought of them makes most people cringe, but being aware of intestinal worms means that you can look after yourself and your family by treating an infestation at the earliest opportunity.

The most common worms (helminths) in developed countries are pinworms (threadworms), but there are many other worms which may infest humans, some of which are very rare.

PINWORM

The pinworm is the most commonly encountered worm in developed countries.

The gut may easily become infested by the 0.5 to 1cm long pinworm (threadworm) *Enterobius vermicularis*. The pinworm lives in the large **intestine**, but migrates to around the anus to lay eggs, from where they may be transferred to the fingers during wiping or scratching, and then re-enter the original patient's mouth or pass to another person, where the cycle starts again. The worm dies after depositing the eggs and passes out with the faeces, where they may sometimes be seen. The eggs can survive for up to three weeks outside the body.

Children are the most commonly affected group, and they spread the infestation to others by poor personal hygiene. It is very easy for all the members of one family to be affected.

Most patients have no **symptoms** but some will experience anal itching at night, mild diarrhoea and minor abdominal pains. In rare cases the worms may migrate to the vagina and urethra of women and girls.

It is diagnosed by microscopically examining the faeces for the presence of worms or eggs.

Treatment should involve all members of the patient's immediate family. A number of anthelmintic medications can be used to kill the worms. Good hygiene involves careful hand-washing after going to the toilet and not scratching the anus. If the patient does not re-infect themselves the worms will die out in six to seven weeks.

The term Nematodes is used to describe any of the thread-like round worms that may be free living, or parasites within humans, other animals and plants.

ANGIOSTRONGYLIASIS

Angiostrongyliasis (eosinophilic meningoencephalitis) is an infestation of the brain and surrounding membranes (meninges) by the nematode worm *Angiostrongylus cantonensis*. It occurs on Pacific islands, in west Africa, south Asia and in the Caribbean.

The worms normally live in the gut of rats. Their eggs pass out with rat faeces, are eaten by snails, prawns or fish, and then pass to humans if these foods are eaten when poorly cooked. They may directly enter humans if food contaminated by rat faeces (e.g. salads) are eaten. The swallowed eggs hatch into larvae which migrate through the bloodstream to the **brain** and meninges. The incubation period is one to three weeks.

Patients develop a severe headache, fever, neck stiffness, nausea, vomiting and abnormal nerve sensations. The worms may spread into the eye and cause blindness. CT and MRI scans may show the presence of worms in brain.

No specific treatment is available. Symptoms persist for several months until the worm dies, and then most patients recover completely. Rarely, there may be permanent brain damage and death.

ASCARIASIS

The roundworm *Ascaris lumbricoides* is one of a group of roundworms (known as nematodes) that may infest the human gut. Infestations are common in Indonesia, South-East Asia and other less developed countries.

Adult roundworms are between 20 and 40cm long, and live in the **small intestine**. After fertilisation, the females release a large number of microscopic eggs that pass out in the faeces and can survive for many years in the soil. In areas where human faeces is used as a fertiliser, it is easy for them to be swallowed again on food; or if sewerage contaminates the water supply, they may be swallowed in a drink. Once swallowed, the eggs hatch into larvae that burrow through the gut wall into the bloodstream and move through the heart into the lungs. There they penetrate into the small air tubes (bronchioles) of the lung, wiggle their way up through larger airways to the back of the throat from where they are swallowed again to enter the small intestine and grow into mature adults that may live for up to a year.

At all stages the larvae and worms can cause **symptoms**, including a cough, shortness of breath, fever, wheezing, chest pain, abdominal pains and discomfort, nausea and gut obstruction. If severe infestations are left uncontrolled, the worms may move into the gall bladder and pancreas, rupture the bowel, and cause other severe complications that may result in death. The diagnosis is confirmed by finding eggs in the faeces.

A number of drugs are available to treat the disease, but they often have side effects. If patients are given the correct treatment at a relatively early stage of the disease, full recovery is normal.

CUTANEOUS LARVA MIGRANS

Cutaneous larva migrans, or creeping eruption, is a **skin** infestation by a larval nematode worm. The rash is caused by the burrowing of hookworm larvae through the skin. The larvae hatch from dog or cat faeces, mature in the soil and then penetrate human skin.

Patients develop several centimetre-long red, very itchy, twisting tracks in and under the skin. Large blisters may form later. Secondary bacterial infection of skin may occur due to damage by both the larvae and scratching.

A skin biopsy is sometimes used to make the diagnosis. Treatment involves medication by mouth and ointment to kill the larvae, and other creams to ease the skin irritation.

The larvae cannot mature in humans, and die after several weeks, then the skin tracks slowly heal.

GUINEA WORM

Dracunculiasis (Guinea worm disease) is a worm infestation that occurs only in west and central Africa, and uncommonly in south Asia and Arabia.

The worm *Dracunculus medinensis* is caught by swallowing water contaminated by microscopic crustaceans (copepods – water fleas) that contain the worm larva. In the stomach these are released, burrow through the stomach wall into the bloodstream, and migrate to the fat under the skin where they mature. After mating the male worm dies, but the mature female worm, which may be 60 to 80cm long, moves to the **skin** surface where it forms a sore, and through this discharges eggs every time the skin comes into contact with water. The eggs are then swallowed by the copepods where the cycle starts again. The worms eventually die and emerge through the skin sore, or occasionally remain under the skin. The full cycle takes nine to 14 months.

> *Native doctors remove Guinea worms by exposing one end*
> *of the worm and slowly pulling it out over several weeks.*
> *If pulled too quickly, it will break and retreat deep into the body.*

Patients experience generalised itching, fever, shortness of breath and nausea when larvae are in the blood. Redness, burning and itching occurs at the site of skin sores, usually on the foot or leg. After the worm dies, a red, tender ulcer forms.

Smears from skin sores show eggs when examined under a microscope to confirm the diagnosis.

The patient should rest with affected leg elevated. Worms can be individually removed by exposing one end and then slowly drawing them out a centimetre at a time over several days. Medications cannot kill worms, but may encourage them to be expelled through a sore. Secondary bacterial infection of an ulcer can spread to the surrounding skin (cellulitis). Abscesses can form under the skin (particularly if a worm is broken during removal), in joints or rarely in other organs that are reached by worms.

The ulcers heal after a month or two and most patients recover eventually.

HOOKWORM

One quarter of the entire population of the world is affected by hookworm (Ancylostomiasis), which is an infestation of the **gut** by the nematode worm *Ancylostoma duodenale*.

The eggs of the adult hookworm, which is 1cm long, pass out in the faeces, and if the faeces fall onto moist ground, the larvae will hatch from the eggs. The larvae remain active in moist soil for up to a week, and during that time, a larva may penetrate the skin of the foot of any person who treads on it. The larva then migrates through the bloodstream to the lung, where it breaks into the air-carrying passageways of the lung. From there it is carried with sputum up into the throat, where it is swallowed, enters the gut, develops into an adult worm and starts the process all over again. It may be caught in all the tropical countries of the world.

Patients develop an itch at the site of skin penetration, a cough, wheeze and fever while the larvae are in the lung, and mild abdominal discomfort and diarrhoea when there are a large number of worms in the gut, but only in patients who are otherwise ill or malnourished does a hookworm infestation cause significant problems

Examination of a sample of faeces under a microscope reveals the worm or its eggs, and drugs are available to successfully destroy the worms.

HYDATID DISEASE

Hydatid disease or echinococcosis, is an infestation of human tissue by the larva of the tapeworm *Echinococcus*.

The normal life cycle of *Echinococcus* requires infested meat to be eaten by a dog or other carnivore. The larva enters the gut and grows into a tape worm, which then passes eggs out in the faeces to contaminate grass and soil. The normal hosts are cattle, sheep and other grazing animals which eat the contaminated grass and are eventually killed by the *Echinococcus* infestation in their body. This allows the carcass to be eaten by meat-eating animals, and the life cycle of the parasite starts again. If a human eats food that has been contaminated by the faeces of an infected animal (usually dogs or other meat-eating animals), the larva migrates to the **liver, lung, spleen** or **brain**, where it forms a cyst that remains lifelong. The disease is rare in developed countries, but widespread in South America, around the Mediterranean, in east Africa and central Asia.

After the cyst forms in the body, it usually remains dormant for many years, often causing no symptoms. Over a decade or more the cyst slowly enlarges, until the pressure it exerts on its surroundings causes problems. With liver cysts, there may be pain in the upper part of the abdomen, nausea, vomiting and jaundice. In the lung, the cysts may cause part of the lung to collapse, pain and shortness of breath. In the brain symptoms occur earlier, and even a small cyst may cause convulsions or severe headaches. If a cyst ruptures, the reaction in the body to the sudden release of a large number of larvae may cause sudden death or severe illness and the formation of multiple cysts in other parts of the body. If multiple cysts are present, the long-term outlook is grave.

> *Because it is imperative to remove the cyst intact, surgery on an hydatid cyst is some of the most delicate ever performed.*

The condition is diagnosed by seeing the cyst on a CT or ultrasound scan. Specific antibody blood tests can be performed to determine whether or not a person has a cyst somewhere in their body, but discovering the actual site of the cyst may then prove very difficult. The blood test remains positive long-term after an infection.

If possible, a cyst should be removed surgically. It is vital for the surgeon not to rupture the cyst during its removal, because the spilled larvae can then spread through the body. In other cases, or as an additional form of treatment, potent medications may be prescribed to kill the larvae, but the cyst will remain. Provided the disease is not widespread, the results of treatment are good. Dogs in affected areas can be treated regularly to prevent them carrying the disease.

STRONGYLOIDIASIS

Strongyloidiasis is an infestation of the human by the tiny 2mm-long worm *Strongyloides stercoralis* that is found throughout the tropics. This worm can live freely in moist soil or its larvae may penetrate the skin of a human, enter the bloodstream, pass through the heart into the lungs, and pass from the blood into the air passages of the lung. From there it moves up into the throat, is swallowed and develops into an adult worm in the **intestine**. It then produces eggs which pass out with the faeces and contaminate the soil. The eggs may also hatch into larvae in the intestine and these larvae can penetrate the bowel wall to enter the blood and reinfect the host human. There are no male and female worms, only a single asexual form.

Many patients have no or minimal **symptoms**, but in long-standing or severe cases symptoms may include itchy buttocks and wrists, raised rashes, belly pains, nausea, diarrhoea and weight loss. Rarely in severe chronic cases the larvae may invade the liver, kidney and brain.

It is diagnosed by finding the eggs or worms in the faeces or by a specific blood test, and then appropriate medication can be prescribed to eradicate the infestation.

TAPEWORMS

Mature tapeworms live in the **gut** of humans or other animals.

Six different types of tapeworm (Taeniasis) can infect man. They vary in length from half a centimetre (dwarf tapeworm) to more than 20m (beef tapeworm) and are members of a class of worms known as Cestodes. Tapeworms were named because they are divided into segments in much the same way as a tape measure. At one end there is a head (scolex) that has a large sucker on it, and this is used to attach the worm to the inside of the gut.

Segments that are full of eggs constantly drop off from the end of the worm, pass out with the faeces and remain in the soil until eaten by another animal. When the egg is swallowed, it hatches an embryo that burrows into the muscle of the animal and remains there for the rest of that animal's life. If the animal's flesh is eaten, the embryo enters the gut of the new host, attaches to it and grows into a mature tapeworm.

The longest tapeworm recorded was 23m. The human
gut is about 10m long from mouth to anus.

Tiny tapeworm embryos may be found in the flesh of cattle, pigs and fish but are destroyed by cooking. Less common tapeworms can be transmitted by fleas and other insects from rats and dogs to man, and another uncommon form passes directly from the gut of one human to another through faeces and contaminated food. Tapeworms may be caught in many parts of the world but are rare in developed countries.

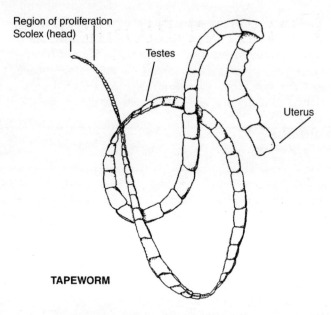

Region of proliferation
Scolex (head)

Testes

Uterus

TAPEWORM

There may be no **symptoms** until the numbers of worms present is quite high, when nausea, diarrhoea, abdominal discomfort, hunger, weight loss and tiredness may occur. Sometimes patients find segments of the worm in their underclothes or bedding. Except for the rare cases where the embryo stage spreads to the brain, there are no long-term complications.

The presence of tapeworms can be confirmed by examining faeces under a microscope for the presence of segments or eggs. It is then cured by the use of appropriate medication.

TRICHURIASIS
Trichuriasis is an infestation of the **large intestine** with the 3 to 5cm-long whipworm *Trichuris*. Adult whipworms live in the colon and produce eggs that pass out with the faeces to contaminate the soil. If contaminated food or water is consumed, the eggs will hatch in the small intestine to form larvae that then migrate to the large intestine and mature into adult worms. The cycle takes a minimum of three months and adult worms may live for three years, and they are found throughout the tropics.

Most patients have no **symptoms**, but with severe infestations abdominal pain, loss of appetite and diarrhoea may occur. Badly infested children may have bloody diarrhoea and become malnourished.

The condition is diagnosed by finding the eggs on microscopic examination of the faeces, then very effectively treated by the drug mebendazole.

CURIOSITY
Extract from an 1821 medical text book:
'An intense itching of the nose is an invariable sign of worms'.

FINAL CURIOSITIES

Pneumonoultramicroscopicsilicovolcaniosis is the longest word used in medicine, and, for obvious reasons, it is used rarely. It is a lung disease caused by breathing in the microscopic particles of ash emitted by a volcano.

Orf is the shortest name of any disease. It is an unusual viral infection of sheep and goats that can infect the skin on the fingers and hands of people (e.g. shearers, abattoir workers, veterinarians) who come into close contact with infected animals.

Von Recklinghausen's disease of multiple neurofibromatosis is not only the disease with the longest name in the medical lexicon, but also a disfiguring condition of skin and nerves that affects one in every 3000 Europeans. Fatty lumps grow from cells that form the soft sheath around nerves.

INDEX

As you lie dying, about to breathe your last, there is no way you will be thinking 'I wish I had spent a few extra hours at the office'.

Look after yourself.

Work to live, don't live to work.